A CENTURY OF
TUBERCULOSIS
SOUTH · AFRICAN
PERSPECTIVES

CW01496557

EDITED BY
HM COOVADIA & SR BENATAR

1991
Oxford University Press
Cape Town

OXFORD UNIVERSITY PRESS

Walton Street, Oxford OX2 6DP, United Kingdom

OXFORD NEW YORK TORONTO
DELHI BOMBAY CALCUTTA MADRAS KARACHI
PETALING JAYA SINGAPORE HONG KONG TOKYO
NAIROBI DAR ES SALAAM CAPE TOWN
MELBOURNE AUCKLAND

and associated companies in
BERLIN IBADAN

A CENTURY OF TUBERCULOSIS

ISBN 0 19 570583 1

Cover design: Mara Singer
House editor: Susan Lawrence

Published by Oxford University Press Southern Africa
Harrington House, Barrack Street, Cape Town, 8001, South Africa

DTP conversion by Theiner Typesetting (Pty) Ltd, Bellville, in 10 on 11 pt Garamond.
Printed and bound by Clyson.

Contents

Section 1
History and epidemiology

Section 2
Clinical aspects

Section 3
Occupational tuberculosis

Section 4
Diagnostic, immunologic and therapeutic considerations

List of Authors

AINSLIE G M; MBChB (Cape Town), FCP (SA). Lecturer, Department of Medicine, University of Cape Town and Groote Schuur Hospital.

BATEMAN E D; MBChB MD (Cape Town), DCH (London), FRCP (London). Associate Professor and Head, Respiratory Clinic, Department of Medicine, University of Cape Town and Groote Schuur Hospital.

BENATAR S R; MBChB (Cape Town), FFA (SA), FRCP (London). Professor and Head, Department of Medicine, University of Cape Town and Groote Schuur Hospital. Chief Physician, Groote Schuur Hospital.

BEYERS J A; MBChB (Cape Town), MMed(Rad), MD(Clin) (Pretoria). Emeritus Professor of Radiology, University of Stellenbosch.

BUCH E; MBChB, MSc(Med), FFCH (SA), DTMH, DOH. Lecturer, Department of Community Health, University of the Witwatersrand.

COLLINS T F B; MBBCh, DPH (Witwatersrand). Director, Community TB Education, South African National Tuberculosis Association.

COMMERFORD PJ; MBChB (Cape Town), FCP (SA). Professor of Cardiology, University of Cape Town and Groote Schuur Hospital.

COOVADIA H M; MBBS (Bombay), MD (Natal), MSc (Immunology) (Birmingham), FCP (SA). Professor and Head, Department of Paediatrics, University of Natal.

COWIE R L; MBChB, MD (Cape Town), MSc (McGill), FCP (SA), MFOM (UK). Associate Professor, Division of Respiratory Medicine, Department of Medicine, and Department of Community Health Services, University of Calgary. Director for Tuberculosis Services, Southern Alberta. Internist, Respiratory Medicine, Foothills Hospital, Calgary.

DONALD P R; MBChB, MD (Stellenbosch), DCh (Glasgow), FCP (SA), MRCP (UK), DTM&H (London). Associate Professor, Department of Paediatrics, Tygerberg Hospital and University of Stellenbosch.

DUBOVSKY H; MBChB, DPH (Cape Town). Consultant and Lecturer, Department of Internal Medicine, University of the Orange Free State.

GINWALA K; MBChB, BAO (Dublin), M.Med (Comm.Health) (Natal), Dip.Hosp.Admin. (London). Acting Head, Department of Community Health, University of Natal.

LALLOO U G; MBChB (Natal), FCP (SA), DOH (Witwatersrand). Senior Specialist, Lecturer and Head of the Respiratory Unit, Department of Medicine, University of Natal and King Edward VIII Hospital.

LEE T; MBChB, BA, BSc, DPHC(Ed). Researcher, Centre for Health Policy, Department of Community Health, University of the Witwatersrand.

METCALF C A; MBChB (Cape Town), BScMed(Hons)(Epidemiology) (Stellenbosch). Medical Researcher, Centre for Epidemiological Research in Southern Africa, South African Medical Research Council.

METS J T; Arts Examen (Leiden), LRCP (London), MRCS (UK), DOM (Stellenbosch), MD (Pretoria), MFOM (UK), FACOM (USA). Formerly Senior Lecturer in Occupational Health, University of Cape Town.

MOODLEY M; MBChB (Natal), FCP(Paeds) (SA), MRCP (UK). Senior Specialist and Senior Lecturer, Department of Paediatrics and Child Health, University of Natal.

PACKARD R M; MBChB (Cape Town), PhD (Wisconsin), MRCP (UK), BA (Wesleyan), MA (Northwestern). Professor of History, Tufts University.

SARKIN T L; MBChB, MDMCh (Cape Town), FRCS (England), FRCS (Edinburgh). Professor of Orthopaedic Surgery, University of Natal.

SAXE N; MBChB (Cape Town), FFDerm (SA). Associate Professor and Head of Department of Dermatology, Groote Schuur Hospital and University of Cape Town.

SEAGER J R; BSc(Hons), PhD (Wales). Specialist Scientist, Centre for Epidemiological Research in Southern Africa, South African Medical Research Council.

STRANG J I G; MBBS, MRCP (London), BSc. Consultant Physician, Cecilia Makiwane Hospital and Honorary Lecturer in Medicine, University of Cape Town.

STREBEL P M; BSc, MBChB (Cape Town), MPH (Johns Hopkins), DCH (SA). Chief Medical Researcher, Centre for Epidemiological Research in Southern Africa, South African Medical Research Council.

Acknowledgements

In addition to the co-authors whose efforts are gratefully acknowledged in the Preface, we would like to thank the following for permission to use copyright material:

American Review of Respiratory Diseases
   Vertebral column found in a Neolithic cemetery near Heidelberg, showing collapse and fusion of 4th and 5th thoracic vertebrae. (Figure 1.1).
   Clay figurine of an emaciated man with a hunchback. (Figure 1.2)
   Hunchback figures from Egyptian tomb inscriptions. (Figure 1.3)
   Hunchback art from America showing rounded deformities. (Figure 1.5)
   The decline in tuberculosis death rates in the United States 1910–80. (Figure 1.8)

Basil Blackwell
   The decline in respiratory tuberculosis death rates in England and Wales since 1938. (Figure 1.7)

Cape Archives, Cape Town
   Workers cooking at a mine compound, Kimberley (Figure 1.9)

Dr V Chrystal, Department of Anatomical Pathology, University of Natal
   Histopathology slide of TBM and TB spinal cord. (Figure 9.3)

Epidemiological Comments
   Annual tuberculosis notification rate, RSA, 1921–85. (Figure 1.13).

Journal of the American Medical Association
   Pictures of Kokopelli, the hunchbacked flute player. (Figure 1.4)

Oxford Medical Publications.
   The pathogenesis of TBM. (Figure 9.1)

Penguin Books
   The comparative mortality factor for respiratory tuberculosis in England and Wales 1905–55. (Figure 1.6)

South African Library, Cape Town
   Kimberley Sanatorium. (Figure 1.11).

South African Medical Journal
   Notified annual tuberculosis death rate, RSA, 1945–77. (Figure 1.12)

Thorax
   Various chemotherapy regimens anbd some recommendations (Table 16.3)
   Doses and side-effects of anti-tuberculosis drugs (Table 16.6)

While every effort has been made to trace and acknowledge copyright holders, this has not always been possible. Should any infringement have occurred, apologies are tendered and any omissions will be rectified in the event of a reprint.

Preface

More than a hundred years after Robert Koch's discovery of the tubercle bacillus, tuberculosis remains a major cause of morbidity and mortality among the world's poor. In the global context 8 to 10 million people, the majority of whom live in developing countries, are afflicted by this disease each year and of these, two to three million die.

Through the ages the burden of tuberculosis has been borne by the most disadvantaged members of society. Indeed the history of tuberculosis is inextricably tied to the misery and wretched social conditions of the poor. It is rightly believed to be the pre-eminent social disease and a useful barometer of the standard of living and equity in any society.

Tuberculosis is a time-bomb in Africa. The high prevalence of infection, which in most people remains dormant and never gives rise to disease, threatens to erupt in response to many causes of reduced immunity. Poverty, malnutrition, overcrowding, alcoholism and measles seem pale shadows against the dark spectre of HIV infection which may trigger millions of people infected with *Mycobacterium tuberculosis* into frank clinical disease, often well before other manifestations of AIDS become evident.

While there are several excellent texts on tuberculosis, there is a disappointing shortage of books written by health professionals in countries where the disease is most prevalent, namely the third world. Available single texts seldom go beyond a restricted medical horizon to address the wider range of issues related to tuberculosis. Tuberculosis is the most common notifiable disease in South Africa with epidemic proportions being reached in some regions. The story of tuberculosis from the South African perspective of the 1990s illustrates, *par excellence*, the interplay between many social forces in determining the balance between disease and health. These considerations influenced our decision to include in the scope of this book descriptions of the historical, social, political, economic and biological influences on this disease.

By bringing together contributions from workers involved in a wide range of medical and other disciplines to describe and analyse its protean manifestations, to unravel the complexities of causal interrelationships, to apply modern medical knowledge to an understanding of the pathophysiology of tuberculosis, and to document the development of a multipronged therapeutic approach – all testimony to intellectual progress in the last 50 years – we have endeavored to broaden perspectives on an old disease.

While we would hesitate to make claims to uniqueness for the South African situation, we feel justified in suggesting that the contours of health and disease have rarely been as profoundly shaped by social and political realities anywhere, as they have been in this country. Accordingly, it seems entirely appropriate that the experience of tuberculosis in South Africa is reflected in a text by individuals from this country who have worked on this subject.

While this book was being written, South Africa was embarking on a political journey that offers hope for progress out of the wilderness created by its apartheid policies into a relationship with the world which could make it a catalyst for sub-Saharan development. South Africa reflects the crossroads in human progress in relation to many conflicts in the modern world – between capitalism and socialism, between individualism and collectivism, between Eurocentric and Afrocentric ideologies, between wealth and poverty, between progress and retrogression, between intercultural belligerence and mutual understanding, and between destruction and conservation of a precious ecology. The potential for successfully meeting these challenges and finding common ground is arguably better here than anywhere else in the world. Time will tell whether we shall follow the high or the low road.

The conquest of tuberculosis in the ensuing years will be one important indicator of progress towards social justice in this new order. Our hope is that this account of tuberculosis will make some, even if a very small, contribution towards finding this high road to freedom from want, poverty and injustice.

We thank our co-authors for their enthusiastic and generous response to our requests for contributions. We are delighted with this collection of essays which goes beyond our original expectations. The accomplishments of this project reinforce our belief in the need for research and scholarship, even in underfunded medical communities in third world countries. We hope that the contents of the book will be of interest to all those professionals and scientists interested in health and disease who wish to acquire a deeper insight into one of humankind's most durable natural enemies.

S R Benatar
H M Coovadia

CHAPTER 1

A history of tuberculosis

C Metcalf

INTRODUCTION

If diseases are to be prevented, it is essential to know the features of their development, features which extend deep not only into individual life, but down the centuries into the history of human development.[22]

The burden of ill-health and death caused by tuberculosis makes it one of the most important diseases in the history of human society. There has been no other single disease which has been so prevalent and widespread over such an extensive period in time. John Bunyon in his seventeenth century book, *The Life and Death of Mr Badman*, wrote of it as 'the captain of all these men of death' while in 1861 Oliver Wendell Holmes named it 'the white plague',[60] both being sombre commentaries on the extent of the disease in England.

Tuberculosis, although contagious, has not produced such acute dramatic epidemics as have the acute infectious diseases such as plague, smallpox and cholera. Consequently, it did not cause nearly as great a degree of public alarm, even though it caused more deaths than these conditions. Coventry, a general practitioner from New York, when speaking in 1856 of the high mortality due to tuberculosis noted:[47]

When a new epidemic disease like the cholera ravages the country, community becomes alarmed and every means is resorted to to stay its progress [although] the actual mortality is less than from this insidious disease.

Tuberculosis tends to have a more protracted course than these acute epidemic diseases, and historically was so universal that many societies did not generally regard it as infectious and so gave it scant, if any,

mention in texts on epidemic diseases. For example, Creighton's massive two volume tome, *A History of Epidemics in Britain*,[21] published in the 1890s, does not even consider tuberculosis.

However, the devastating effect of tuberculosis was well-recognized in European society:[24]

There is no other more dangerous disease than pulmonary phthisis, and no other is so common … It destroys a very great part of the human race,

according to the French medical professor, Antoine Portal (1742–1832), while Thomas Young wrote in London in 1815 that:

Of all hectic affections, by far the most important is pulmonary consumption, a disease so frequent as to carry off prematurely about one fourth part of the inhabitants of Europe, and so fatal as to deter the practitioner from even attempting a cure.

It is thought that pulmonary tuberculosis killed more people in nineteenth century Britain than did smallpox, measles, whooping cough, scarlet fever and typhus combined.[16] According to one estimate tuberculosis accounted for nine million deaths in France during the nineteenth century, compared with two million deaths due to war and 400 000 cholera deaths.[55] As late as 1889 it was still responsible for a quarter of all deaths in Paris.[55] Although tuberculosis incidence and mortality has subsequently declined to low levels in these countries, tuberculosis remains an important disease in many parts of the world, including South Africa, and globally it still causes an estimated two to three million deaths each year.[83]

The history of tuberculosis is not just the history of an infectious disease, but is intrinsically linked to demographic changes and to historical variations in social and environmental conditions. Thus, processes such as urbanization, industrialization, European colonization and war have been major determinants of the course of tuberculosis in different populations. The close historical relationship between tuberculosis incidence and mortality and social and environmental conditions highlights the continuing importance of these factors, and stresses the need for attempts to combat this disease to look beyond medical interventions. This has been emphasized by the physician Sir William Osler.[60]

In order to give a more complete appreciation of the subject, this chapter summarizes what is known about the origin of tuberculosis and its presence in early cultures. The pitfalls of interpreting historical data on tuberculosis are discussed in order to encourage readers to interpret historical material with due caution, and to recognize limitations in our knowledge of its history. At the same time, historical processes and conditions influencing the occurrence of tuberculosis are outlined. As these factors were common determinants of tuberculosis in different parts of the world, and as historical statistics tend to be inaccurate, detailed regional accounts of the history of tuberculosis are not given. The chapter concludes with a focus on the origins and development of tuberculosis in South Africa to illustrate the importance which socio-economic, demographic and political factors have had in determining the historical course of tuberculosis within a society.

ORIGINS OF TUBERCULOSIS

Where and when humanity first became afflicted by tuberculosis is unknown, but from the available evidence it appears that tuberculosis predates written records and has had a widespread occurrence for several millennia.

Evolution of *Mycobacterium tuberculosis*

The close genetic similarities between *Mycobacterium tuberculosis*, the usual causative organism in human tuberculosis, and *Mycobacterium bovis*, which causes tuberculosis in cattle and other animals as well as in humans, has led to speculation that cattle were the original source of tuberculous infection in humans, and that *M. tuberculosis* evolved from a mutant of *M. bovis*.[39, 58] The spread from cattle to humans rather than *vice versa* is suggested by the bovine bacillus *M. bovis* having a broad host range,[34] while the human bacillus *M. tuberculosis* is non-pathogenic in cattle.[19]

Cattle first became domesticated in the Neolithic period,[48–9] which is also the earliest period showing evidence of tuberculosis in humans. There is evidence of cattle domestication on a large scale in the northeastern Mediterranean basin between 5000 and 7000 BC, and milking of cattle is thought to have started in the Middle East between 4000 and 5000 BC. Consequently, Neolithic people may have first become infected by drinking milk from infected cows or by eating infected cattle flesh, but it has not been established when tuberculosis first became a disease of cattle. The earliest clear evidence of tuberculosis in domesticated animals comes from India where elephants have been shown to have suffered from tuberculosis prior to 2000 BC.[48–9]

Early evidence of tuberculosis from human remains

The earliest evidence of tuberculosis in humans comes from the study of skeletal remains, although most people dying of tuberculosis do not leave evidence of their condition, as disease of the bones is an uncommon manifestation of tuberculosis and, even when the body is mummified, the lungs and other organs are rarely well-preserved.[58]

A characteristic site for skeletal tuberculosis is the spine, where the infection erodes one or more of the spinal vertebrae, typically resulting in a hunchback deformity, but it is important to bear in mind that there are several other causes of bone lesions that resemble tuberculous spondylitis. These include other bacterial as well as fungal infections, trauma, bone tumours and certain types of arthritis.[58] Thus,

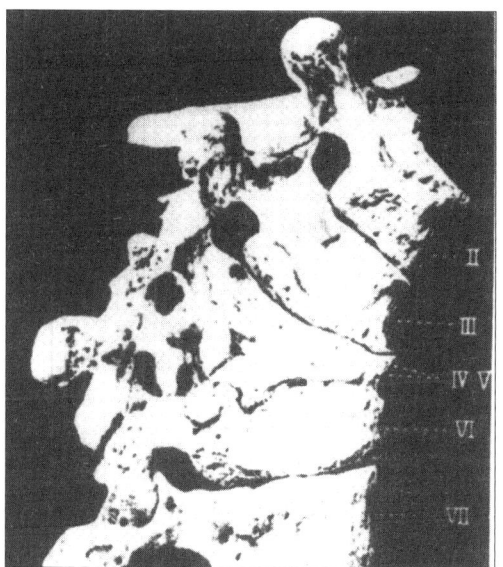

Figure 1.1. Vertebral column found in a Neolithic cemetery near Heidelberg, showing collapse and fusion of 4th and 5th thoracic vertebrae. Thought to be the first evidence of human skeletal tuberculosis. (Source: Morse D, 1961. Prehistoric tuberculosis in America. *American Review of Respiratory Diseases.* 83, 490)

palaeopathological evidence for tuberculosis is often suggestive but rarely unequivocal. Furthermore, even when bone lesions are due to tuberculosis it is possible that they were caused by *M. bovis*, which is a common cause of skeletal tuberculosis but rarely causes pulmonary tuberculosis.[39]

Skeletal deformities suggestive of tuberculosis have been found in ancient skeletons from several parts of the world, the earliest possible case being the skeleton of a Neolithic man found near Heidelberg in Germany[73] and which dates from about 5000 BC (Figure 1.1). Although the vertebral lesions in this skeleton are suggestive of healed spinal tuberculosis, there is some doubt about the validity of this diagnosis.[49]

Apart from this one example, the earliest palaeopathological evidence of human tuberculosis comes from Egypt, where several studies of early skeletal remains, spanning the period 3700 to 1000 BC, show evidence of possible tuberculosis.[58] The earliest definitive evidence for tuberculosis in Egypt dates back to the Dynastic period (which

started about 3400 BC), and an example is the mummy of a five year old child with evidence of pulmonary and vertebral tuberculosis. Acid-fast bacilli (presumed to be *M. bovis* or *M. tuberculosis*) in vertebral bone on microscopy support the diagnosis.[96] A further well-known example, dating from about 1000 BC, is Nesperehan, the mummy of a young man with spinal lesions and an associated large psoas abscess.[58] Examples of possible skeletal tuberculosis, dated between 3150 and 2200 BC, have also been found in early Bronze Age Jordan.[61]

However, extensive studies of ancient Egyptian mummies have not provided much evidence of pulmonary tuberculosis,[11] but this is not surprising as mummies are rarely well-preserved.[58]

Apart from the Heidelberg skeleton (in which the diagnosis of tuberculosis is disputed), palaeopathological evidence for tuberculosis in northern Europe and the British Isles is considerably more recent.[49] The earliest evidence of possible tuberculous spondylitis from Scandinavia was found in Denmark in the skeleton of a young woman dated between 2500 and 1500 BC.[73] In Britain the earliest palaeopathological evidence of possible tuberculosis dates back to between the third and fifth centuries AD, and very few specimens pre-date the Norman Conquest (1066 AD).[49]

The presence or absence of tuberculosis in the Americas prior to Columbus' arrival in 1492 has been the subject of much debate.[5, 27, 56-7, 63-4] The early American peoples were cut off from the Old World after the submersion of the Bering land bridge between Siberia and Alaska in about 8000 BC, several thousand years prior to the earliest evidence of tuberculosis in Asia and Europe. Evidence of tuberculosis in pre-Columbian America has thus been used to infer an even earlier origin to human tuberculosis than can be established from Asian and European sources. However, participants in this debate tend to give scant consideration to the possibility that tuberculosis might have been brought to the Americas by other seafarers (such as the Vikings) prior to Columbus.

While much of the palaeopathological evidence for pre-Columbian tuberculosis in various parts of the Americas is tentative and has been questioned,[56] definitive evidence has recently emerged.[5, 48, 64] A convincing example is the mummy of a child from the Nazca culture dated about 700 AD found in southern Peru.[5] This child had a spinal deformity typical of tuberculosis, with an associated psoas abscess and miliary tuberculosis in several organs. The diagnosis of tuberculosis was confirmed by the demonstration of acid-fast bacilli on histological examination of tissue specimens.

Palaeopathological studies of spinal deformities have provided evidence of the antiquity of tuberculosis in several parts of the world, but do not give an estimate of the occurrence of pulmonary tuberculosis in early cultures. The frequency of pulmonary tuberculosis in relation to skeletal tuberculosis is likely to have varied in different societies according to whether the

human or the bovine bacillus, or both, were endemic. Pulmonary tuberculosis is of far greater importance than skeletal tuberculosis, as it is the communicable form of the disease, and the form that causes the most deaths.

It must be remembered that failure to demonstrate lesions resembling tuberculosis in collections of human remains does not establish its absence in any particular culture or time period.

Evidence from primitive art

Artistic representations of figures which appear to have hunched backs have been put forward as evidence of skeletal tuberculosis in several early cultures. However this evidence is of limited scientific value in establishing the presence of tuberculosis as, in addition to the possibility that the deformities had a non-tuberculous cause, the

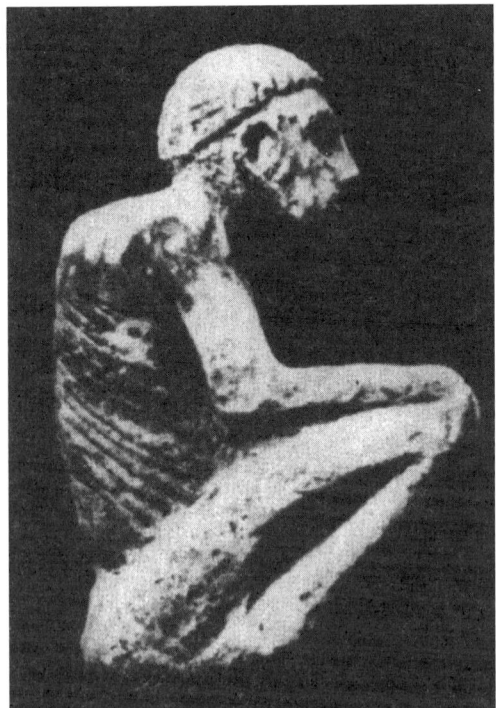

Figure 1.2. Clay figurine of an emaciated man with a hunchback. Thought to be Predynastic. (Source: Morse, D, Brothwell D R & Ucko P J, 1964. Tuberculosis in Ancient Egypt. *American Review of Respiratory Diseases*. 90, 525)

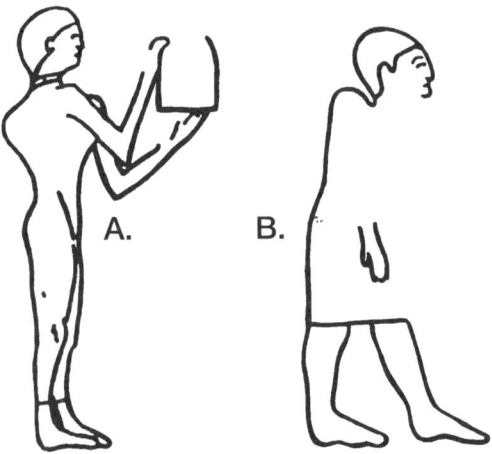

Figures 1.3 a & b. Hunchback figures from Egyptian tomb inscriptions. Dynastic Period. (Source: Morse, D, Brothwell D R & Ucko P J, 1964. Tuberculosis in Ancient Egypt. *American Review of Respiratory Diseases*. 90, 526). **Figure 1.3a:** Bas-relief of a serving girl. From Gizeh Tomb no. 45, IVth Dynasty. **Figure 1.3b:** Painting of an attendant. Found in tomb at Beni Hasan, XIIth Dynasty.

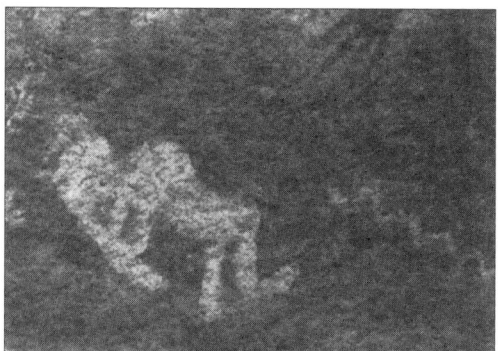

Figure 1.4a

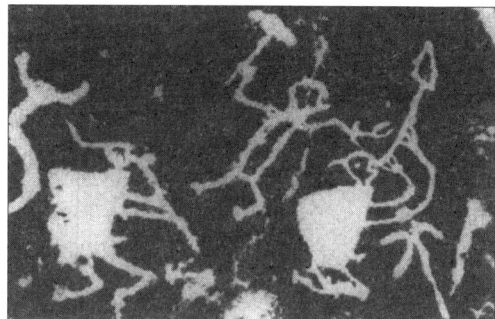

Figure 1.4c

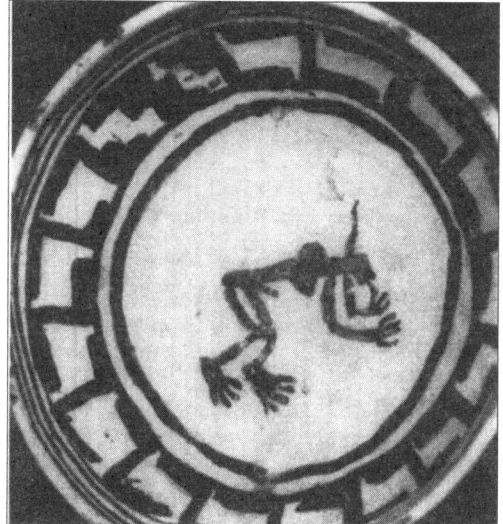

Figure 1.4b

Figures 1.4 a, b & c. Pictures of Kokopelli, the hunchbacked flute player. (Source: Wellmann K F, 1970. Kokopelli of Indian Paleology. Hunchbacked Rain Priest, Hunting Magician & Don Juan of the Old Southwest. (*Journal of the American Medical Association.* 212 (10), 1680–1). **Figure 1.4a:** Pictograph of a hunchbacked flute player. From a rock shelter in Arizona, United States. Possibly dating to before 700 AD. **Figure 1.4b:** Kokopelli on a pottery bowl. Great Pueblo Period (before 1300 AD). **Figure 1.4c:** Two hunchbacked flute players and a figure with a tomahawk. From a cave in New Mexico. Pueblo Culture, circa 1450 AD.

deformities may be apparent rather than real as a result of stylistic conventions of the culture.[57–8]

Many artistic relics with hunchbacks were left by the ancient Egyptians, the earliest examples being figurines, of which some may date back to before the Dynastic period (before 3400 BC) (Figure 1.2). Hunchback figures occur frequently in ancient Egyptian tomb inscriptions from the Dynastic period (Figure 1.3).

Hunchback artistic relics have also been put forward as evidence of tuberculosis in early Central and South American peoples, including the Pueblo and the Inca cultures.[93] Kokopelli, a hump-backed rain priest and a hunting magician in the Pueblo culture (Figure 1.4), is a well known exam-ple, but he was a mythical character and his hump had a mythical function.[93] The hunchbacks in early American prehistoric art tend to have smooth, rounded backs (Figure 1.5) which do not resemble the more angular deformity resulting from tuberculous spondylitis[58] and thus do not provide additional evidence for the presence of tuberculosis in pre-Columbian America.[57]

Early written accounts

Since human remains and primitive art provide very little information on the presence and distribution of the pulmonary form of tuberculosis in early cultures, evidence has been sought in early writings. However, many cultures did not have written records,

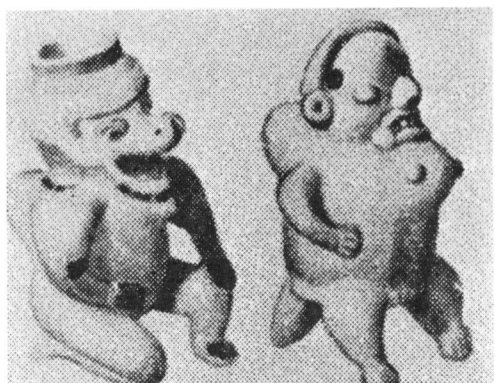

Figure 1.5a

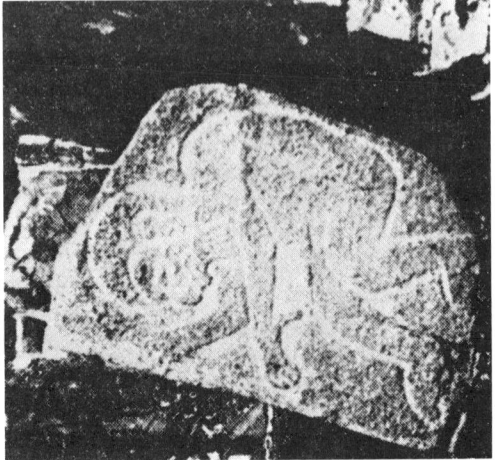

Figure 1.5b

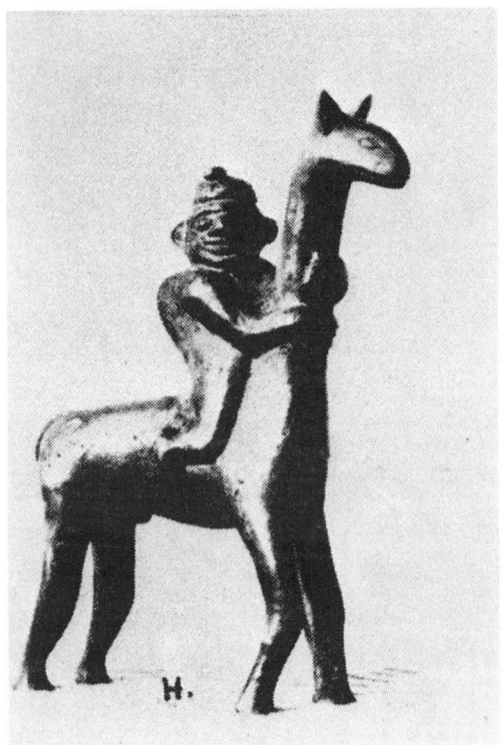

Figure 1.5c

Figures 1.5 a, b & c: Hunchback art from America showing rounded deformities. (Source: Morse D, 1961. Prehistoric tuberculosis in America. *American Review of Respiratory Diseases.* 83, 495). **Figure 1.5a:** Clay figurines from Costa Rica. **Figure 1.5b:** Figure on a stone block from Mexico. **Figure 1.5c:** Mounted silver figurine from Peru. Inca culture (pre-Spanish).

and where records have survived, diseases described are often difficult to identify with any certainty as historical conceptions of disease were very different from modern understanding. Lacking modern diagnostic aids, earlier observers diagnosed diseases largely on the basis of symptom complexes. As the symptoms of tuberculosis are non-specific, descriptions of consumption and phthisis (the terms commonly taken as denoting tuberculosis in historical writings) do not allow tuberculous and non-tuberculous disease to be separately identified. Historical terms for different forms of tuberculous disease are given in Table 1.1.

Some of the oldest surviving medical documents are the Egyptian medical papyri, which do not contain any clear reference to tuberculosis,[41] which is surprising given the numerous skeletal remains with lesions suggestive of tuberculosis from ancient Egypt.[57-8] The Ebers papyri refer to two different types of cervical lymphadenopathy and it is possible that one of these types was tuberculous scrofula.[39]

The earliest written evidence of pulmonary tuberculosis comes from Asia.[41, 57] However many of these writings have been difficult to date with any degree of precision.[57] Early Chinese writings dated about

Table 1.1
Terms used previously to denote tuberculosis

TYPE OF TUBERCULOSIS	HISTORICAL SYNONYMS*
Acute progressive tuberculosis	Galloping consumption[24]
Pulmonary tuberculosis	Consumption
	Phthisis
	Tabes pulmonalis
	Tissic[16]
	Hectic fever
	Gastric fever
	Asthenia
	Lupus
Cervical adenitis	Scrofula
	Struma[2]
	King's evil[16]
Abdominal tuberculosis	Tabes mesenterica
Tuberculosis meningitis	Acute hydrocephalus[54]
	Infantile encephalitis[54]
Vertebral tuberculosis	Pott's disease[2]

*Also applied to non-tuberculous conditions

2700 BC mention the conditions 'lung fever' and 'lung cough', and these probably included pulmonary tuberculosis, as they had symptoms of cough, wasting, and the expectoration of blood and sputum.[41] The Vedas (hymns) of the Hindu Indo-Aryan civilization, which were written in Sanskrit, contain many references to tuberculosis, and suggest that these people had become familiar with pulmonary tuberculosis by 1500 BC, the approximate date of the Rig-Veda, which is the earliest surviving record.[41, 57]

As with India and China, the early writings from Babylonia and Assyria are difficult to date accurately and there have also been difficulties in translating Mesopotamian medical texts.[57] The Code of Hammurabi (Babylonia 1700 BC) does not have any clear reference to tuberculosis.[57] More recent Mesopotamian medical texts dating from about 675 BC describe a condition which is suggestive of pulmonary tuberculosis with its symptoms including cough, haemoptysis and excessive sweating.[57]

It is unclear whether tuberculosis was present among the ancient Hebrew people. The books of Leviticus (1490 BC) and Deuteronomy (1451 BC) in the Bible contain threats of punishment with what Rashi in the twelfth century translated as consumption, if people were to invoke God's wrath.[79] However, neither the Old nor the New Testaments give any clear description of a disease resembling pulmonary tuberculosis[18, 57] and there was no word for 'cough' in the ancient Hebrew language.[79] The Talmud, on the other hand, provides a description of lesions in the lungs of animals, suggestive of tuberculosis,[18] and according to Mosaic Law such animals are not fit for human consumption.[79]

The early Greek literature has several references to consumption, the earliest being in the writings of Homer, dated 800 BC.[57] The word 'phthisis' is thought to have been introduced by Hippocrates in the fifth century BC,[60] and his description of phthisis, given in volumes one and two of *de Morbis*[79] include the symptoms of persistent cough, fever, excessive perspiration, wasting and haemoptysis (coughing up blood). He noted the presence of nodules in the lungs and commented that deceased people with high spinal curvatures usually had nodules in their lungs.[79] It can thus be inferred that the condition he described included tuberculosis. Aristotle (384–322 BC) was the first to suggest the contagious nature of phthisis,[45] stating that with close contact 'one takes the disease because there is in the air something disease-producing'.[60] Galen (131–200 AD), the Greek physician who practised in Rome, also considered phthisis to be contagious.[45] Aretaeus, who lived in Alexandria in the second century AD, gave a clear account of phthisis, distinguishing it from empyema,[76] and describing the presence of cavities in the lungs.[79]

Many Roman writers referred to tuberculosis, the earliest being Plautus in 184 BC.[57] Written accounts of tuberculosis from other cultures are more recent and include the writings of the Byzantine physician, Alexander of Thalles (*c.* 600 AD) and Arabian medical literature such as that of Rhazes (900 AD) and Avicenna (1000 AD).[57]

Thus there is evidence dating back several millennia of the presence of forms of tuberculosis in many parts of the world. While many people believe that tuberculosis originated in ancient civilizations in the Near East after the domestication of cattle, and these beliefs are plausible in the light of current knowledge, evidence on the origin and spread of tuberculosis is still fragmentary and no clear picture has yet emerged.

DIFFICULTIES IN DETERMINING THE HISTORICAL EPIDEMIOLOGY OF TUBERCULOSIS

Absence of data

Knowledge of the historical epidemiology of tuberculosis depends on the presence of written records. A major problem when trying to assess tuberculosis trends in many parts of the world is the absence of data. The greatest volume of historical writings and the earliest reliable vital statistics are European, and so the history of tuberculosis is largely undocumented except in Europe and in those parts of the world colonized by Europeans. However, it cannot be inferred from the absence of records that tuberculosis did not exist in a society.

Knowledge of the presence and extent of tuberculosis in pre-colonial societies is limited as most did not have written records, while in the case of the Aztec culture, records were destroyed by the invading Spanish colonists. The earliest knowledge of tuberculosis in the indigenous peoples of North and South America, Africa and Australasia comes from reports by early European travellers and missionaries, the reliability of which is sometimes questionable as they were based on superficial encounters with native people and tend to be biased by beliefs prevailing in their culture at the time.

The problem of the absence of data is not only a historical one, as it is still a major problem in developing countries. Figures are still generally either unavailable or totally unreliable for much of Africa, Asia (including China) and Latin America, which together account for about three-quarters of the world population.[83] The availability and validity of reported tuberculosis statistics are highly correlated with national wealth, and so international statistics are likely to be weakest in those areas where the tuberculosis situation is worst.[20] Consequently, not much is known about the history of tuberculosis in those parts of the world where tuberculosis is far from being a historical problem.

Unreliability of historical statistics

Major difficulties are confronted when trying to establish an accurate picture of historical trends in tuberculosis incidence and mortality, even in countries for which historical information is available.

The London Bills of Mortality which were first compiled in 1532 are one of the oldest sources of death statistics. These Bills have been used by researchers (including the well known work of Brownlee[12]) to try to determine trends in tuberculosis mortality in England. However, in addition to the problem of inaccurate certification of the cause of death,[17] the approach of drawing inferences about mortality rates from the proportion of deaths attributed to consumption has other major flaws, and cannot be reliably used to determine historical mortality trends. This approach does not take into account the population size, changes in the age-structure of the population, or changes in competing causes of death, and is very unsatisfactory for those periods when acute epidemic diseases such as plague, typhus and cholera caused a high mortality.

The first census in Britain was carried out as relatively recently as 1801, and earlier population statistics are controversial.[33] It is not possible to obtain reliable estimates of tuberculosis mortality rates in Britain prior to the mid-nineteenth century as there are no accurate death statistics for England and Wales before the introduction of death registration in 1838. Even after the introduction of death registration, tuberculosis mortality figures are unreliable as many people were reluctant to have deaths registered as consumption, while in Wales deaths were easily misregistered initially as a medical certificate was not required.[80]

In Australia no reliable figures for tuberculosis mortality prior to 1865 can be determined as phthisis was classified with bronchitis and pneumonia.[86] Thus, the apparent increase in tuberculosis mortality in the late nineteenth century is exaggerated.

In the United States vital statistics were still fragmentary during the last century, and so tuberculosis mortality rates prior to this century cannot be reliably determined.[6] The geographical regions from which United States mortality figures were derived has changed over time, with mortality rates in 1900 being based on returns from only 10 states. From then on states were incorporated serially until 1933, by which time all the states had been included.[36] The secular trend in tuberculosis incidence and mortality may have been distorted by changes in the geographical area from which the figures were derived prior to 1933.

Estimates of tuberculosis incidence are not available for any country prior to the twentieth century, as notification of tuberculosis has only been introduced relatively recently. Some dates when compulsory notification of tuberculosis was introduced are: New York 1897, Norway 1901, the Cape and Natal Colonies in South Africa in 1904, Denmark 1905, the United States by 1906, England 1913, Scotland 1914.[13, 90]

In England notification remained patchy until after the 1921 Tuberculosis Act,[80] and failure to notify tuberculosis remained a major problem in some districts into the 1940s despite repeated legislative attempts to enforce notification.[13] The high proportion of tuberculosis notifications made posthumously during the 1920s to 1940s[13] implies that a high proportion of non-fatal cases escaped notification.

In South Africa there was resistance to notification on the part of local authorities as they deemed the notification fee (of two shillings and sixpence) to be a waste of money.[90] Variation in criteria used to notify tuberculosis, both within a country and between countries, is an ongoing problem when trying to make regional comparisons and to establish secular trends.

Under-reporting

Under-reporting of tuberculosis deaths was a serious problem historically. In England, France and the United States the belief that tuberculosis was caused by a 'hereditary taint' persisted through most of the nineteenth century, and thus placed a stigma on the family and decreased eligibility for marriage, certain occupations and life insurance among members of affected families.[24] Family members were also reluctant to have the cause of death recorded as tuberculosis lest it interfere with the collection of death claims from insurance companies.[29] Many tuberculosis deaths were thus attributed to other causes such as pneumonia and bronchitis,[13, 29, 84] a reversal of the situation that had existed some centuries earlier in London, when many plague deaths were recorded as consumption in the Bills of Mortality because of the stigma of plague![17] In 1918 Sir Robert Philip said of English tuberculosis mortality statistics:[65]

... mortality statistics as published by the Registrar-General include only deaths certified by the patients' doctors as having occurred from tuberculosis. It is common knowledge that many deaths occur from tuberculosis which are not thus certified, either because the disease has not been recognized, or because it has been

Table 1.2

Conditions commonly confused with tuberculosis

TYPE OF TUBERCULOSIS	CONDITIONS CONFUSED WITH TUBERCULOSIS
Consumption	Conditions causing weight loss (e.g. cancers and diabetes mellitus)[24]
Pulmonary tuberculosis	Pneumonia and its complications (lung abscess, gangrene, empyema, purulent pericarditis)[9] Heart conditions (mitral stenosis, aortic aneurysm and aortic incompetence)[9] Lung cancer (primary & secondary) [9] Silicosis ('Miner's phthisis') [24]
Cervical adenitis	Other infections (including syphilis & leprosy)[85] Lymphoma and secondary cancers[85] Sarcoidosis[85] Goitre[2]
Abdominal tuberculosis	Crohn's disease (regional ileitis) [3] Appendix mass[3] Cancer of the colon (right-sided) [3]
Tuberculous meningitis	Other bacterial meningitides[54] Encephalitides[54]

described euphemistically. What the patient died of, and what he is said to have died of are not always one and the same thing. Many deaths are labelled as from pneumonia, bronchitis, measles, whooping-cough, or influenza, which are really referable to tuberculosis.

In the United States the tuberculosis statistics for blacks during the nineteenth century are an underestimate, as blacks often presented with acute pulmonary tuberculosis, which tended to be misdiagnosed as pneumonia. Tuberculosis in black Americans was also widely believed to be a different disease to consumption in whites and was thus often excluded from tuberculosis mortality figures, being classified under names such as 'Negro consumption', 'Negro poisoning', 'struma Africana' and 'cachexia Africana'.[88]

Overdiagnosis

Overdiagnosis of tuberculosis because of a lack of diagnostic precision and an inability to distinguish it from other conditions which produce a similar clinical picture, occurs on a significant scale in the twentieth century, and is likely to have been more frequent in previous centuries.

Evidence of overdiagnosis comes from a number of autopsy series of patients hospitalized for tuberculosis, published between 1915 and 1920.[9, 29] Although the autopsy cases were a select group and were not a representative sample of deaths attributed to tuberculosis, they do provide an indication of conditions that were misdiagnosed as tuberculosis. Conditions commonly confused with the different forms of tuberculosis are shown in Table 1.2.

The high frequency of 'sputum negative' tuberculosis in patients admitted to sanatoria early this century has led to the suggestion that a high proportion of sanatorium patients had non-tuberculous conditions.[29] In this connection it is interesting to note that in Ash's autopsy series referred to above, several patients without evidence of active tuberculosis at autopsy had had sputum confirmation of tuberculosis prior to death![9]

HISTORICAL CONCEPTIONS OF TUBERCULOSIS

Failure to recognize the different forms of tuberculosis as a single disease

Until late in the nineteenth century tuberculosis in different organs was not widely recognized as being different manifestations of one disease, a fact which, however, had limited significance from an epidemiological viewpoint as pulmonary tuberculosis has always accounted for the majority of deaths, and non-pulmonary forms are generally not transmissible.

The association between vertebral and pulmonary tuberculosis alluded to by Hippocrates seems to have been suspected in western Europe during the eighteenth century.[38] However, scrofula was long thought to be independent of phthisis[60] although several people, including Englishman Richard Morton (1689) and Sylvius of Leyden (seventeenth century), had proposed that consumption and scrofula were different manifestations of the same disease.[2, 60] Prior to 1836, when Green, on noting the presence of tubercles on inflamed meninges, introduced the term 'tubercular meningitis', cases of tuberculous meningitis were given non-specific diagnoses.[54]

The French physician, Laënnec (1781–1826), who invented the stethoscope, recognized the unity of tuberculosis in different organs in 1804. However, his unitarian theory of tuberculosis was not generally accepted at the time, being rejected by influential people such as Virchow, the pathologist.[24] In 1839 Schönlein, a Professor of Medicine at Zürich, proposed the use of the word 'tuberculosis' for all manifestations of phthisis, as the tubercle was the basic underlying pathology.[24] However, it was to be some time before this word was to come into general use.

The heredity versus contagion debate

In Europe, different beliefs about the cause of tuberculosis prevailed in different regions for more than three centuries.[59] Southern Europeans in Italy, Spain and the south of France gradually came to regard tuberculosis as contagious from the mid-sixteenth century, and by the second half of the eighteenth century there was a widespread movement throughout southern Europe to prevent contagion.[60]

The theory of contagion was proposed by the Florentine physician Fracastorius, who in 1546 published the first modern description of tuberculosis.[60] He believed that tuberculosis was caused by invisible *seminaria* which could live outside the body for many years, and wrote:

> *These seeds are the carriers of contagion and that they are the first origin of the disease there can be no doubt.*

As a result of their belief in the contagiousness of tuberculosis, Italian anatomists, including Valsalva (1666–1723), refused to perform autopsies on people who had died from the disease.[60]

The Italian Republic of Lucca was the first place in the world to take legislative action to control tuberculosis when, in 1699, it passed an edict which made the reporting of consumption compulsory and ordered the burning of clothing and personal effects of those who had died of the disease.[60, 91] Later edicts contained orders to air the house of consumptive patients and to take precautions with the disposal of their sputum.[60] Similar laws were passed in Spain in 1751 and in Naples in 1782.[60, 91] These edicts were later revoked as a result of adverse public opinion and the economic losses entailed in destroying property.[91]

In England and northern France the belief that tuberculosis was due to a hereditary disposition (sometimes termed a 'tubercular diathesis') prevailed until the late nineteenth century, and was based on the observation that the disease tended to run in families. The belief that tuberculosis was contagious was generally not accepted in this region or the European colonies until late in the nineteenth century.

The Englishman Richard Morton, whose book *Phthisiologia* was published in 1689, devoted several pages to discussion of heredity, but he did not even mention contagion.[59] However, in 1720 the English physician Benjamin Martin in his book entitled *A New Theory of Consumptives, more Especially of a Phthisis or Consumption of the Lungs* proposed that pulmonary tuberculosis was infectious.[59] In this work he stated that: 'The original and essential cause [of phthisis] … may possibly be some certain species of animalculae or wonderfully minute living creatures'. He also correctly proposed that sustained close contact with a case of tuberculosis was necessary for the transmission of a sufficiently infectious dose to cause disease, and that transmission was airborne. However, these theories were ignored by his contemporaries.

It is now accepted that genetic factors play a very minor role in determining susceptibility to tuberculosis and are overshadowed by environmental factors. The frequent occurrence of tuberculosis in families can be explained by the transmission of infection within the home, as well as by family members being subjected to the same environmental risk factors.

The domination of anticontagionism (i.e. the belief that tuberculosis was not contagious) was brought to an end by microbiological discoveries in the second half of the nineteenth century.[2] The French military surgeon, Villemin, carried out experiments from 1865 to 1868 in which he transmitted tuberculosis to animals by serial inoculation of tuberculous material.[2] The discovery of *Mycobacterium tuberculosis*, the causative organism, has been attributed to Koch, who in 1882 demonstrated the bacillus under the microscope using special staining techniques.[2] However, Koch's discovery took about a decade to find general medical acceptance in Britain.[80]

As tuberculosis incidence and mortality rates in the different European countries are not known for this period, the contribution that these different beliefs about the cause of tuberculosis may have made to possible regional differences in mortality cannot be determined.

Race, epidemic waves and the notion of a virgin population

Much has been written about the role of race in determining susceptibility to tuberculosis because of the large disparities that have been observed between people of different ethnic groups living within a region. However, the association between race and tuberculosis need not imply that certain races are intrinsically more susceptible to tuberculosis, as race is usually associated with socio-economic status, which is an important determinant of disease risk.

The theory of differences in racial susceptibility to tuberculosis has been shown historically to be unsound, as under adverse environmental conditions, ethnic groups that are apparently relatively resistant to tuberculosis have rapidly become susceptible. This has been strikingly demonstrated in Jewish communities in Europe. Of all ethnic groups, European Jews (both Sephardim and Ashkenazim) had a reputation for having had the greatest degree of 'racial resistance' to tuberculosis,[2, 24, 46, 67, 74] as in several European cities recorded tuberculosis mortality rates were lower in Jews than in Gentile inhabitants. However, this situation was rapidly reversed during the period of intense Jewish persecution and environmental disruption at the time of the Second World War, when tuberculosis mortality in Jewish people increased several fold in places such as Warsaw and came to exceed the rates in Gentiles.[24]

During the process of European colonization the native inhabitants of colonized territories developed much higher rates of tuberculosis than did the colonizers. This included racially diverse people such as the Inuit and American Indians in North America, Aborigines in Australia, and Africans in African colonies. Native groups were generally more prone to the rapidly progressive form of tuberculosis referred to in historical texts as 'galloping consumption'.

A popular theory in the late nineteenth and early twentieth centuries to explain these racial disparities was the notion of a 'virgin population', which, because of lack of previous exposure to infection, had not had a chance to acquire resistance and was therefore susceptible. This theory had two variations: a Lamarckian approach, in which acquired resistance was thought to be passed from one generation to the next; and a Darwinian approach, in which 'natural selection' was thought to weed out those who were genetically most susceptible over several generations.

The 'virgin population' theory suited the ideology of European colonizers, who were its main proponents. When confronted by the ravages of tuberculosis among native inhabitants of the colonies, this theory conveniently allowed them to underplay or ignore the role of adverse changes in environmental factors brought about by colonization.

The notion of a 'virgin population' is applicable to some infectious diseases such as smallpox (which also decimated native populations in many parts of the world during the period of European colonization), as individuals acquire permanent immunity following disease or immunization. However, with tuberculosis, the immunity is relative and can be reversed by environmental factors; thus the 'virgin population' notion does not make biological sense.

Some people still subscribe to the Darwinian view that natural selection is an important determinant of racial differences in tuberculosis disease rates.[10] The proponents of this theory believe that natural selection has accounted for epidemic waves of tuberculosis, often lasting several decades, in different ethnic groups and geographical regions. They explain racial differences in susceptibility to tuberculosis in terms of phase differences in the epidemic wave.[10, 68] However, the theory of epidemic waves is based on extremely thin evidence,[24] epidemic cycles in tuberculosis being largely due to environmental factors, which can be modified by human intervention. Although age-specific tuberculosis rates have declined in successive birth cohorts in the United States since 1880,[30] this decline was too rapid to be explained on the basis of natural selection. As many people who developed tuberculosis had already produced offspring, it is unlikely that natural selection has played a role in the decline of tuberculosis in developed countries. Phase differences among different racial and ethnic groups, both within and between regions, are determined by lifetime environmental exposures, and are not an inherited phenomenon passed down from generation to generation.

Tuberculosis as a disease of famous people

There have been many accounts of tuberculosis in famous people. Two groups which

Table 1.3
Famous creative people alleged to have suffered from tuberculosis

PERSON	LIFE PERIOD	VOCATION
Henry Purcell[1]	1659–95	English composer
Antoine Watteau[18]	1684–1721	French painter
Niccoló Paganini[45]	1782–1840	Italian violinist
Percy Bysshe Shelley[45]	1792–1822	English poet
John Keats[26, 28, 45, 81]	1795–1821	English poet
Elizabeth Barrett Browning[43, 45]	1806–61	English poet
Frédéric Chopin[45, 59]	1810–49	Polish pianist and composer
The Brontë Sisters[44]		English writers
Charlotte	1816–55	
Emily	1818–48	
Anne	1820–49	
Edvard Grieg[1]	1843–1907	Norwegian pianist and composer
Robert Louis Stevenson[45]	1850–94	Scottish writer
Anton Chekhov[25]	1860–1904	Russian playwright
Amedeo Modigliani[8, 18]	1884–1920	Italian painter
D H Lawrence[18]	1885–1930	English writer
Katherine Mansfield[45]	1888–1923	New Zealand/English writer

have received special attention in the literature are medical people and artists.

Until the present century tuberculosis was commonly believed to be associated with creativity and genius,[1] people with consumption being alleged to possess a special creative energy which the Greeks called 'spes phthisica'.[1] Some examples of famous creative people in history who are alleged to have suffered from tuberculosis are shown in Table 1.3. However, it should not be inferred from the prominence given to these people that they were more prone to tuberculosis than were less-distinguished members of society. There is also no evidence that the disease breeds genius. Dubos[24] has speculated that the association between tuberculosis and genius (if it has ever truly existed) may be explained by 'eagerness for achievement [leading] to a way of life that renders the body less resistant to infection.'

Many medical figures famous for their work in connection with tuberculosis, including Laënnec, and Dr Trudeau, have themselves had the disease. This is hardly surprising as tuberculosis was widespread and a leading cause of death in their times, and this association was therefore not necessarily due to occupational exposure. Some doctors were prompted to take an interest in tuberculosis because of their personal experience of the disease. Doctors were also more likely to provide a lucid account of their symptoms and have their disease diagnosed.

HISTORICAL PROCESSES AND CONDITIONS INFLUENCING TUBERCULOSIS OCCURRENCE AND MORTALITY

The risk factors for tuberculosis infection and disease are discussed in Chapter 4. These risk factors seldom occur singly, and a number of historical processes, such as urbanization, industrialization, colonization, and war, have led to changes in risk factor profiles in communities and populations, resulting in increases in tuberculosis. Population movements have also affected the occurrence and distribution of this disease.

Possible changes in the virulence of *Mycobacterium tuberculosis*

Secular trends in some infectious diseases are affected by changes in the genetic structure and virulence of the organism. An example is the virulent strain of the influenza virus, which in 1918 caused an influenza pandemic that led to extensive global mortality, causing more deaths than the First World War. The tubercle bacillus is a relatively stable organism and possible changes in virulence are believed not to have contributed to secular or regional variations in tuberculosis mortality rates.[24]

Urbanization and industrialization

An American physician, Dr Edward Livingstone Trudeau, performed a classic experiment which demonstrated the important role played by the environment in modifying an individual's susceptibility to tuberculosis.[50] He inoculated ten rabbits with identical doses of tubercle bacilli, and then set five of them free while confining the remainder in damp, sunless conditions, feeding them a poor diet. The confined rabbits soon died, while the unconfined rabbits, when recaptured some time later, showed evidence of healing. Although such experiments are not ethically possible in humans, the process of urbanization which is closely associated with industrialization, replicates the conditions of the confined malnourished rabbits with consequent increases in tuberculosis mortality.

As pulmonary tuberculosis was so common and, on the whole, not believed to be infectious, no precautions were taken to avoid transmission, and so infection spread unchecked. The industrial revolution, which started in Britain during the eighteenth century and spread to other countries during the nineteenth and twentieth centuries, led to the rapid growth of towns and often to severe overcrowding. People were thus exposed to high doses of infection, and as the risk of developing tuberculosis is directly related to the infecting dose, it is not surprising that the disease was rife.

Tuberculosis death rates have repeatedly been shown to be related to economic factors. For example, in Hamburg early this century, tuberculosis death rates were shown to be inversely related to the amount of income tax paid; in Paris tuberculosis mortality was shown to be lowest in the rich district Elysée and highest in the very poor Vingtième Arrondissement.[29] The higher rates in poorer sectors of society were due not only to the poor housing and overcrowding brought about by urbanization, but also to poor diets which lowered resistance to the disease.

There is a strong association between tuberculosis mortality and industrialization.[24] In most developed countries, tuberculosis mortality peaked during the phase of rapid industrialization. There is thus a close relation between the sequence in which countries industrialized and the sequence in which tuberculosis declined in these countries.

Migration

As a result of the widespread emigration of Europeans in the nineteenth and early twentieth centuries, the changing population in several countries contributed to secular trends in tuberculosis mortality. Population movements led not only to the rapid growth of urban centres and conditions favouring the development of tuberculosis, but also to changes in the composition of the population at risk. Thus, the large scale immigration of susceptible Irish settlers to the United States after the Irish famine of 1848 led to increased tuberculosis mortality in American cities such as Boston where many Irish people settled.[36]

Climate and altitude therapy for tuberculosis were very popular in the last century (from about 1830) and places with high altitudes and sunny dry climates were promoted extensively in both medical and lay publications.[31, 37, 75, 87, 92] This led to the large-scale migration of people with tuberculosis to favoured locales. Initially most health resorts were in Europe, but with the development of European colonies in North America, Africa and Australia, and with the improvements in sea travel, increasing numbers of consumptives travelled to the United

States and the colonies in the second half of the nineteenth century. For example, it has been estimated that consumptives who had immigrated for health reasons constituted one-third of the population of Colorado by 1880.[70] This selective migration increased tuberculosis mortality in Colorado,[70] Cape Town and Beaufort West in South Africa,[90] and Melbourne in Australia.[86] These immigrants also indirectly increased the tuberculosis incidence and mortality by acting as sources of infection to local residents. Examples of this happening can be found in the Alps[7] and Karoo towns in South Africa.[90]

As the numbers of people who emigrated from Britain and Europe on account of tuberculosis is not known, the extent to which the exportation of the disease may have contributed to the decline in tuberculosis mortality in these countries has not been assessed.

Colonialism

Historically, indigenous people in those parts of the world undergoing colonization have been very susceptible to tuberculosis. In the past this was attributed to racial susceptibility because of their being virgin populations. However, a more likely explanation is the adverse changes in demography, lifestyle and environment brought about by colonization. The prime motivation for colonization was the commercial exploitation of territory by the colonizers. In general this led to impoverishment of native people through loss of land (which led to overcrowding and loss of food sources) and a transition to wage labour. Colonizers tended to have a better environment than those colonized. The increased susceptibility of newly-colonized people to tuberculosis can thus be ascribed to a deterioration in environmental conditions rather than to racial susceptibility.

Several people have documented the association between European colonization and the emergence of tuberculosis in Africa. Tuberculosis is thought to have been uncommon in tropical Africa until late in the nineteenth century. However, European colonization brought about rapid increases in tuberculosis in the late nineteenth and early twentieth centuries in African colonies.[69] In 1867 the English epidemiologist William Budd, who was a friend of the missionary Dr David Livingstone, wrote:[14]

Everywhere along the African sea-board, where blacks have come into contact and intimate relations with the whites, phthisis causes a large mortality among them. In the interior, where intercourse with the whites has been limited to casual contact with a few great travellers or other adventurous visitors, there is reason to believe that phthisis does not exist.

Some years later Calmette (after whom the Bacillus Calmette-Guérin vaccine was named), expressed similar opinions in his 1912 review of tuberculosis in the French colonies.[15] He stated that the spread of tuberculosis in the colonies was directly associated with commercial development and that Europeans were the principal vehicle in the worldwide dissemination of tuberculous infection. He had found that tuberculosis was still rare in places where European penetration had been relatively recent. He observed that bovine tuberculosis contributed minimally to the incidence of the disease in the French colonies, as local cattle were free of infection and many native children did not drink cow's milk. He claimed that bovine tuberculosis was non-existent in the east African interior.

However, African people had not been living in isolation from the world prior to European colonization, as Arab traders had settled along the eastern seaboard of Africa and had established trade routes into the interior.

A possible explanation for the rise in tuberculosis following European colonization is the demographic change that took place.[69] In pre-colonial days Africans generally lived in small tribes and clans which had infrequent contact with the outside world, and so tuberculosis may have occurred sporadically without being widely disseminated to neighbouring tribes. European colonization resulted in the development of urban centres, and the people who migrated to these centres initially kept close contact with their rural homes, thus disseminating infection to rural areas.

Native people on other continents also experienced very high tuberculosis mortality rates following colonization. The excessive tuberculosis morbidity and mortality rates experienced by the American Indians following colonization is now acknowledged as having been solely due to unfavourable environmental conditions rather than to a hereditary lack of resistance.[57] A dramatic example of the importance of change in environmental conditions following European colonization is provided by the Indians of the Qu'Appelle Valley in Canada.[66] These people had been nomadic buffalo hunters until 1881, when they were confined to locations, after which their annual tuberculosis death rate is reported to have risen precipitously from 10 per 1 000 in 1881 to 90 per 1 000 in 1886. Although black Americans have consistently had higher rates of tuberculosis than their white counterparts, it has been shown that both groups have comparable incidence, morbidity and mortality within a similar environment.[40]

War

In the past, tuberculosis mortality rates have increased in times of war. Thus, during the First World War, tuberculosis mortality increased in several countries including Germany, Austria, France, England, Poland and Holland.[29]

Although housing and working conditions are thought to have contributed to the rise in tuberculosis mortality rates during this war, circumstantial evidence suggests that poor nutrition was the most important factor.[13, 29] In Germany, tuberculosis death rates increased dramatically after food consumption was limited by a tightening of the blockade,[13] while in Denmark, which did not participate directly in the war, tuberculosis mortality increased transiently, but declined after exportation of meat and dairy products were blocked by submarine warfare in 1917.[13, 24] Mortality did not increase in the United States where there were no food shortages.[29] In Britain tuberculosis mortality fell directly after the war at a time when nutrition had improved but overcrowding was still prevalent.[13] Because of the bombing, there were greater housing

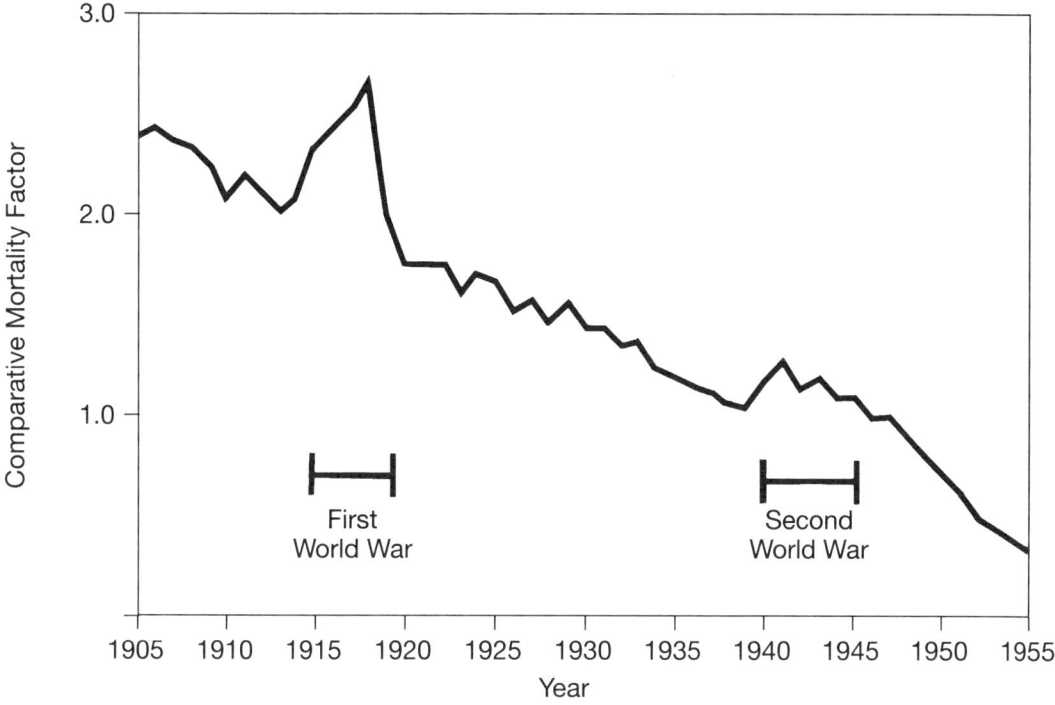

Figure 1.6. The comparative mortality factor for respiratory tuberculosis in England and Wales 1905–55, using the 1938 population as the standard (=1). This shows the relative increase in deaths from respiratory tuberculosis during the two world wars. (Source: Gale A H, 1959. *Epidemic Diseases.* Middlesex: Penguin Books.)

shortages in Britain during the Second World War than in the First World War, but nutrition was better as a result of effective rationing. The increase in tuberculosis mortality in Britain was less marked in the Second World War than in the First World War.[13] (Figure 1.6).

Elimination of infected milk

Infection takes place either by inhalation of the organism through contact with a case of pulmonary tuberculosis, or by ingestion of infected milk. The role of milk in spreading infection was only demonstrated late last century, and the need to prevent the sale of infected milk did not come to be appreciated until early this century.[16] Therefore, until recently milk was an important source of tuberculous infection, but measures were taken to eliminate this source of infection in several countries during the first half of this century including pasteurization of milk and the tuberculin-testing of cattle. These

measures have greatly reduced the incidence rates of non-pulmonary forms of tuberculosis such as scrofula, but have not affected the incidence of pulmonary tuberculosis as this is transmitted by droplet infection.[16]

The elimination of milk as a source of infection probably did not make a significant contribution to the overall decline in tuberculosis mortality in most developed countries, as most deaths have always been due to pulmonary disease. However, in the United States death rates from non-pulmonary forms of tuberculosis decreased rapidly after 1917, when a rigorous policy to eliminate bovine tuberculosis and the consumption of infected milk was introduced.[13]

THE DECLINE OF TUBERCULOSIS IN DEVELOPED COUNTRIES — WITH A FOCUS ON BRITAIN

The incidence of tuberculosis in Europe throughout the mediaeval period is

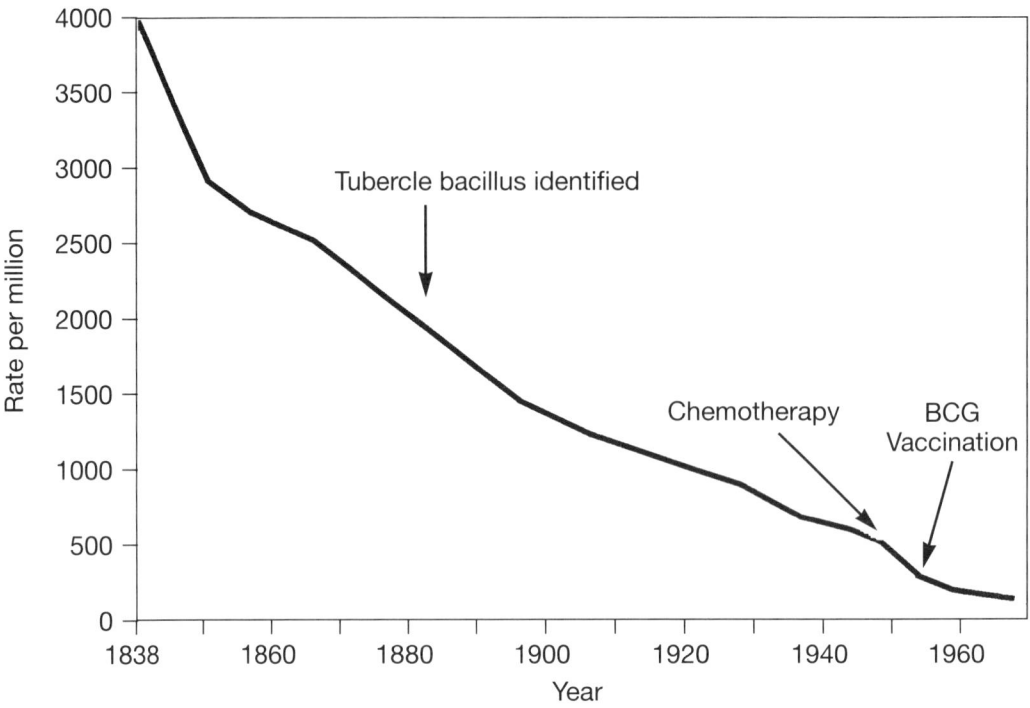

Figure 1.7. The decline in respiratory tuberculosis death rates in England and Wales since 1838. Standardized to the 1901 population. (Source: McKeown T, 1979. *The Role of Medicine: Dream, Mirage or Nemesis?* Oxford: Basil Blackwell.) The effects of the two world wars are not shown on this graph, as the points on which the curve is based were plotted at intervals, resulting in a smoothed curve.

unknown. An indication of the high prevalence of scrofula in France and England during the fourteenth to seventeenth centuries can be gleaned from records of the number of people who were touched by French and English kings in the hopes of being cured[41, 60] — King Charles II of England being reputed to have given the royal touch to 92 000 people with scrofula between 1660 and 1682![17, 60] However, the term 'scrofula' included non-tuberculous conditions,[17] and many cases are likely to have been due to bovine tuberculosis.

Of the developed countries, the history of tuberculosis has been best documented (in English texts) in Britain, although the course of the tuberculosis epidemic in Britain prior to 1838 is speculative because of the absence of reliable statistics, as explained earlier.

It has been claimed that there was an increase in tuberculosis in Britain in the eighteenth century, before the start of the industrial revolution in about 1780.[17, 71] This is quite possible as the English population is thought to have grown rapidly in the eighteenth century, due to a decline in infant and childhood mortality,[33] a decrease in deaths due to plague, typhus and malaria[2] and the immigration of the Huguenots, followed by immigrants from eastern and central Europe.[17] This population growth led to the enlargement of urban centres which in turn facilitated the spread of tuberculous infection. Changes in the age composition of the population may also have led to increases in tuberculosis mortality rates during this period. Gilbert Blane claimed in 1815 that tuberculosis had increased in young adults, and he attributed this increase to a fall in rates of acute childhood infectious diseases, which resulted in an increasing proportion of children surviving to adulthood.[68]

In England the industrial revolution brought about major social and demographic changes which favoured an increase in tuberculosis.[32] Agricultural reforms, despite their increasing overall food yield, led to fewer families being able to produce their own food. Industrialization led to large scale urbanization and the development of industrial slums. Houses were dark and poorly-ventilated as a result of the existence of a window tax and the belief that draughts spread disease.[2] The labouring class worked excessively long hours in crowded factories, and children were also exploited as a source of cheap labour. The newly urbanized working class was distanced from food sources and generally had a very poor diet. The concomitants of industrialization thus created environmental conditions that were conducive to the development of tuberculosis.

There is no consensus as to tuberculosis trends in Britain during this phase of rapid industrialization, and it is not known when tuberculosis mortality rates reached their peak. Environmental conditions in the early nineteenth century favoured high mortality, as by the second decade of the nineteenth century poverty was more widespread than ever (largely as a result of agricultural and industrial change),[71] and housing was poor with much overcrowding and poor sanitation and hygiene.[17]

Although it is not known when tuberculosis mortality rates began to fall in Britain, they have shown an overall downward trend, apart from transient wartime increases, since the introduction of death registration in 1838 when they were first recorded. The reasons for the decline are not fully understood (Figure 1.7).

The introduction of death registration coincided with a period of sanitary and labour reform in Britain, heralded by the 1833 Factory Act, which prohibited the employment of children under nine years and limited working hours for people under 21 years, and the Poor Law reform of 1834.[71] Further legislation, including the Public Health Act of 1848 and the establishment of voluntary groups for improving living conditions among the urban labouring classes, led to improvements in living conditions during the second half of the

nineteenth century, even though urban population growth exceeded the increase in available housing during this period. However, tuberculosis death rates were declining even before the improvements in housing and working conditions, brought about by these reforms, could exert any effect.[16]

In the late nineteenth century many tuberculosis sanatoria were established, based on the belief that fresh air and exercise could cure tuberculosis; dispensaries were introduced for diagnosis and for the provision of education in environmental hygiene.[13] The National Association for the Prevention of Tuberculosis was established in 1898, with the aims of providing health education, eliminating tuberculosis in cattle, and promoting the expansion of treatment facilities.[13] Although much attention has been focused on these interventions as factors that contributed to the decline in tuberculosis mortality rates, it is difficult to measure their true contribution. Their role may have been overemphasized, as the rate of decline did not increase after these developments.

Tuberculosis mortality rates continued to decrease in the twentieth century and had

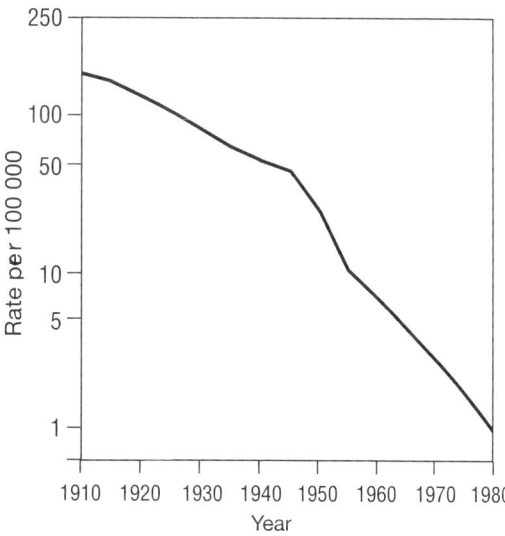

Figure 1.8. The decline in tuberculosis death rates in the United States 1910–80. (Source: Comstock G W, 1982. Epidemiology of tuberculosis. *American Review of Respiratory Diseases.* 125 (3 pt. 2), 9.

already fallen to low levels by the time that effective chemotherapy was introduced in the 1950s.[13] In Britain the BCG vaccination was only introduced on a wide scale in the 1950s[13] and thus did not make a significant contribution to the lowering of tuberculosis mortality. The gradual reduction in tuberculosis mortality rates appears to have been similar in pattern in other developed countries — the decline in the United States is shown in Figure 1.8.

THE HISTORICAL DEVELOPMENT OF TUBERCULOSIS IN SOUTH AFRICA

The history of tuberculosis in South Africa illustrates the importance of socio-economic, political and demographic factors in determining its incidence. What follows is an overview of those factors which played an important role in determining the course of tuberculosis in South Africa prior to the introduction of anti-tuberculous drugs in the 1940s and 1950s. Some recent work on the determinants of tuberculosis in South Africa is discussed in Chapter 4. For an in-depth discussion of the political and economic factors associated with the development of tuberculosis in South Africa, readers are recommended to consult Packard's authoritative book on the subject.[62]

Knowledge of the extent and prevalence of tuberculosis in South Africa prior to this century is very limited as the compilation of health statistics is a relatively recent innovation, and there are no written accounts by ethnic groups native to the region. What is known of the early history of tuberculosis in South Africa comes from the writings of travellers and missionaries.

The introduction of health statistics at the turn of the century led to an increased awareness of the problem and drew attention to the extent of tuberculosis in South Africa as well as to its racial and geographical distribution.[90] The introduction of compulsory registration of deaths in the Cape Colony in 1895 enabled tuberculosis mortality rates to be estimated for the first time.

In 1904 notification of tuberculosis was made compulsory in the Cape and Natal but met with resistance, with the result that reported figures underestimated the

problem.[90] There are no notification figures for the country as a whole prior to the 1920s. In 1943 it was stated that notification figures:

> *… cannot be relied upon to give an accurate estimate of the incidence of the disease in South Africa [as] notification of tuberculosis … is very poorly observed [and] is often erroneous, being based on purely clinical and not radiological or bacteriological grounds.[23]*

Notification rates should be interpreted with caution not only because of undernotification, but also because of distortions due to changes in the intensity of case-finding and in diagnostic criteria over time. It is difficult to obtain an accurate picture of secular trends in the black population because of incomplete mortality data and uncertainty in black population estimates, especially in rural areas.[4, 89, 90]

Tuberculosis is established following European colonization

Tuberculosis is a relatively new disease in southern Africa. Although it had been endemic in Europe and Asia for millennia, it is unlikely that it had occurred to any great extent among races native to southern Africa prior to the era of European colonization.[90]

European colonization of southern Africa began in the south-western Cape in the mid-seventeenth century, with the purpose of providing provisions for ships following the trade route between Europe and Asia. Colonization was thus limited at first, but over a period of 200 years European settlement spread, so that by the late nineteenth century the whole of southern Africa was under European control.

Reports of tuberculosis in South Africa first appeared around the end of the eighteenth century, when several travellers noted that consumption was common among European colonists,[90] which is not surprising, considering the high incidence in their Continental counterparts at the time.

From historical accounts it appears that the initial spread of tuberculosis among the different people native to South Africa was closely related to their degree of European contact.[52, 90] In the early nineteenth century tuberculosis was reported to be a problem among the Khoikhoi (Hottentots) who lived in the south-western parts of South Africa which had been colonized early, while those black peoples who remained geographically separate for a longer period were apparently relatively free of tuberculosis until later in the century.

The San, colloquially known as 'Bushmen', were ravaged by tuberculosis following European contact. Dr John Polson, in the late nineteenth century stated that he could not recall any case of tuberculosis in blacks but that it occurred frequently among 'Bushmen'. The dehumanizing effect that colonization had had on these people can be inferred from his statement:[52]

> *These interesting creatures are dying out, and do not seem to thrive in civilized condition ... when tamed and civilized by the Boers [Dutch speaking colonists] and cooped up in close houses ... they contracted phthisis!*

The scarcity or absence of tuberculosis among different black groups was noted in a number of eighteenth and early nineteenth century writings.[52, 62, 90] Although the view that black peoples were a virgin soil for tuberculosis has been widely accepted in the past, the disease had probably existed at a low level of endemicity prior to this century.[62] Oral history and linguistic studies suggest that the disease was of long standing among some black peoples such as the Zulus, but that other groups were not familiar with the disease.[52] Dr Peter Allan, who did extensive surveys in the Ciskei and Transkei regions of South Africa in the 1920s, believed that tuberculosis had a long history among black people in these regions.[62]

The role of the mining industry in the spread of tuberculosis

The mining industry has played a key role in the spread of tuberculosis in southern Africa. The high tuberculosis mortality rates in black mine workers early this century led to an inquiry into the health of black mine

workers in the Witwatersrand area being included in the brief of the 1912 Tuberculosis Commission. This was to be the first of many investigations into the problem.

The discovery of diamonds in 1867, and gold in 1886, created a demand for cheap labour which led to the development of an extensive migrant labour system in southern Africa. Labour for the mines was drawn not only from within the South African colonies, but also from other southern and central African colonies and protectorates including Basutoland (Lesotho), Bechuanaland (Botswana), Swaziland, Portuguese East Africa (Mozambique), Southern Rhodesia (Zimbabwe) and Nyasaland (Malawi).[89] Mine workers were employed on a contract basis and housed in mine compounds.

For many years medical examinations were cursory and failed to weed out those physically unfit to work on the mines. New recruits were often susceptible to tuberculosis at the time they started their contracts.[62] They were often in a poor state of health, with scurvy, malaria and pneumonia being common. At the time of the 1912 Tuberculosis Commission high rates of tuberculosis were being experienced, with a high proportion of recruits developing the disease within the first few months of service.

Conditions in the mines favoured the spread of infection from miners with tuberculosis.[62] The stopes were poorly-ventilated and very humid, and mine workers worked for long hours in close proximity to each other. They were housed in overcrowded mine compounds without partitions between the bunks (Figure 1.9).

Tuberculin tests conducted in mine recruits at the time of the 1912 Tuberculosis Commission showed a higher prevalence of infection in men who had previously been employed in the mines than in new recruits from the same area of origin (Table 1.4).[90] A tuberculin survey in Lesotho produced similar evidence — adult males who had been out of the territory (mostly to work in the mines) had an infection prevalence of 36,0 per cent, compared to a prevalence of 15,5 per cent in those who had remained within the territory.[90]

Mine workers who developed tuberculosis had their contracts terminated and were repatriated as soon as possible. Official figures of tuberculosis mortality among mine workers, although high, greatly underestimate the true mortality rate, as those who died after being repatriated were not included in mine mortality statistics.[62] The high mortality rate among repatriated workers was demonstrated in a follow up study of mine workers sent back from the Witwatersrand to the Transkei and Ciskei territories during the years 1926 to 1929 (Table 1.5).[89]

The practice of repatriating mine workers who developed tuberculosis played a key role in disseminating the disease to rural areas. The hut tax led to overcrowding in rural areas and facilitated the spread of tuberculosis among the families of returning mine workers.[62] The 1912 Tuberculosis Commission found that the distribution of tuberculosis in rural areas was directly related to the extent to which the area's population had been involved in migrant labour.

Conditions on the mines lowered resistance to disease, so that those infected with tuberculosis often succumbed rapidly. Mine workers tended to have very inadequate diets[62] — for example, those working in the diamond mines in Kimberley had to provide their own food, but the cost of an adequate diet was beyond their means. (The 1912 Tuberculosis Commission estimated that an adequate diet would have used up one third of the average wage paid to black mine workers at the time.) Mine workers on the Witwatersrand were provided with food, but also had inadequate diets during

Table 1.4

The prevalence of tuberculosis infection in new recruits compared to workers with previous mine experience*

| | AREA OF ORIGIN | | |
MINE EXPERIENCE	NYASALAND (MALAWI)	MOZAMBIQUE	NOT SPECIFIED
New recruits	6 / 129 (4,7 %)	7 / 415 (1,7 %)	
Workers at the end of first contract			26 / 131 (19,7 %)
Re-employed workers (with previous mine experience)	10 / 52 (19,2 %)	11 / 63 (17,5 %)	

* Source: Tuberculosis Commission Report, 1914, 113–4.

Table 1.5

Survival of mine workers repatriated from the Witwatersrand to the Transkei and Ciskei*

| | YEAR OF REPATRIATION | | | |
	1926	1927	1928	1929
Number repatriated	123	148	186	237
Follow up period (approximate)	3 yr	2yr	1 yr	6 mo
Number traced	85	122	141	127
Number dead	49	76	71	51
Percentage of those traced dead at follow up	57,6	62,3	50,4	40,2

* Source: Report of the Tuberculosis Research Committee, 1932, p. 236.

this period as the staple food provided was mealie meal, leading to a diet that was lacking in protein and vitamins. There was a high prevalence of scurvy in both diamond and gold mine workers as a result of the lack of fresh fruit and vegetables in mine diets. Vitamin C deficiency has been shown to lower resistance to tuberculosis.[62] It has also been suggested that deficiencies of other dietary factors in mine diets, such as vitamin A and calcium, may have lowered resistance.

Other factors which may have increased mine workers' susceptibility to tuberculosis were the physically demanding nature of their work and the long working hours, shifts sometimes being as long as 18 hours in times of labour shortage.[62] Tuberculosis repatriation and mortality rates in coal miners increased during periods when workers were made to work longer shifts,[62] although this may also have been due to less healthy recruits being accepted in times of labour shortages.

The combination of overcrowding, poor diet and long workshifts endured by mine workers bears similarity to conditions experienced by workers in England a century earlier. These conditions accounted for the high tuberculosis mortality rates demonstrated by both these groups. The members of the 1912 Tuberculosis Commission, two of whom were closely associated with the mines, were strongly divided over the role of housing, diet and working conditions in causing tuberculosis in black mine workers, and failed to reach consensus in their recommendations.[90] However, the chairman of the Commission, Dr Gregory, concluded that the mining industry was one of the most important factors in the cause and spread of tuberculosis in the black population.

Surgeon-General W C Gorgas, the Chief Sanitary Officer of the Isthmian (Panama) Canal Commission, paid a visit to South Africa in 1914 and published recommendations for improving the health of mine

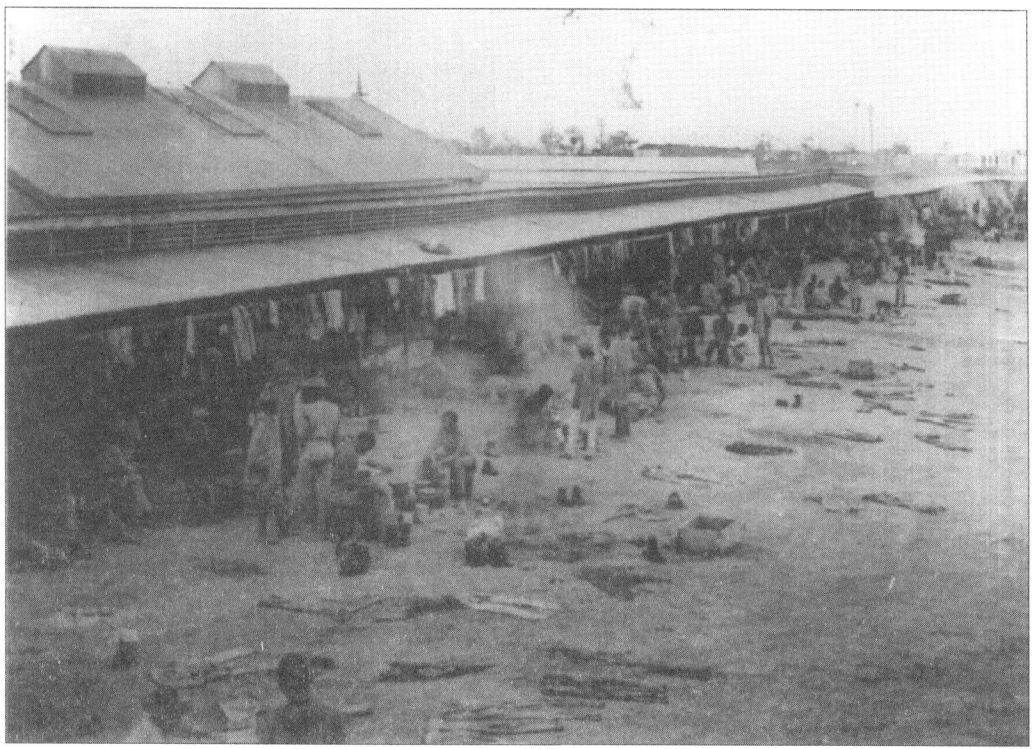

Figure 1.9. Workers cooking at a mine compound, Kimberley (Source: Jeffreys Collection, Cape Archives, Cape Town).

employees.[89] He expressed concern about the high tuberculosis incidence and mortality among black mine workers, and strongly criticized the conditions to which they were being subjected, including the overcrowded barracks and the provision of a predominantly mealie meal diet. He recommended the establishment of a village hut system to accommodate mine workers and their families, but this recommendation was never taken up.

However, improvements in diet, working and living conditions were gradually introduced as a result of public pressure. The incidence of tuberculosis in black mine workers declined between 1913 and 1935, in contrast to increasing tuberculosis incidence and mortality rates in other South African blacks during this same period.[62] Although this decline has been attributed to improved conditions in the mines, it was also partially due to the stricter screening of recruits and the weeding out of those most susceptible to disease.[62]

In Zimbabwe the repatriation of mine workers played a similar role in promoting the spread of tuberculosis.[77] Tuberculosis was first noticed in the mines, then in urban centres, and finally in rural areas.[78] From 1907 onwards workers who developed tuberculosis while working in the mines were repatriated, and the spread of tuberculosis to rural areas has been attributed to returning mine workers.[77] Tuberculosis death rates in Zimbabwe fell once the migrant labour policy had been abandoned and facilities provided for the families of mine workers to settle at the mines.[78]

The effect of the importation of tuberculosis: the promotion of South Africa as a health resort (c. 1875–1900)

Although it is unlikely that tuberculosis was ever absent from Europeans in South Africa, the pool of infection was boosted by the large number of consumptive people (predominantly English and Scottish in origin) who came to South Africa in the last quarter of the nineteenth century hoping to be cured by the climate.[90] The towns where

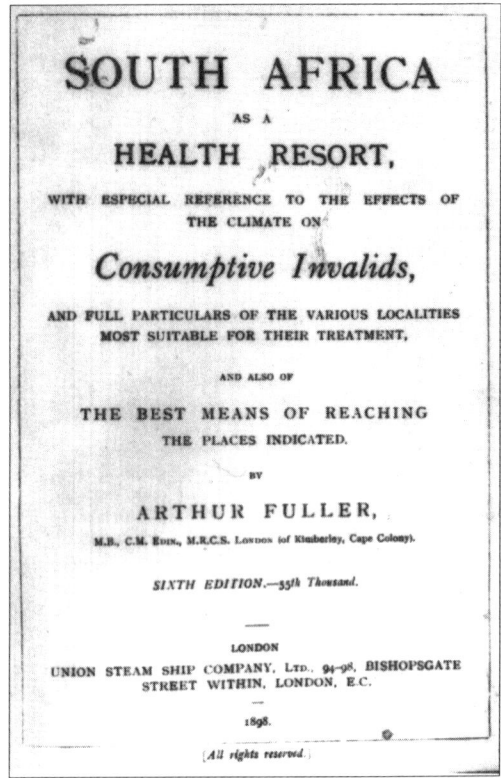

Figure 1.10. Bookplate of the 6th edition of the book *South Africa as a health resort,* published in 1898.

consumptive immigrants collected formed foci from which the disease spread.[90] However, although this contributed to the spread of the disease, tuberculosis had already become established in the Cape prior to this time and Drs Gregory and McVicar, who carried out some of the earliest definitive work on the development of tuberculosis in South Africa, were both of the opinion that consumptive immigrants were not the main source of the disease.[89]

South Africa's popularity as a health resort increased during the late nineteenth century as a result of improvements in shipping, as well as of the economic development which led to extensions to the railway network (which improved access to favoured localities), improvements in accommodation facilities, and to a strengthening of English colonial culture in the region. The benefits of the South African climate for

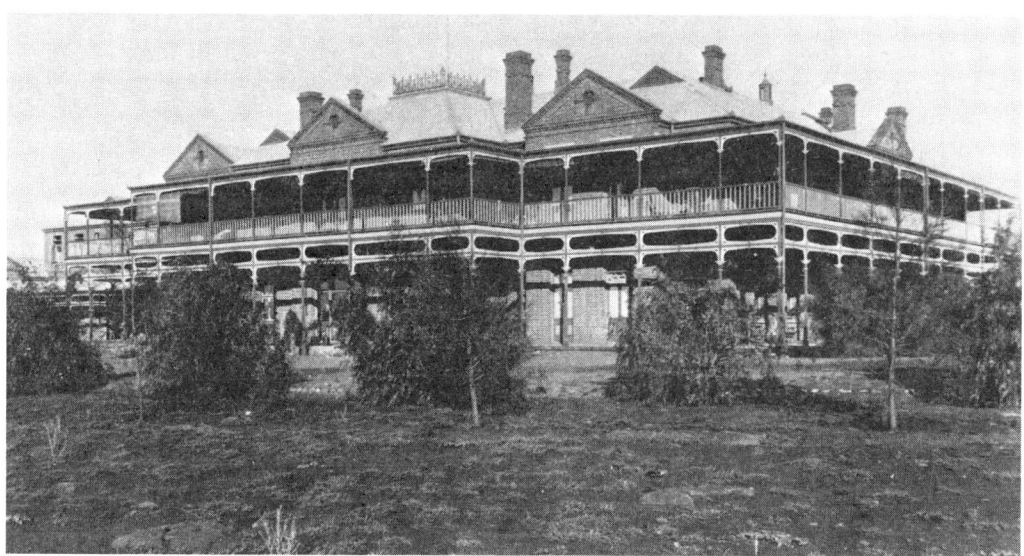

Figure 1.11. Kimberley Sanatorium. (Source: Postcard collection, South African Library, Cape Town.)

those with consumptive complaints were publicized extensively in books[31, 72, 75] and articles[37, 87, 92] during this period. During the 1890s the following appeared in a local newspaper:[75]

> *South Africa, the land of the High Veldt [sic] and the Karroo [sic]! The land of soaking sunlight, and crisp dryness, and the cool night-wind! The land of elevated plains, which join the virtues of the desert, for which sick men flee to Egypt, with the virtues of the mountain, for which they seek Switzerland! The Cape which cures consumption; the Cape which is of Good Hope to all weak chests; the Cape which offers life and health and a career to the Englishman suddenly confronted by that modern absolutist, the doctor, with the cold sentence of death or exile!*

Among those promoting South Africa as a health resort was the Union Steamship Company, which benefited directly from the increased number of people seeking a passage to South Africa. It printed more than 50 000 copies of a book entitled *South Africa as a Health Resort* (Figure 1.10) between 1886 and 1898.

The Karoo (whose name is derived from a Khoikhoi word meaning 'dry') was acclaimed for its sunny dry climate and acceptable altitude. Towns in South Africa which were popular among consumptive immigrants included Beaufort West (in the Karoo), Kimberley, Bloemfontein, Harrismith, Cradock and Middelberg,[31, 75, 90] with Cape Town being the main port of entry. However, many people arrived in such an advanced stage of tuberculosis that they were not able to travel into the interior.[75]

Several sanatoria were established in the late nineteenth century, coincident with the growing sanatorium movement in Europe.[31, 75] The mining industry, which played a key role in the dissemination of the epidemic (see above), also made a direct contribution to South Africa's popularity as a health resort by supplying the capital for the building of a prestigious sanatorium outside Kimberley (Figure 1.11), described by Dr Fuller as 'a first class hotel for invalids'.[31] This was done on the instigation of the mining magnate Cecil John Rhodes, who is himself alleged to have come out to South Africa on account of tuberculosis.

As a result of the selective immigration of tuberculotics, the tuberculosis mortality rate among Europeans in the Cape is thought to have exceeded that of their British counterparts in the late nineteenth century, and for some time the proponents of South Africa as a health resort did not consider the impact that the importation of tuberculosis would have on the spread of the disease. Paradoxically Dr Scholtz raised the problem in his book promoting South Africa as a health resort:[75]

> *It might in future seriously affect the population of South Africa — namely the almost daily wholesale influx of phthisical and scrofulous cases, especially of the poorer classes, into the country from Europe.*

Dr Scholtz's concern was apt, as early this century towns such as Beaufort West and Cradock, which had been frequented by consumptive people seeking a climatic cure, had the highest tuberculosis mortality rates of all South African towns, in both their white and coloured populations.[90] Concern about the importation of the disease led to the 1913 Immigrants Regulation Act, which prohibited the entry of people with clinically recognizable tuberculosis, except by permit and subject to certain conditions.[23] However, this Act came too late and had little effect, as the popularity of seeking a climatic cure had already waned by this time,[52] and by 1911 the tuberculosis incidence and mortality rates among whites in South Africa were generally lower than in England, although Cape Town was an exception.[90]

The role of urbanization and economic recession

Urbanization, housing shortages, economic recession and droughts have all contributed to the South African tuberculosis epidemic. In the early phase of the epidemic, disease rates were closely associated with urban development, early observers noting that the epidemic started in coastal regions,[52] in keeping with early urban development being centered around ports. Tuberculosis also appears to have become established at an early date among coloured people living in the early inland urban centres such as Graaff-Reinet and Oudtshoorn.[90]

The discovery of diamonds and gold led to rapid industrial development and stimulated urban growth in the late nineteenth and early twentieth centuries. New cities such as Johannesburg developed in the

mining areas, and port cities such as Cape Town grew as a result of increased trade and an influx of people. Until the 1870s the black population of South Africa was mainly rural, and few lived in large settlements or in the vicinity of urban centres.[62] However, industrial development led to a rapid urbanization of blacks and coloureds in the late nineteenth century. Although tuberculosis incidence and mortality rates are not available, anecdotal evidence suggests that these rates rose rapidly during this period.[52, 90]

In the late nineteenth century, when tuberculosis was first seen to be a problem among blacks, it was noted that the disease was more common among those who adopted European dress than among those rural blacks who retained a more traditional lifestyle.[90] Although the adoption of European clothing was blamed for the increased incidence of tuberculosis among blacks at the time,[90] any change in the mode of dress was generally associated with other changes and a greater degree of urbanization, which was more likely to have been the reason for their increased susceptibility to tuberculosis.

Depression in the mining industry during the first decade of this century led to a more generalized economic recession which also affected the shipping industry, with consequent increases in unemployment. At the same time rural areas were severely deprived as a result of drought, the Anglo-Boer War, and a rinderpest epidemic which eliminated over 90 per cent of African cattle. These factors caused many indigent rural people to drift to towns, which in turn led to the development of multiracial slums.[62] Tuberculosis mortality rates increased in Johannesburg and the port cities (Cape Town, Port Elizabeth and Durban) at this time.[62]

The 1912 Tuberculosis Commission found that tuberculosis was three times as prevalent in towns as in rural areas, and that it was most prevalent in the large coastal and industrial towns, on the mines, and in those places previously favoured by consumptives.

During the First World War the demand for labour led to continuing black urbanization, with the growth of urban slums.[62]

Tuberculosis mortality rates of blacks in Johannesburg continued to rise during this period.[4]

The economic recession of the early 1920s led to further urbanization as a result of decreased economic opportunities in the rural areas. The influx of blacks to towns during the 1920s exceeded the construction of new housing, and tuberculosis rates rose during this period as living conditions deteriorated.[62] Dr Peter Allan, in his 1924 report,[4] identified poor living conditions as an important factor contributing to the high tuberculosis mortality in urban locations.

Deteriorating conditions in locations and periurban slums led to the 1934 Slum Clearance Act, and the population removals

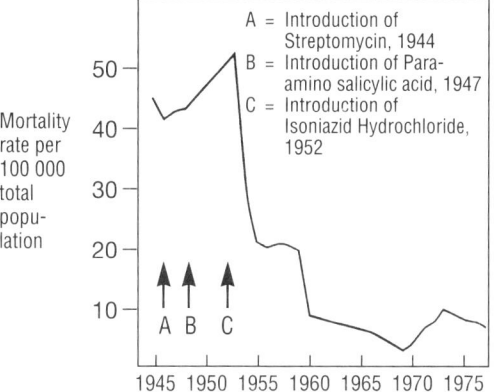

Figure 1.12. Notified annual tuberculosis death rate, South Africa, 1945–77. (Source: Kustner H G V, 1979. Trends in four major communicable diseases. *South African Medical Journal.* 55, 460–73)

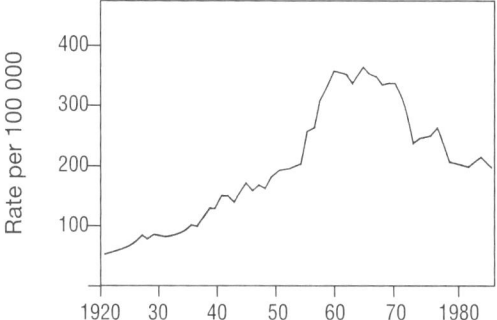

Figure 1.13. Annual tuberculosis notification rate, South Africa, 1921–85. (Source: Epidemiological Comments 1985, 12, 9)

which followed this Act were associated with a fall in tuberculosis rates in the major urban centres.[62] However, this fall was apparent rather than real, because tuberculosis was simply relocated rather than overcome.[62] Black people who were moved beyond municipal boundaries were excluded from municipal health statistics although they continued to have high rates of disease. Thus, for example, black tuberculosis mortality dropped in the Port Elizabeth Municipality in the late 1930s, but increased in the nearby periurban location of New Brighton. Urban tuberculosis death rates in blacks continued to rise steeply during the 1940s, in contrast to white South Africans, whose tuberculosis mortality was among the lowest in the world by this time.[94]

Droughts have led to periodic food shortages, which in turn have contributed to the incidence of tuberculosis. However, the drought at the turn of the century was but one of many factors contributing to an increased incidence of tuberculosis at the time. There is more recent evidence that the incidence of tuberculosis has increased in times of drought. For example hospital admissions for pulmonary tuberculosis in the Ciskei rose in 1919–20, and again in 1929–30 following droughts.[53]

Although accurate statistics of tuberculosis rates in blacks living in rural areas are not available, tuberculosis was generally felt to be less prevalent in rural areas than in urban centres. While Dr Allan found that tuberculosis had become prevalent in rural areas such as the Transkei and Ciskei by the 1920s, he also commented that blacks living in their 'natural surroundings' in these territories had a considerable degree of resistance to tuberculosis.[4] Dr Wiles[94] noted that in the towns tuberculosis often took on an acute rapidly fatal form, previously known as 'galloping consumption', while in the reserves the disease tended to take on a more chronic indolent form. He attributed the acute form of the disease to 'a complete breakdown of resistance due to inadequate food and severe living conditions.' The (apparently) lower rate of disease in blacks living in rural areas compared to those living in urban areas, despite high levels of infection in both settings, has been cited as evidence against them being intrinsically (racially) susceptible to tuberculosis.[23]

Conclusion

The introduction of anti-tuberculosis drugs in the 1950s was followed by a sharp decline in tuberculosis mortality rates (Figure 1.12), but incidence rates continued to increase (Figure 1.13). The fall in notification rates in the 1970s was partially due to undernotification from states within South Africa after their attainment of nominal 'independence'. However, recent notification figures suggest that the incidence rate is rising in some areas.[51, 95]

Large disparities still exist between tuberculosis incidence and mortality rates in different racial groups in South Africa, because of continuing differences in economic and environmental circumstances. Factors such as urbanization, inadequate housing, unemployment and poverty, which contributed to the high incidence of tuberculosis in the past, still operate to make tuberculosis an ongoing problem in this country.

REFERENCES

1 Abbott E C, 1982. Composers and tuberculosis: the effects on creativity. *Canadian Medical Association Journal.* 126 (5), 534, 536–8, 543–4.

2 Ackernecht E H, 1965. *History and Geography of the Most Important Diseases.* New York: Hafner.

3 Addison V, 1983. Abdominal tuberculosis — a disease revisited. *Annals of the Royal College of Surgeons of England.* 65 (2), 105–11.

4 Allen P, 1924. *Report of Tuberculosis Survey of the Union of South Africa.* Cape Town: Cape Times.

5 Allison M J, Mendoza D & Pezzia A, 1973. Documentation of a case of tuberculosis in pre-Columbian America. *American Review of Respiratory Diseases.* 107 (6), 985–91.

6 Anderson G W, 1977. In: Myers J A: *Captain of All These Men of Death: Tuberculosis Historical Highlights*, Introduction. St Louis: Warren H Green.

7 Anonymous, 1892. The communicability and spread of phthisis. *British Medical Journal.* Jan 30, 256.

8 Anonymous, 1986. *The Great Artists. Their Lives, Works and Inspiration. Part 76: Modigliani.* London: Marshall Cavendish Ltd.

9 Ash J E, 1915. The pathology of the mistaken diagnoses in a hospital for advanced tuberculosis. *Journal of the American Medical Association.* 64 (1), 11–5.

10 Bates J H, 1982. Tuberculosis: susceptibility and resistance. *American Review of Respiratory Diseases.* 125 (3), 20–4.

11 Brothwell D, 1967. In: Brothwell D, Sandison A T (eds): *Diseases in Antiquity*, Chapter 5. Springfield: Charles C Thomas.

12 Brownlee J, 1918. *An Investigation into the Epidemiology of Phthisis in Great Britain and Ireland.* London: National Health Insurance Medical Research Committee, Special Report Series no. 18.

13 Bryder L, 1988. *Below the Magic Mountain. A Social History of Tuberculosis in Twentieth Century Britain.* Oxford: Clarendon Press.

14 Budd W, 1867. The nature and mode of propagation of phthisis. *Lancet.* II, 451–2.

15 Calmette A, 1912. Enquête sur l'épidémiologie de la tuberculose dans les colonies françaises. *Annals de l'Institute Pasteur.* 26 (7), 497–514.

16 Cartwright F F, 1977. *A Social History of Medicine.* New York: Longman.

17 Chalke H D, 1962. The impact of tuberculosis on history, literature and art. *Medical History.* 6, 301–18.

18 Chalke H D, 1959. Some historical aspects of tuberculosis. *Public Health.* 74, 83–95.

19 Clark G A, Kelley M A, Grange J M & Hill M C, 1987. The evolution of mycobacterial disease in human populations. A re-evaluation. *Current Anthropology.* 28 (1), 45–62.

20 Comstock G W, 1982. Epidemiology of tuberculosis. *American Review of Respiratory Diseases.* 125 (3 Pt 2), 8–15.

21 Creighton C, 1891–4. *A History of Epidemics in Britain*, vols I and II. Cambridge: Cambridge University Press.

22 Davydoskii I V, 1962. Problems of causality in medicine. English translation from: *Federal Proceedings.* 24 (2), 225–30.

23 Dormer B A, Friedlander J & Wiles F J, 1943. A South African team looks at tuberculosis. Reprint of *Proceedings of the Transvaal Mine Medical Officers Association*, 23 (557).

24 Dubos R & Dubos J, 1953. *The White Plague: Tuberculosis, Man and Society*. London: Victor Gollancz.

25 Dubovsky H, 1979. Anton Chekhov (1860–1904). Writer, physician and tuberculosis patient. *South African Medical Journal*. 55 (17), 682–6.

26 Dubovsky H, 1981. John Keats (1795–1821) — poet, physician and tuberculosis patient. *South African Medical Journal*. 59 (24), 875–8.

27 El-Najjar M Y, 1979. Human treponematosis and tuberculosis: Evidence from the New World. *American Journal of Physical Anthropology*. 51, 599–618.

28 Evans, Lord of Hungershall, 1969. Keats — the man, medicine and poetry. *British Medical Journal*. 3 (661), 7–11.

29 Fishberg M, 1922. *Pulmonary Tuberculosis*. 3rd ed. Philadelphia: Lea and Febiger.

30 Frost W H, 1939. The age selection of mortality from tuberculosis in successive decades. *American Journal of Hygiene*. 30, 91–6.

31 Fuller A, 1898. *South Africa as a Health Resort with Especial Reference to the Effects of Climate on Consumptive Invalids, and Full Particulars of the Various Localities Most Suitable for their Treatment, and also of the Best Means of Reaching the Places Indicated*. 6th ed. London: Union Steamship Co.

32 Galdston I, 1942. The dynamics of epidemiology in relation to epidemic tuberculosis. *American Review of Tuberculosis*. 45, 609–15.

33 Gale A H, 1959. *Epidemic Diseases*. Middlesex: Penguin.

34 Grange J M & Collins C H, 1987. Bovine tubercle baccilli and disease in animals and man. *Epidemiology of Infections*. 92, 221–34.

35 Grigg E R N, 1958. The arcana of tuberculosis. Part II. Theoretical considerations regarding the epidemiology of tuberculosis. *American Review of Tuberculosis*. 78, 157–72.

36 Grigg E R N, 1958. The arcana of tuberculosis. Part III. Epidemiologic history of tuberculosis in the United States. *American Review of Tuberculosis*. 78, 426–453.

37 H.L., 1879. Notes on South Africa for invalids. *Cape Monthly Magazine*. 18, 272–9.

38 Hanefeld G T, 1980. Pott's disease before Pott. *Netherlands Journal of Surgery*. 32 (1), 2–7.

39 Hare R, 1967. In: Brothwell D & Sandison A T (eds): *Diseases in Antiquity*, Chapter 8. Springfield: Charles C Thomas.

40 Katz J & Kunofsky S, 1960. Environmental versus constitutional factors in the development of tuberculosis among Negroes. *American Review of Respiratory Diseases*. 81, 17–25.

41 Keers R Y, 1981. Laënnec: his medical history. *Thorax*. 36 (2), 91–4.

42 Keers R Y, 1978. *Pulmonary Tuberculosis: A Journey Down the Centuries*. London: Balliere Tindall.

43 Leavesley J H, 1985. Elizabeth Barrett Browning. *Medical Journal of Australia*. 142, 365–7.

44 Leavesley J H, 1985. The Brontë family. *Medical Journal of Australia*. 143, 415–7.

45 Leff A, Lester T W & Addington W W, 1979. Tuberculosis. A chemotherapeutic triumph but a persistent socio-economic problem. *Archives of Internal Medicine*. 139 (12), 1375–7.

46 Long E R, 1941. Constitution and related factors in resistance to tuberculosis. *Archives of Pathology*. 32, 122–62.

47 Long E R, 1953. Tuberculosis in Modern Society. *Bulletin of Historical Medicine*. 27, 306.

48 Manchester K, 1984. Tuberculosis and leprosy in antiquity: an interpretation. *Medical History*. 28 (2), 162–173.

49 Manchester K, 1983. *The Archaeology of Disease*. Bradford: University of Bradford.

50 Marais D P, 1932. Tuberculosis. *South African Medical Journal*. 6, 519–25.

51 McDonald K D, 1984. A rise of tuberculosis among coloureds. *Epidemiological Comments*. 11, 2–43.

52 McVicar N, 1932. The prevalence of certain diseases amongst the natives of the Ciskei. *South African Medical Journal*. 6, 721.

53 McVicar N, 1908. Tuberculosis among the South African natives. *South African Medical Record*. 6, 161–76, 181–5, 197–208, 213–22, 229–35.

54 Meindl J L & Meindl C O, 1982. Tuberculous meningitis in the 1830s. *Lancet*. 1 (8271), 554–5.

55 Mitchell A, 1988. Obsessive questions and faint answers: the French response to tuberculosis in the Belle Epoque. *Bulletin of Historical Medicine*. 62 (2), 215–35.

56 Morse D, Brothwell D R & Ucko P J. Tuberculosis in ancient Egypt. *American Review of Respiratory Diseases*. 90, 524–41.

57 Morse D, 1967. In: Brothwell D & Sandison A T (eds): *Diseases in Antiquity*, Chapter 19. Springfield: Charles C Thomas.

58 Morse D, 1961. Prehistoric tuberculosis in America. *American Review of Respiratory Diseases.* 83, 489–504.

59 Mullan F, 1973. The sickness of Frédéric Chopin: A study of disease and society. *Rocky Mountain Medical Journal.* 70 (9), 29–34.

60 Myers J A, 1977. *Captain of all These Men of Death: Tuberculosis Historical Highlights.* St Louis: Warren H Green.

61 Ortner D J, 1979. Disease and mortality in the early Bronze Age people of Bab edh-Dhra, Jordan. *American Journal of Physical Anthropology.* 51 (4), 589–97.

62 Packard R M, 1989. *White Plague, Black Labour. Tuberculosis and the Political Economy of Health and Disease in South Africa.* Berkeley: University of California Press.

63 Paulsen H J, 1987. Tuberculosis in the native American: Indigenous or introduced? *Review of Infectious Diseases.* 9 (6), 1180–6.

64 Perzigian A J and Widmer L, 1979. Evidence for tuberculosis in a prehistoric population. *Journal of the American Medical Association.* 241 (24), 2643–6.

65 Philip R, 1918. Present day outlook on tuberculosis. Inaugural address delivered on the institution of the chair of tuberculosis in the University of Edinburgh, 16 April 1918. *Edinburgh Medical Journal.* 20 May, 289–306.

66 Pinner M, 1940. Epidemiological trends of tuberculosis. *American Review of Tuberculosis.* 42, 385.

67 Rakover J, 1953. Tuberculosis among Jews. *American Review of Tuberculosis.* 67, 85–93.

68 Roberts F, 1955. The effects of epidemics on population and social life. *Proceedings of the Royal Society of Medicine.* 48, 785–9.

69 Roelsgaard E, Iversen E & Bløcher C, 1964. Tuberculosis in Tropical Africa. *Bulletin of the World Health Organization.* 30, 459–518.

70 Rogers F B, 1969. The rise and decline of the altitude therapy of tuberculosis. *Bulletin of Historical Medicine.* 43 (1), 1–16.

71 Rosen G, 1958. *A History of Public Health.* New York: MD Publications.

72 Ross J A, 1876. *Consumption: Its Treatment by Climate with Reference Especially to the Health Resorts of the South African Colonies.* London: H Renshaw.

73 Sager P, Schalimtzek M & Møller-Christensen V, 1972. A case of tuberculosis spondylosa in the Danish Neolithic Age. *Danish Medical Bulletin.* 19 (5), 176–80.

74 Sawchuk L A & Herring D A, 1984. Respiratory tuberculosis mortality among the Sephardic Jews of Gibraltar. *Human Biology.* 56 (2), 291–306.

75 Scholtz W, 1897. *The South African Climate including Climatology and Balneology and Discussing the Advantages, Peculiarities and Capabilities of the Country as a Health Resort — More Particularly with Reference to Affections of the Chest.* London: Cassell.

76 Sharpe W D, 1962. Lung disease and the Greco-Roman physician. A review. *American Review of Respiratory Diseases.* 86, 178–92.

77 Shennan D H, 1960. The evolution of tuberculosis in Southern Rhodesia. Part I — History: The introduction and spread of infection. *Central African Journal of Medicine.* 6 (8), 352–5.

78 Shennan D H, 1960. The evolution of tuberculosis in Southern Rhodesia. Part II — Pathogenesis: The relation of infection to disease. *Central African Journal of Medicine.* 6 (9), 395–8.

79 Smith E R, 1960. Chest diseases in Biblical times. *British Journal of Diseases of the Chest.* 54, 226–33.

80 Smith F B, 1979. *The People's Health 1830–1910.* New York: Holmes and Meier.

81 Smith H, 1984. John Keats: poet, patient, physician. *Review of Infectious Diseases.* 6 (3), 390–404.

82 Styblo K & Rouillon A, 1981. Estimated global incidence of smear-positive pulmonary tuberculosis. Unreliability of officially reported figures on tuberculosis. *Bulletin of the International Union against Tuberculosis.* 56 (3–4), 118–26.

83 Styblo K, 1988. Overview and epidemiological assessment of the current global tuberculosis situation: with an emphasis on control in developing countries. *Bulletin of the International Union against Tuberculosis.* 63, 39–44.

84 Swan P, 1985. The romantic's death. *Nursing Times.* 81 (11), 47–9.

85 Talmi Y P, Finkelstein Y, Shem Tov Y, Zohar Y & Laurian N. Scrofula revisited. *Journal of Laryngology and Otolaryngology.* 102 (4), 387–8.

86 Thomas B & Gandevia B, 1959. Dr Francis Workman, emigrant, and the history of taking the cure for consumption in the Australian colonies. *Medical Journal of Australia.* 46 (II), 1–10.

87 Thompson S, 1889. South Africa as a health resort. *Proceedings of the Royal Collegiate Institution.* 20, 4–51.

88 Torchia M M, 1977. Tuberculosis among American Negroes: medical research on a racial disease, 1830–1950. *Journal of Historical Medicine.* 32 (3), 252–79.

89 Tuberculosis Research Committee, 1932. *Tuberculosis in South African Natives with Special Reference to the Disease amongst the Mine Labourers on the Witwatersrand.* Johannesburg: South African Institute for Medical Research.

90 Union of South Africa, 1914. *Report of the Tuberculosis Commission 1914.* Cape Town: Cape Times.

91 Warring F C, 1981. A brief history of tuberculosis. *Connecticut Medicine.* 45 (3), 177–85.

92 Weber H, 1885. The hygienic and climatic treatment of chronic pulmonary phthisis. *British Medical Journal.* 4 & 11 April, 688–90, 725–7.

93 Wellmann K F, 1970. Kokopelli of Indian Paleology. Hunchbacked rain priest, hunting magician, and Don Juan of the old southwest. *Journal of the American Medical Assocation.* 212 (10), 1678–82.

94 Wiles F J, 1947. *The Effect of Environment on Tuberculosis in the Bantu. Tuberculosis in the Commonwealth 1947: Complete Transactions of the Commonwealth and Empire Health and Tuberculosis Conference.* London: National Association for the Prevention of Tuberculosis.

95 Yach D, 1988. Tuberculosis in the western Cape health region of South Africa. *Journal of Social Science and Medicine.* 27 (7), 683–9.

96 Zimmerman M R, 1979. Pulmonary and osseous tuberculosis in an Egyptian mummy. *Bulletin of the New York Academy of Medicine.* 55 (6), 604–8.

CHAPTER 2

The management of tuberculosis in the pre-chemotherapeutic era

H. Dubovsky

THE ANCIENT MIDDLE EAST

The literature of the biblical Hebrews makes no mention of recognizable tuberculosis, and their nomadic existence and religiously motivated hygienic laws would militate against the group establishment of this disease. Tuberculosis is also not documented in the writings of Mesopotamia or ancient Egypt. Indirect evidence of the disease in Egypt emanates from figurines and drawings on tombs that depict the typical angular deformity of bone tuberculosis of the upper thoracic spine, and similar deformities in mummies. Ancient Egyptian remains were first examined by pathologists at Cambridge University in 1962, using specimens[18] originally uncovered by Sir Flinders Petrie in 1895 in an anthropological survey of an ancient cemetery at Nagada. Carbon-dated 3700 to 1000 BC, they showed the typical spinal changes of tuberculosis — extensive destruction and fusion of two or more vertebral bodies without involvement of the posterior neural arch that caused the typical angular deformity of the spine. With disease in this era considered to have had a supernatural cause, usually as punishment by God or other deities, treatment would have been by prayer, animal sacrifice and measures to drive out evil spirits with vile concoctions or flagellation.

THE ERA OF RATIONAL MEDICINE

The first description of tuberculosis comes from the works of Hippocrates[16] (400–375 BC) in Classical Greece. Hippocrates describes it as a disease of the 18 to 35 year-old age group presenting in spring 'with a smoothness of the skin, slight pallor, freckles, a slight flush, sparkling eyes, white phlegm and winging of the shoulder-blades'. Hippocrates dissociated magic from medicine, thus initiating a rational approach. He considered that disease was due to an altered state of four body fluids or humours (blood, phlegm, yellow bile and black bile), which resulted in irritative substances being the cause of disease which had to be removed before medication was applied. Known as the treatment of depletion this entailed venesection, emetics and purgation and the application over the affected part of leeches, blistering agents and various measures to produce a discharging skin ulcer. This humoral theory of disease formed the basis of western medicine for 2 500 years, largely because of the image of Hippocrates as being the father of medicine with his ethical approach, accurate clinical observation and attention to the patient's way of living.

Thomas Sydenham[22] (1624–79), known as the English Hippocrates, drew on humoral theory when he observed that 'the frequency of consumptives in London' was due to 'a perpetual mist mixed with fumes that arise from several trades managed there, but especially the sulphur and fumes of sea coals being sucked into the lungs causing the blood to be hot and acrid'. He treated early tuberculosis with 'pectorals', tablets containing sugar candy and liquorice. Where this did not help and for advanced cases he used venesection and purging, but concluded that 'of all the remedies for phthisis, long and continued journeys on horseback bear the bell'. This exposure to fresh air as well as open carriage riding for ladies was to feature in tuberculosis treatment for the following 200 years.

Strong support for a variation of the humoral theory was to come from an aggressive and flamboyant Frenchman, Francois Broussais (1772–1838), who proposed that disease entities did not exist, but that disease resulted from organ irritation by toxins absorbed from the gastrointestinal tract. Vigorous measures of depletion with starvation, purgation, venesection and leeches, which he designated as *antiphlogistic*, were used to counteract the hypothetical irritative *phlogiston* released from the heat of inflammation, according to the *Vitalism* theory of the previous century. However, doubts about the humoral theory in tuberculosis did begin to emerge in Paris early in the nineteenth century when Gaspard-Laurent Bayle (1774–1816), who discussed the issue in his *Recherches sur la Phthisie Pulmonaire* (1810) based on 900 autopsies. He found that tuberculosis was a specific disease entity and not a morbid degeneration resulting from 'tissue irritation' due to a neglected 'pulmonary catarrah'. This was confirmed by his co-worker at the Charité Hospital, René-Theophile Laënnec (1781–1826) who, besides establishing the varied appearances of tuberculosis as being progressive stages of one disease, found[11] that 'the growth of tubercles in the lungs most commonly takes place without any previous inflammation'. John Forbes,[11] who translated Bayle's work, added that 'from the anatomical character of tubercular phthises, it is evident that we have little or nothing to expect from the employment of venesection or other antiphlogistic measures'. Besides inventing the stethoscope and the art of auscultation, Laënnec[11] also brought hope of cure in an era when tuberculosis was considered incurable when he described cavitation as being a process of healing 'the efforts of nature in maturing and evacuating the tuberculosis matter'. He also described cicatrization as a healing process.

Broussais' wide influence is shown in William Stokes'[21] textbook of chest diseases (1837). While lauding Laënnec for his discovery of auscultation, the theories of Broussais were adopted in the treatment of tuberculosis which Stokes regarded as 'preceded by irritation … an ordinary cold, an attack of influenza … '. While Stokes paid attention to regimen in diet, winter residence in a temperate climate and horseback riding, he advocated 'the principle of the local depletion of Broussais' in the application of leeches over the affected area as determined by auscultation 'to diminish irritation of the lung as the true method of arresting the disease in its early stages'.

THE SANATORIUM MOVEMENT

This movement which lasted for 100 years up to the middle of this century, formed the basis of tuberculosis treatment before chemotherapy. It can be divided into four phases.

The experimental phase c. 1840–84

The originator of this concept was George Bodington[3] (1799–1882), a country practitioner who advocated a special institution for the disease 'with a certain class of practitioner to exclusively pursue this practice as a distinct branch', who would treat 'not with anti-phlogistics but with moderate quantities of nourishing diet and wine'. He advocated constant outdoor exposure by increasing walking distances irrespective of weather conditions, and he established a home for the supervision of patients. Medical thought at the time was far too greatly influenced by Broussais for the acceptance of his ideas, and he lost interest after a blistering attack by the *Lancet* of 1840 for his 'beefsteak and porter treatment' and for his 'very crude and unsupported ideas'. This journal had the good grace to record in his obituary notice of 11 March 1882 that 'it was remarkable that a village doctor should have arrived in 1840 at those conclusions which anticipated some of our most recent teaching. It is less remarkable that he met with the fate of those who question authority'.

Bodington's principles of treatment were used in the development of the institutions in Germany, then known as *sanitaria* (L. *sanitas*, meaning health). Hermann Brehmer (1826–89) chose the mountains at

Goebersdorf for his pioneer sanatorium in 1859, on the grounds that tuberculosis was rare at high altitudes and according to the theory that the disease was caused by patients having small hearts that yielded a poor pulmonary circulation. He therefore recommended graduated walking exercises up mountain slopes to strengthen the myocardium. His former patient Peter Dettweiler (1837–1904), in his institution at Falkenstein, emphasized 'rest', introducing the concept of 'rest periods' in the open on reclining chairs — the *liegekur* — in 1876. This practice developed as a ritual of an hours' complete physical and mental rest a few times a day and gained wide acceptance as the 'cure de silence' or 'rest hour'. Otto Walther (1853–1919), at his sanatorium at Nordrach-in-Baden in 1888, used hyperalimentation and enforced a discipline which excluded entertainment and discouraged visitors.

These basics of treatment were generally adopted, especially in private sanatoria in the mountains of Switzerland, after the first sanatorium had been established at Davos in 1866 by the German trained Alexander Spengler (1827–1901). A unique medico-social entity existed in these closed communities made up mainly of the young on the threshold of life's activities. Long hospitalization, a slow decline with a 60–70 per cent mortality; enhanced mental activity due to low grade fever, boredom, loneliness, frustration and fear provided the essential ingredients for the vivid articulation of life's joys and sorrows. This found expression in a genre of fiction, sanatorium literature, with the classic in this field being *Der Zauberberg*[17] (*The Magic Mountain*, 1924) by Thomas Mann (1875–1955). Based on a three-week visit in 1912 to the *Wald* sanatorium at Davos where his wife was a patient (the *Berghof* of the novel), the account affords a penetrating insight into the psychology and philosophy of chronic disability. Mirrored in the characters of the novel is the daily running of these luxury private institutions. Mann, in a postscript to the work, reveals that he developed a fever there and that 'the professor with an eye to profit declared me obviously tubercular … and that I would be acting wisely to remain

for six months. If I had followed his advice I might still be there. I wrote *The Magic Mountain* instead'.

The public and sanatoria personnel of Davos protested about the image of commercialism and the eccentricity of its doctors that were projected by the book. Krokowski, the assistant director, holds spiritualism sessions with patients and disappears with selected ones in a cellar for psycho-analysis. Behrens, the director, dining with patients, cheerfully explains at table the process of decomposition: 'You lie there in your sawdust and shavings and the gases distend you, you swell enormously and your belly explodes. Hurray! You are much relieved'.

The developmental phase c. 1885–1910

As the fact that tuberculosis was curable became accepted, *sanataria* became *sanatoria* (L. *sanare* meaning to heal). Following the discovery of the tubercle bacillus in 1882 by Robert Koch (1843–1910), and the belief that oxygen was harmful to the germ, exposure to fresh air was emphasized. This phase heralded the sanatorium doctor, often recruited from patient ranks, as a specialist, laboratory research worker and academician in a new discipline. This applied particularly in the United States where the sanatorium movement, pioneered by Edward L Livingstone Trudeau (1848–1915), was extensive. Two years after graduation, he himself contracted tuberculosis while in general practice in New York, and deteriorated to a near-moribund state. As a lover of nature he decided to spend his last days at Saranac Lake in the Adirondack mountains where, surprisingly, he improved and returned to his practice but relapsed. After a third repetition of the cycle he moved to Saranac permanently and, influenced by the writings of Brehmer, established a cottage in 1885 for five patients maintained by public subscription. This developed into an internationally known institution where distinguished persons such as Robert Louis Stevenson were treated. The Saranac Laboratory, started by Trudeau in 1890, where research on tuberculosis immunity was undertaken, also became a prestigious investigating unit in this field. The American Thoracic Society has, since 1926, awarded the Trudeau Medal to eminent workers in tuberculosis, and, of the first 30 recipients, at least 21 had had the disease and worked in sanatoria.

The British equivalent pioneer sanatorium was also inspired by an individual. Robert Philip[8] (1857–1939), a recent graduate, hearing Koch lecture on *Mycobacterium tuberculosis* in Vienna in 1882, when the discovery had not yet been accepted, was inspired to return to Edinburgh to make a career of tuberculosis studies, despite contrary advice from former tutors who considered the subject exhausted and the outlook hopeless. Financed by friends, he founded the Royal Victoria Hospital near the city in 1883. This service broke new ground when it became part of a local tuberculosis administrative unit, the Edinburgh Scheme (Figure 2.1), with the dispensary as the control unit. The dispensary was the prototype of the modern tuberculosis clinic — it established contact-tracing and examination, together with documentation

EDINBURGH ANTI-TUBERCULOSIS SCHEME

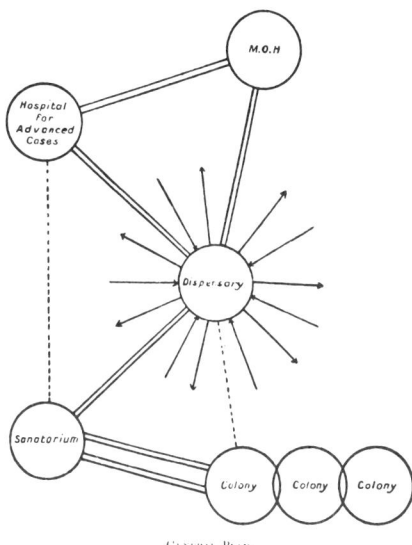

Figure 2.1. The Edinburgh Scheme. The dispensary treated its own patients in addition to those from the sanatorium and farm colony, as well as the advanced cases from the local authority.

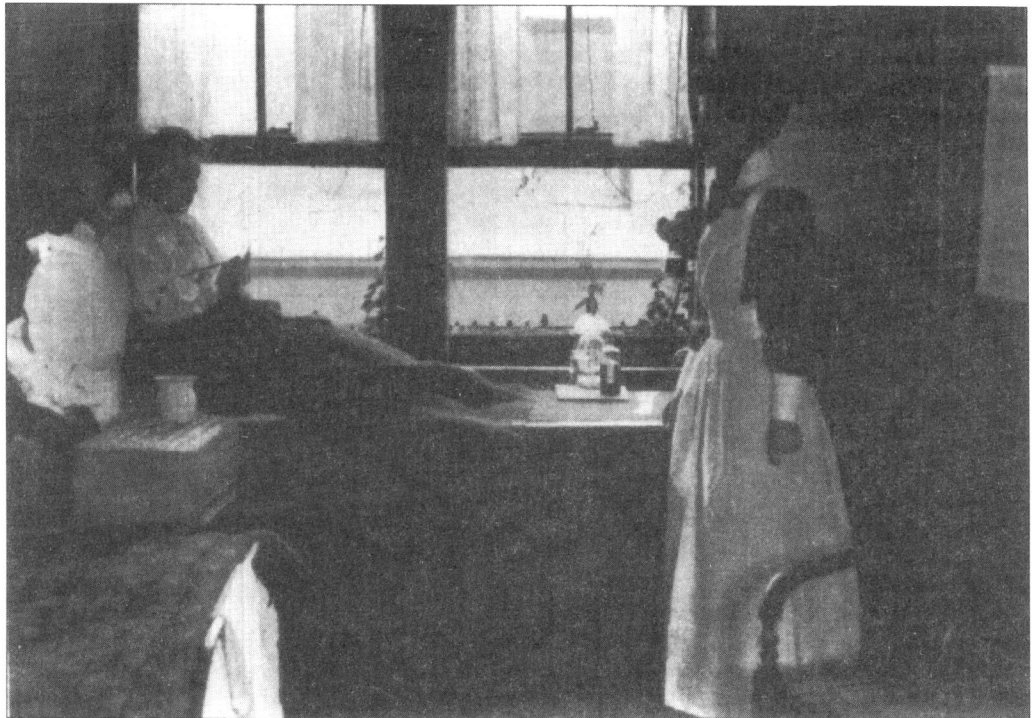

Figure 2.2. A health visitor from the dispensary supervising home treatment. Note the maximum exposure to fresh air.

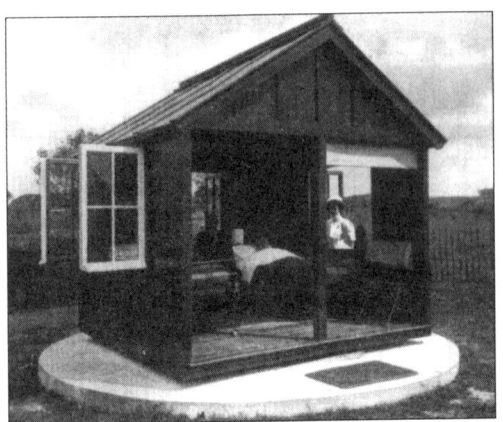

Figure 2.3. Cabin-like shelters mounted on a concrete base which allowed for rotation so as to obtain maximum sun and air exposure. These were set in the grounds of institutions or homes in Edinburgh.

of case and home conditions by the first-ever appointed health visitors (Figure 2.2). Constant exposure to fresh air was stressed (Figure 2.3). The Edinburgh Scheme was maintained by public subscription and attracted world wide interest.

The supplementation of treatment phase (1910–50)

This progressive era was characterized by a unique, long and close doctor-patient relationship. X-ray plates were explained and sedimentation rates and sputum results discussed. The patient was kept fully informed both of his or her progress and of decisions made at staff meetings attended by occupational therapist, physiotherapist, radiographer and thoracic surgeon. The emotional problems of a sequestered existence, of insecurity, of fear and of hostility were sympathetically handled by doctors and nurses who were often themselves at a more advanced stage of recovery. However, at this time the outlook for tuberculosis was still gloomy. William Farr[9] (1885) quotes the hospital case mortality rate as 62 per cent in the first year, 85 per cent in the second year and 95 per cent in the fifth year after presentation. Artificial pneumothorax (APT), the induction of a temporary and selective collapse of the affected part of the lung by the introduction of air into the pleural space, was the first specific treatment of tuberculosis that resulted in patient improvement. APT was initiated by Carlo Fornalini[12] (1847–1918) in 1894 after he had observed that the complication of pneumothorax in tuberculosis often resulted in patient improvement. Stokes[21] (1837) describes 'a gentleman in whom a phthisical cavity opened into the right lung ... After recovery from the first violence of the disease he gradually regained his flesh, strength and appearance ... and took horse exercise every day. He assured me that he could trot or canter his horse, only for the splashing in his chest which annoyed him'.

The theory of APT must be credited to James Carson[6] (1772–1843), a practitioner in Liverpool. Establishing the elasticity of the lungs in animal experiments, he concluded that when a lesion occurs in the lungs 'the sides of the divided substances recede in opposite directions' and that 'the divided surfaces would be brought into close contact ... by admitting a small quantity of air into the chest ... as favourable to the healing process'. However, his attempt in 1822 to induce an APT by open inter-costal incision failed as the patient had an adherent pleura.

Whereas Carson intended APT as a single completed treatment, Fornalini used several injections of small amounts of nitrogen (200 to 250 ml) given at intervals of a few days. The latter employed frequent refills within a closed method of APT. He used two connected bottles, one containing water and the other nitrogen. Raising the bottle of water forced nitrogen through a tube connected to the needle into the pleural space. However, Fornalini's work aroused little interest.

In 1899, John Benjamin Murphy (1857–1916), Professor of Surgery at Chicago, better known for 'Murphy's Button', a device for anastomosing hollow abdominal viscera, independently published a paper[19] in which he advised 'collapse and enforced rest of the lung ... [to cause] ... cicatrization and encapsulation of the tubercular foci ... '. Using an induction needle, he introduced nitrogen gas in large quantities (one to three litres), relying on the degree of mediastinal displacement for control. By 1906 he and his assistant A F Lemke had treated 358 patients with equivocal results, but after that interest in APT ceased in the United States.

From about 1910 APT gradually gained acceptance in Europe, starting in the Nordic countries. Fornalini's method was employed in effecting collapse, but with air instead of nitrogen and manometric control of pleural pressure. The apparatus used was simple and portable and was based on the gravitational displacement of air by water between two connected containers (Figure 2.4). However, the ease of induction disguised the potential danger of cerebral air embolism, and APT could only be done on patients with unilateral infiltrative disease limited to an apex or upper lobe. A preliminary period of bed rest for about a month was needed for reducing disease activity.

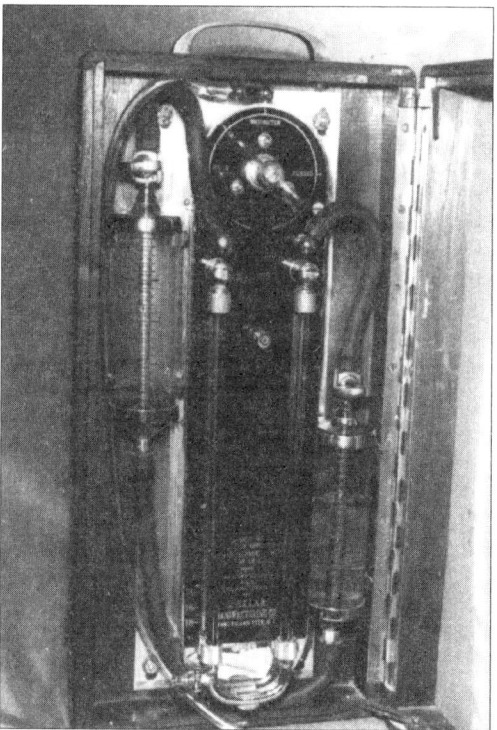

Figure 2.4. The Davidson (APT) Artificial Pneumothorax 'box' with manometer was commonly used in South Africa. The lever interchanges the levels of two 100 ml cylinders thereby allowing a measured quantity of water in one to enter the other and so displace air via the tubing and needle into the pleural space.

Using a needle of the trocar and cannula type, the fourth or fifth inter-costal space in the mid-axillary line was selected to establish the patency of the pleural space by obtaining a 'negative swing' of between 4 and 12 ml of water with respiration. Thereafter air in quantities of 300 to 500 ml at intervals of a few days was introduced, maintaining a negative pressure.

An APT was continued for an average of two years, including out-patient follow up treatment, but could be stopped at any stage due to atelectasis caused by endo-bronchial tuberculosis, pleural effusion or activation of disease.

Noting Farr's mortality figure in 1885 of 80 per cent, there had really been no change in outlook since Laënnec's time. Brieger,[5] analysing survival rates in Europe and England, found that improvement only began after 1920 with the increasing use of sanatorium treatment and APT, and that towards the end of the 1930s the survival rate was 20 per cent better than without this treatment. Alexander,[1] comparing results of APT in the Michigan State Sanatorium in the early 1930s (where APT was done on 87 per cent of patients) with a group of other sanatoria (where only 10 per cent of patients had an APT), found that the former discharged 47 per cent of its patients as 'arrested', compared with 17 per cent from the other sanatoria. This difference was achieved despite the fact that the latter group had more early cases (16 per cent) than the Michigan institution (nine per cent).

A variation of 'relaxation therapy' for basal tuberculosis was the division of the phrenic nerve in the anterior triangle of the neck. This was devised by Sauerbruch and Schepelman in 1913 to paralyse and raise one diaphragm. A later development produced temporary muscle paralysis by crushing the phrenic stem for about 1 cm or by injection with alcohol. A related procedure, more frequently used in South Africa for raising both diaphragms, was a pneumoperitoneum, which had been introduced in the United States by A L Banyai[2] in the 1930s. Using an APT apparatus, half to one litre of air was introduced into the peritoneal space, reducing both lung volumes by one quarter or a third, and affording patients a sense of well-being with less risk of air embolism.

The logical development of an APT was permanent lung collapse, which was indicated in patients where the pleura was adherent. This was done by thoracoplasty with the removal of ribs. Brauer and Friedrich in 1907 removed the entire length of the 2nd to the 10th ribs at the para-vertebral level in one operation. Three of the first seven patients died of respiratory and circulatory failure due to paradoxical movement of the resected chest wall and pendulum movement of the mediastinum, but from this drastic procedure thoracoplasty evolved so that by 1937 it was limited to the removal of restricted lengths of the upper five to seven ribs. This was performed in two or three stages and was carefully quantitated so as to collapse a persistent cavity with apicolysis (the dissection of the lung apex from its attachments in the extra fascial plane to ensure a concentric collapse). Carl Semb[20] of Oslo, who perfected the latter technique, reported a sputum conversion of 90 per cent with an operative mortality below three per cent. A suitable thoracoplasty candidate was a 'stable chronic'

with a persistent upper zone cavity and positive sputum, with limited non-progressive disease in the other lung. Thoracoplasty was used with success in South Africa as it was safer than lung resection, but it was unsuitable for manual workers as it resulted in a weakened shoulder on the operated side.

Illustrative case

A coloured woman was diagnosed in 1967. When admitted to a tuberculosis hospital in April 1973 for the fourth time, this recalcitrant patient had had a total of two and a half years of unsuccessful institutional chemotherapy. She was in poor general condition, weighing 33 kg and with a positive sputum. The x-ray (Figure 2.5) showed a large cavity in the left upper zone surrounded by extensive fibrosis. A five rib thoracoplasty was done in December 1973, obliterating the cavity (Figure 2.6) and converting the sputum to negative. At discharge she had gained 10 kg. The justification for operating on this patient, who was unlikely to take medication after discharge, was proved by the maintenance of her improved clinical and radiological state up to August 1975.

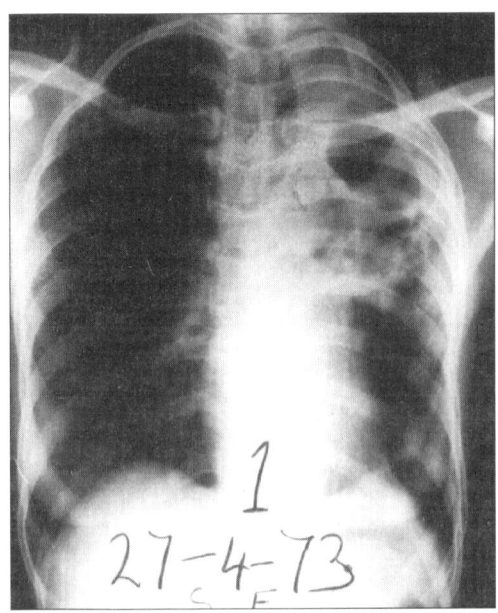

Figure 2.5. Admission plate of AF: extensive chronic cavitation in the left upper zone.

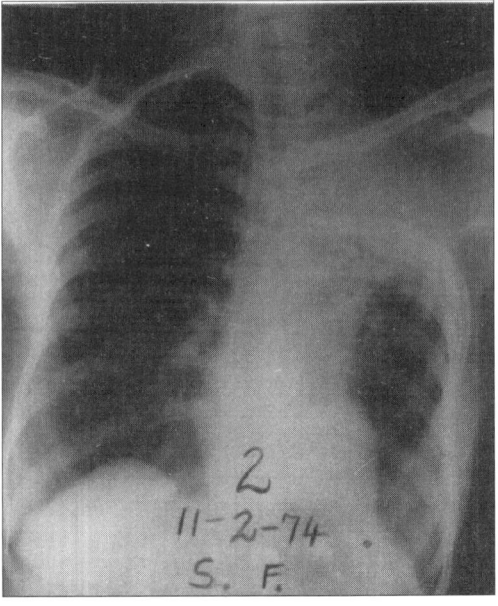

Figure 2.6. Plate of AF eight months later, after a five-rib thoracoplasty: obliteration of the cavity.

Over some 50 years during which thoracoplasty was being developed, lung resection had been largely abandoned after the poor results of the removal of apical lesions in the 1880s in Germany. Heaf[14] quotes mortality rates of 45 per cent for pneumonectomy and 25 per cent for lobectomy in 1940. However, from 1943 there was a gradual improvement in mortality and complication rate with more selective lobectomy in unilobular lesions; an improved operative technique of meticulous hilar dissection with separate bronchial and blood vessel ligature, and the cover of chemotherapy. A later refinement of resection was Chamberlain's[7] removal in 1953 of affected pulmonary segments, particularly the apical and posterior segments of the upper lobes, and the posterior segments of the lower lobes, where chronic tuberculosis was mainly located.

Using this approach Brewer and Bai[4] in 1955 reported a series of 129 patients with a recovery rate of 98 per cent and a mortality rate of 0,9 per cent. This series had the benefit of streptomycin (SM), para-amino salicylic acid (PAS), and isoniazid (INH). By about 1958, these drugs had replaced thoracic surgery for tuberculosis treatment in the western world.

The discovery of the tubercle bacillus by Koch in 1882 and Ehrlich's *salvarsan* in 1909 (an arsenical that killed spirochaetes in syphilis) stimulated an intensive search for a similar preparation for tuberculosis. Commonly tried compounds were creosote, calcium chloride and mercury perchloride, given orally or by injection. The inhalational route for a combination of iodoform, eucalyptus, chloroform and ether was used in New York and was described by the *Medical Annual* of 1890 as being 'formidable but rational'. Some treatments were bizarre; the subcutaneous injection of dog's serum in Italy was reported by the *British Medical Journal* of 1890 as 'very encouraging'.

The *Medical Annual* of 1922 reported the use in the United States of a course of chest radiation to promote fibrosis and healing. Katherine Mansfield, the novelist (1888–1923), received this treatment in Paris, which probably caused progressive heart failure in her. The agent that had the longest run (1925 to 1931) was *sanocrysen*,[15] an inorganic gold salt given by injection and introduced by Hollger Mollgaard of Copenhagen. Despite early evidence of renal and hepatic toxicity, the treatment had authoritative support until 1931, when in the United States the only controlled trial found it to be not only ineffective but also dangerous. Reviewing the situation that year, Gideon Wells[24] commented that 'we have come to realize that chemotherapy in the sense that Ehrlich introduced the term is more of a dream than a reality'.

The period of the decline of sanatoria *c.* 1950–8

Contrary to Wells' prediction, tuberculosis chemotherapy did arrive and it accelerated the decline of sanatoria in the western world by shortening hospitalization.

Ferrebee and Palmer[10] conducted trials of 26 hospitals in the United States from 1947, involving more than 10 000 patients. Assessing results of treatment *after a year* in various groups, they found that patients who had had no anti-microbial treatment had a mortality of 21 per cent; 54 per cent were still sputum positive and 25 per cent were sputum negative. A combination of SM and PAS in the early 1950s reduced mortality to three per cent; 32 per cent remained sputum positive and 65 per cent became non-infectious. By 1963, mainly through the impact of INH and SM, PAS and pyrazinamide, the mortality rate had dropped to one per cent, sputum-negatives increased to 95 per cent and only four per cent remained sputum positive.

Other factors responsible for the decline of sanatoria were the gradual decrease of tuberculosis mortality from about 1850 as a result of improved social conditions and the use of mass miniature radiography as a screening measure of populations after the Second World War. The latter brought cases suitable for out-patient therapy to early attention. By 1958 sanatoria, at that stage state-owned, were running out of patients and had begun to close down. Private sanatoria had bowed out in the depression years of the 1930s while the philanthropic institutions like Saranac Lake ceased functioning in the early 1950s as they were unable to meet the rising costs of tuberculosis treatment, advances in thoracic surgery, more sophisticated radiography, occupational therapy and the greater number of nursing and specialist staff employed.

Sanatoria in South Africa

The climatic treatment

From about 1850 South Africa was a recognized venue for overseas visitors for the 'cure'. Burney Yeo's *Manual of Medical Treatment* (1893) recommended its dry interior as being suitable for 'limited non progressive disease'. The influx of immigrants warranted a government commission[23] in 1912 which reported that 'the primary factor in its [tuberculosis] introduction into many centres until then free from it has been the immigration of consumptive persons', and cited Beaufort West and Cradock as examples.

The matter was also of concern to Bloemfontein's Medical Officer of Health, D M Tomory, in 1911. In his annual report he noted that tuberculosis presented no problem in the white population, with only 10 deaths from tuberculosis in a white population of 10 968, but he did express concern at the number of deaths (13) in visitors from overseas from as far afield as Russia, New Zealand, Wales and Scotland. He added, 'I have seen cases taken out of the train and unable to walk, and straight to the National Hospital, to be tended in life and buried after death at the expense of a state and town on which they have not the slightest claim …. Some die in outside rooms, in backyards among conditions favouring the transmission of disease to others in lonely misery …. Many hotels and boarding houses have rooms that have been infected and other people occupy the same rooms ignorant of the fact'.

Small 'sanatoria', in reality guest farms, run by doctors or nurses exploited the putative therapeutic potential of the Karoo air. Purceval Gibbon[13] used this setting in his 1911 novel, *Margaret Harding*. The character of the title arrives from London to join a group of ex-Londoners at a farm sanatorium

in the Karoo. The patients include a monocled clubman and an ex-army officer. Typical of sanatorium literature, the occupants also have in their midst a seedy couple, the doctor and his wife from Clapham Junction, who are in charge. The pervasive boredom of their daily existence, punctuated by class and personal conflicts, with fresh air the only treatment, conveys a vivid impression of life in a sanatorium.

Sanatoria

The Nelspoort Sanatorium, established on a farm in the Karoo near Beaufort West in 1924, was the only example in this country of the prototype sanatorium of this era. It had the typical geographic isolation and self-containment, with power from its own station and food supply from farming. Established as a gift from John Garlick of Cape Town, it was maintained by the state. *Die Huisgenoot* of 30 May 1941 described the daily regimen of graduated activity with maximum exposure to fresh air of its 174 white and black patients. Some patients received APT, courses of calcium or *sanocrysen* injections. Four 'rest hours' of complete relaxation and silence were practised. Recreational facilities were well-structured and included a concert hall, gardening, croquet, miniature golf and a newspaper, the *Rest Hour*.

Tuberculosis hospitals run on sanatorium lines were developed by the state at major centres after the Second World War. Unlike overseas sanatoria, they increased and progressed for the next 25 years to meet the demand of heavy new case loads. Work was demanding as most of these patients had extensive or moderately extensive disease. The sanatorium regimen was ideally suited for the newly introduced and successful prolonged chemotherapy of 18 to 24 months' duration. Collapse therapy and thoracic surgery were mainly practised in South Africa within this framework, but these limited interventions made little impact on the country's tuberculosis problem because of the extensive spread of the disease. As chemotherapy became increasingly effective, collapse therapy ceased after about 1958 and thoracic surgery was used only to salvage failed cases of conservative treatment or to remove damaged lung tissue which was acting as a source of chronic pyogenic infection.

Under the guidance of B A Dormer, a major contribution made by these state institutions was the training of young doctors. They made a career in this field, acted as regional consultants and supervised the extensive state subsidized scheme of rural mission hospitals and settlements of the South African National Tuberculosis Association.

REFERENCES

1 Alexander J, 1937. Quoted in Kayne G G *et al.*, 1939. *Pulmonary Tuberculosis.* London: Oxford University Press.
2 Banyai A L, 1946. *Peritoneum Treatment.* St Louis: The C V Mosby Company.
3 Bodington G, 1840. *An Essay on the Treatment and Cure of Pulmonary Consumption.* London: Simpkin, Marshall, Hamilton and Kent, 1840. Quoted from Keers R Y, 1978. *Pulmonary Tuberculosis. A Journey down the Centuries.* London: Balliere Tindall.
4 Brewer L A & Bai A F, 1955. Quoted from Keers R Y, 1978. *Pulmonary Tuberculosis. A Journey down the Centuries.* London: Balliere Tindall.
5 Brieger E, 1937. Quoted in Kayne G G *et al.*, 1939. *Pulmonary Tuberculosis.* London: Oxford University Press.
6 Carson J, 1821. *On the Elasticity of the Lung* and *On the Lesions of the Lung.* Quoted in Cummins S L, 1949. *Tuberculosis in History.* London; Balliere, Tindall and Cox, 69–78.
7 Chamberlain J M *et al.*, 1953. Quoted from Keers R Y, 1978. *Pulmonary Tuberculosis. A Journey down the Centuries.* London: Balliere Tindall.
8 Dubovsky H, 1973. Robert W. Philip (1857–1939). Pioneer of the holistic approach to tuberculosis and its voluntary movement. *South African Medical Journal* 1973; 1007–10.
9 Farr W, 1885. *Vital Statistics.* London: Noel A Humphreys. Quoted from Kayne G G *et al.*, 1939. *Pulmonary Tuberculosis.* London: Oxford University Press.
10 Ferebee S H & Palmer C E, 1965. The epidemiological bonus. *American Review of Tuberculosis.* 91, 104–7.
11 Forbes J, 1979. *A Treatment of Diseases of the Chest* (1821). tr. of Laënnec R T H. *De l'auscultation médiate (1819).* Special edition. Birmingham, Alabama: The Classics of Medicine Library.
12 Fornalini C, 1894. First attempts at artificial pneumothorax in pulmonary phthisis. *Gazetta Medica di Torino.* tr. 1934 by Lafacono S. *Tubercle.* 16, 121–5.
13 Gibbon P, 1911. *Margaret Harding.* London: Methuen & Co. 1983 reprint by Africa South Paperbacks. Cape Town: David Philip.
14 Heaf F R G, 1957. *Symposium of Tuberculosis.* London: Cassel and Co Ltd.
15 Keers R Y, 1980. The gold rush 1925–35. *Thorax.* 35, 844–89.
16 Lloyd G E R, 1978. *Hippocratic Writings.* London. Pelican Classics.
17 Mann T, 1924. *Der Zauberberg.* Berlin: S Fischer Verlag. tr. 1980 as *The Magic Mountain.* London: Secker and Warburg.
18 Morse D *et al.*, 1964. Tuberculosis in ancient Egypt. *American Review of Respiratory Diseases.* 90, 524–41.
19 Murphy J B, 1898. Surgery of the lungs. *Journal of the American Medical Association.* 31, 151, 208, 281.
20 Semb C, 1935. Quoted from Keers R Y, 1978. *Pulmonary Tuberculosis. A Journey down the Centuries.* London: Balliere Tindall.
21 Stokes W, 1837. *Diseases of the Chest*, 1837. Dublin: Hodges and Smith.
22 Sydenham T, 1979. *The Works of Thomas Sydenham, M D.* Special edition of the Sydenham Society's 1848 edition. Birmingham, Alabama: The Classics of Medicine Library.
23 Union of South Africa, Tuberculosis Commission, 1912. *First Report Dealing with the Question of the Admission of Tuberculosis Immigrants into the Union.* Pretoria: Tuberculosis Commission.
24 Wells H G, 1931. The chemotherapy of tuberculosis. *Yale Journal of Biology.* 4, 611–26.

CHAPTER 3

Holding back the tide: TB control efforts in South Africa

R M Packard*

INTRODUCTION

Prior to the end of the nineteenth century tuberculosis was a relatively rare disease in South Africa, but by the beginning of the present century it had become a major cause of both morbidity and mortality in the urban centres of the country, and was rapidly making inroads in the countryside. As in Europe and the United States, the rise of TB in South Africa was clearly associated with the growth of industrial capitalism and took its heaviest toll among workers and their families, both black and white. The appalling living and working conditions associated with the early stages of industrial development and urbanization in South Africa created an ideal environment for both the spread of infection and the development of disease.

Yet the tuberculosis experience of newly industrialized workers in South Africa was not identical to that of their European and American counterparts. To begin with, the TB epidemic in South Africa did not fall evenly on the working class as a whole, but rather fell most heavily on black workers. While many workers fell victim to the 'white plague' at the turn of the century, their mortality rates were uniformly lower than those of black workers. For example, TB mortality in the port cities of Cape Town and Port Elizabeth approached 10 deaths per 1 000 inhabitants among blacks, but only one or two per 1 000 among whites.

This pattern can also be seen in American cities after 1850, though the differences between blacks and other immigrant white communities is not so great as in the South African case. Moreover, the difference between white and black workers in South Africa persisted and has in fact increased over the last 50 years.

Secondly, while the TB epidemic among white workers paralleled the experience of their counterparts in Europe and the United States, with both morbidity and mortality falling off dramatically after an initial epidemic wave, rates for blacks have shown little sign of replicating this downward trend. As a result, only one per cent of the 50 to 60 000 new cases that are currently reported each year occur among whites.

While black TB deaths declined dramatically after the development of effective anti-tuberculosis drugs in the early 1950s, there is little evidence that this decline in TB deaths reflected a significant reduction in the level of TB morbidity. There are those who have argued, in fact, that given inefficient treatment programmes, chemotherapy simply produced a growing pool of half-cured and therefore potentially infectious cases which have contributed to a rising tide of TB.

It may be argued of course that it is too early to assert that the western pattern is not being repeated in Africa. The average length of a TB wave from early rise to decline in Europe and the United States was

---

*The editors of this book originally intended to have this chapter written by David Webster. His tragic death at the hands of a right wing death squad prevented this from happening. My work on the history of TB in South Africa was greatly informed by David's research on this and other critical social issues and I was honoured to be asked to take up the task of writing this chapter. It is not the chapter that David would have written. But I trust that it reflects his critical perspective on life in South Africa.

42

roughly 200 years. In many African countries we are still in the early or middle stages of such a long term curve. It must be remembered, however, that the fall in TB mortality in Europe and the United States was generated in large part by improvements in living and working conditions and that these in turn reflected the convergence of political and economic interests in support of health reform.

The present chapter explores the efforts on the part of the white medical profession and the South African state to stem the tide of tuberculosis in South Africa and why these efforts have led to such disparate results for blacks and whites.[30]

TB CONTROL EFFORTS IN THE PRE-CHEMOTHERAPY ERA

Historical forces governing the spread of tuberculosis

Medical critics of South Africa's system of apartheid have frequently pointed to inequalities in the availability of medical resources (as reflected in the distribution of physicians, nurses, clinics, and hospital beds) as playing an important role in the creation of the wide gulf that exists between the health status of whites and that of blacks. While there is no doubt some truth to this assertion, differences in the allocation of medical resources probably played a minimal role in determining the contrasting TB experiences of whites and blacks prior to the Second World War. This is partly because health resources in South Africa were generally inadequate for the needs of all but the most well off members of society, but, more importantly, differences in access to western medical treatment were unimportant before the development of anti-tuberculosis drugs in the late 1940s because available medical interventions against TB were of little value in controlling the spread of the disease.

Students of the history of TB in Europe and the United States have observed that much of the decline in tuberculosis mortality that occurred from the middle of the nineteenth century was a product of forces that were largely independent of medical efforts.[12, 25] Isolating existing cases and providing them with rest and a healthy diet may have slowed the pace of the epidemic, but did not, by themselves, cause its decline. Instead, it is argued, exposed human populations developed increased resistance to the disease as a result of the death of genetically susceptible individuals and the survival of more resistant hosts. Of equal or greater importance were improvements in living and working conditions which reduced the opportunities for the transmission of infection and also increased host resistance to the disease.

Neither of these processes were naturally occurring phenomena, although they are often presented as such. The growing biological resistance of human populations in Europe and the United States was clearly encouraged by the creation of a more or less permanent class of urban working and non-working poor who lived in constant contact with the TB bacilli. Had the proletarianization of the workforce been less extensive, and the movement of labour into industrial centres more temporary in nature, it is likely that this 'seasoning' process would have been delayed. Grigg, in fact, argues that the steady decline of TB in American cities was disrupted at several points by the introduction of new unexposed immigrant populations.[18]

Similarly, reforms in living and working conditions did not occur by accident, but resulted from a growing convergence of class interests over the need for improved workers' health. A long history of worker activism and the gradual political enfranchising of the working class, together with a recognition on the part of dominant segments of the bourgeoisie that health reforms were essential for the reproduction of capital, led to a gradual movement toward better living and working conditions in Europe and the United States.[30]

Both of these processes also affected white workers in South Africa, but were slow to develop among blacks. This difference accounts in large measure for the differences in the trajectory of TB mortality among blacks and whites prior to the development of effective anti-tuberculosis drugs.

The development of biological resistance to TB among white workers and their families was encouraged, as it was among their counterparts in Europe and the United States, by their rapid proletarianization. From the end of the nineteenth century, white mine and factory workers emerged as a permanent working class totally dependent on wage employment for their survival. By contrast black workers, first by choice and later by law, were largely, though by no means exclusively, migrant workers who moved back and forth between the urban workplace and their rural homes. As a result, their exposure to tuberculosis was more intermittent and their ability to develop a biological balance with the TB bacillus more tenuous. On the other hand, this same pattern of migrant labour contributed to a more rapid dissemination of infection among rural blacks than among rural whites. As a result of this rapid spread from urban to rural communities, genetic susceptibility gradually decreased as a factor in black TB mortality, becoming relatively unimportant by the 1930s.

Similarly, improvements in living and working conditions occurred more rapidly among white workers than among blacks. This reflected marked differences in the extent to which class interests converged around the issue of workers' health.

The achievement of health reform for white workers and their families did not evolve easily. However racist South Africa was to become later in the twentieth century, the alignment of political and economic interests at the beginning of the industrial revolution did not automatically ensure white privilege or white worker health and safety.

Political power during the period of early industrialization, prior to the South African War, lay primarily in the hands of farming and commercial interests. This was particularly true in the Transvaal where the discovery of gold had created a boom town environment along the Rand. The Kruger government, representing the concerns of Afrikaner farmers, had little interest in implementing health reform or other improvements to ensure the well-being of the rapidly expanding industrial workforce, but were primarily concerned with maintaining order and rent-seeking activities.

For its part, capital, working under severe financial constraints, had no more inclination to invest in the health of white workers than in that of blacks, and silicosis took a dreadful toll among white mineworkers during the early years of underground mining.[5, 20]

In the end, the ability of white workers to mobilize and fight for reforms,[20, 23] their growing representation within the state (particularly after 1924) and the mine owners' fear that failure to provide improvements for white workers would lead to the development of a broad-based multiracial labour movement, encouraged the mine owners, with the support of the state, which was committed to the ideal of a white settler society in South Africa, to gradually develop a discriminatory system of wages and benefits.[19] This led to the emergence of the colour bar in industrial relations and to a growing disparity in the working and living conditions of white and black workers.[49] In effect, the interests of white labour, capital and the state came together in an uneasy alignment of political and economic interests which ensured that significant improvements were instituted in white working and living conditions.[20, 23]

Symbolic of the role of the state in implementing a pattern of labour stratification was its provision of housing for white workers in newly constructed working class suburbs around Johannesburg during the first decade of this century, in order to prevent white workers from living in close proximity to Africans and other blacks in boarding houses and slum tenements.

By contrast, black workers found it much more difficult to assert their demands for health workers. The destabilizing effects of the migrant labour system on efforts to organize black labour, combined with the absence of black worker representation within the state, greatly hampered the development of worker-driven health reforms. Moreover, while there were moments during the 1940s, as well as later during the 1970s, when the interests of black labour converged with those of certain segments of industrial capital and the state, over the question of health reform for urban blacks, these were temporary in nature, fragile in terms of the level of commitment exhibited by either capital or the state, and weakened by the opposition of other powerful sets of economic and political interests within white South African society. As a result, much less was achieved or even attempted in the way of fundamental reforms in the conditions which contributed to high rates of TB among black workers and their families.

Compared to these historical forces, the TB control efforts of medical authorities played a very limited role in determining the disparate disease experiences of blacks and whites in South Africa, prior to the development of effective chemotherapeutic interventions in the late 1940s. It is nonetheless instructive to examine briefly the main lines of these control efforts, for they reveal certain patterns that have persisted up until the present.

Medical control of tuberculosis

Although tuberculosis was a recognized health problem among whites, and to a lesser extent blacks, by the middle of the nineteenth century, little effort was made to control the spread of the disease prior to 1900. Faith in the healing effects of South Africa's sunny, healthful climate was widespread and medical authorities went so far as to encourage European consumptives to migrate to South Africa during the last quarter of the century.

Hundreds of such immigrants settled within communities in the drier inland regions of the Karoo during the 1870s and 1880s, but the threat which these imported cases of TB represented for the native-born populations of the colony, both black and white, was not appreciated prior to 1895. The infectious nature of tuberculosis was only discovered by Koch in 1882 and even then was not widely accepted within the western medical establishment. In addition, the absence of legislation requiring the registration of deaths in the Cape Colony or elsewhere in South Africa made it impossible to assess the force of tuberculosis on mortality rates.

Unaware of the potential consequences of the immigration of consumptives, town officials in the Cape Colony made no effort to curtail the spread of infection among the town's non-infected inhabitants. However, with the establishment of compulsory death registrations in 1895, medical authorities in the Colony came to recognize the high toll that tuberculosis was taking. Compulsory registration of TB cases became mandatory in the Cape and Natal in 1904 (three years before Massachusetts and nine years before England), and in 1907 the country's first accommodation specifically for TB patients was provided in the City Infectious Disease Hospital in Cape Town.[1]

In 1912 a commission was established to look into the state of tuberculosis in South Africa. The commission's report was extensive and clearly indicated the seriousness of the problem. It made numerous recommendations for the implementation of measures for controlling the spread of infection, including a proposal to tightly control the immigration of European tuberculotics. Many of the recommendations were incorporated into the Public Health Act of 1919, which called for improvements in housing and sanitation, education, enforcement of precautions against the spread of the disease, the provision of facilities for the early diagnosis of cases, tuberculosis dispensaries, hospitals and sanatoriums. However, few of these recommendations were acted upon, and Cape Town's 32 beds in the City Infectious Diseases Hospital remained the only such accommodation in the Union until the 1920s, and it was not to be until 1924 that the first public sanatorium would be constructed at Nelspoort. In general, there was much more discussion of the TB problem in South Africa than action.

Lack of accommodation affected both whites and blacks during the early years of TB control, yet it is clear that the few resources allocated by the state and local authorities for TB treatment and prevention prior to the Second World War went primarily to whites. For example, while the initial allocation of spaces at Nelspoort called for the accommodation of 56 white and 56 coloured and black cases, both the overall population and the number of cases

Table 3.1
Provision of beds for tuberculosis patients by race 1907–39[14]

YEAR	WHITE	OTHER RACES
1907	16	16
1924	72	52
1927	88	52
1933	131	191
1934	181	191
1935	181	191
1936	234	191
1937	286	191
1938	426	311
1939	426	430

needing treatment was much larger among the latter than the former. This pattern continued until the Second World War, as indicated in Table 3.1.

Even where space was available for black TB cases, it was often difficult for them to get treatment. The Public Health Act placed responsibility for treatment of persons who could not afford health care (and thus the majority of blacks) on the shoulders of the local authority within which the patient resided, with the government reimbursing the authority for half the resulting expenses. This system led to frequent arguments between local authorities concerning who was responsible for treatment since the authorities in the area in which a patient was diagnosed could, and frequently did, claim that the patient's real home was elsewhere. As a result of these disputes treatment was delayed and many cases were not treated. While the majority of these disputes involved black cases, similar obstacles existed for poor whites during this period.[46]

Lack of accommodation and unwillingness to bear the cost of treatment meant that the primary response of urban medical authorities to black TB cases was to report them to the Native Affairs Department for repatriation to their home area. This policy, initially developed in the mining industry, was rationalized on the grounds that the 'native' patient disliked staying in hospitals, was eager to get home to his family, and in any case stood a better chance of gaining a cure in the 'healthful' surroundings of his rural home. There was no doubt some truth to all these claims. Given the high mortality rate suffered by hospitalized blacks, their aversion to hospitals and their desire to return home were well reasoned. Moreover, given the relative impotence of western medical interventions against TB, a black might do just as well at home. It is important to recognize, however, that the concept of the 'healthy reserve' that pervaded much white medical and popular thinking about black rural life, was little more than a myth by the 1930s, widespread malnutrition and other infectious conditions being pervasive in most rural areas. The returning TB patient, therefore, had little to look forward to in terms of treatment or support and, as Peter Allen discovered in the late 1920s, some 60 per cent of them were likely to die within two years of their return.[48]

Forced removals

Exclusionary policies also marked the few efforts that were made to limit the spread of the disease among blacks through improvements in living and working conditions. The main weapon in this fight was sanitary segregation enforced by slum clearance laws. As in England at the end of the nineteenth century, slum clearance in South Africa prior to the Second World War entailed the clearing of slum properties located in the centre of urban areas and the forced removal of their occupants to locations on the periphery of these centres. Also, as in England, this process was more effective in removing slums than in providing a healthy environment for those who had been removed, despite legislation that required the construction of alternative housing. White urban ratepayers consistently rejected the notion that they should contribute to the welfare of the black work force that served their needs and required that any improvements in location conditions be paid for out of location revenues. This short-sighted vision meant that location housing was inadequate for the needs of the removed populations and soon developed into slums that were as bad or worse than those that had been cleared. The exclusion of location areas from the purview of the various slum clearance acts, moreover, meant that there was little control exercised over housing in the locations. As the Smit Committee would later observe:

Many of the houses being built for Natives under the Housing Acts, themselves primarily designed to prevent or eradicate slums, are from the first day of their occupation overcrowded and therefore slums as defined by the second schedule of the Slum Act and escape condemnation as such only by reason of the specific purview of the Act.[41]

While exclusionary policies could be expected to have little positive affect on the conditions that fostered the spread of TB, statistically they contributed to a significant decline in urban black TB rates. For locations were seldom provided with the medical oversight needed to identify new cases of TB and so were conveniently excluded from urban mortality statistics.

Commenting on the overall effect of slum clearance on the health of blacks in 1931, the Medical Officer of Health in East London observed:

Though slums may disappear from white urban areas, segregation has resulted in overcrowded unhealthy slum areas in locations, hot beds of tuberculosis and venereal disease removed at some distance from the town, or separated from it, and under the eyes of officials alone.[36]

Unable or unwilling to provide the medical or public health resources needed to support the health of black workers and their families, urban authorities, along with private church and civic organizations, devoted considerable energy to educating blacks and poor whites about the dangers of overcrowded housing, improper sanitation and non-nutritious diets. Such efforts, however well-intentioned, had little impact, since the unhealthy conditions under which the urban poor lived resulted primarily from economic rather than social and cultural forces.

The failure of early efforts to control the actual spread of TB in South Africa was dramatically highlighted in the 1940s. The immigration of thousands of blacks into the major urban centres of the country, in response to both the demands of the wartime economy and the collapse of the rural reserves, highlighted the failure of efforts to cope with the rising tide of black TB by pushing it out of the view of white taxpayers. The limited medical resources available to urban authorities, combined with a continued unwillingness of the state, industry or local authorities to provide for the welfare of the growing population of black workers and their families, and high rates of inflation produced a major upsurge in urban TB mortality.

As noted above, these conditions contributed to a renewed awareness on the part of many medical authorities, certain segments of capital and the state, of the need for serious urban environmental reform in order to attack the root causes of TB. Yet, as before, this awareness produced more rhetoric than action. Moreover, consciousness of the need for reform was soon to be dampened by the Nationalist victory of 1948 and the discovery of streptomycin, INH and other anti-tuberculosis drugs that promised to eradicate tuberculosis through purely medical means.

TUBERCULOSIS AND APARTHEID

Tuberculosis control efforts in South Africa since the late 1940s have been impressive in terms of the scale of the attack mounted by both government and private voluntary organizations. Government expenditures for TB control have increased steadily since the Second World War and by the early 1980s amounted to R50 million a year. In terms of their effectiveness, however, these efforts have fallen far short of their goal. While the prevalence of TB among whites continued to decline, virtually disappearing as a health problem by the early 1980s, TB levels among blacks remained high. Thus, despite the availability of the medical means to eliminate TB among all population groups within South Africa, major disparities continued to exist. As before the war, these differences reflected the continuation of oppressive living conditions among blacks, but inequalities in access to medical treatment now also played a much more important role.

While South Africa is not alone in its inability to bring TB under control, there are specific conditions within South Africa that have contributed to this failure. These conditions reflect the subordination of TB control efforts to the overriding political and economic designs of the Nationalist government.

Effects of segregation policies on tuberculosis

Contrary to what is often assumed by critics of apartheid, the Nationalist government did not scrap efforts at urban reform. In fact a good deal more was accomplished in terms of eliminating slums and providing alternative housing during the 1950s than had been done during the 1940s under the more reform-minded United Party. While this difference was partly due to the strict financial limitations that existed during the war, this should not detract from the real accomplishments of the early Nationalist period. However, what needs to be recognized is that urban reform under the Nationalists represented a return to the exclusionary policies that had marked TB control efforts prior to the Second World War, and reflected the Nationalists' overwhelming ideological interest in solidifying white privilege, rather than a serious concern for improving the health of the blacks.

Under the Group Areas Act, slums and squatters settlements that had sprung up during and after the Second World War, along with more established black freehold townships, such as Newclare and Sophia-

town, were eliminated to make room for white residential housing. Those who were considered necessary for the labour needs of whites were removed to hastily constructed housing estates or to site and service schemes which quickly became overcrowded as the rising demand for black labour during the 'apartheid boom' of the 1960s and declining conditions in the rural reserves created a flood of job seekers that quickly overwhelmed available accommodation. Official townships turned rapidly into slums and sprawling squatter camps located in and around the major metropolitan centres. Within this environment, problems of overcrowding and lack of sanitation persisted. On top of this a rapidly rising cost of living combined with only moderate increases in black wages encouraged overcrowding and undermined the ability of urban workers to adequately feed and clothe their families. The estimated cost of adequately feeding a black family of five in Johannesburg in 1954 equalled 94 per cent of the family's household income.[41] Moreover, while wages increased by 14 per cent between 1962 and 1967, the percentage of families living below the poverty datum line remained stationary at 68 per cent.[42]

For blacks who were defined as superfluous to the needs of white society, including large numbers of women, children and old men, a more tragic fate awaited. They were forced to join hundreds of thousands of blacks removed from rural lands coveted by white farmers in desolate resettlement camps in already overcrowded homelands. Minimal efforts at agricultural 'betterment' and the provision of local health services were quickly overwhelmed by the influx of three to four million displaced blacks.

In short, efforts to attack the underlying causes of TB in South Africa after the Second World War did little to improve black living conditions, and represented a continuation, on a grander and ultimately more tragic scale, of the policies of exclusion that had marked earlier control efforts.

Access to health services

Despite the ineffectiveness of the control measures noted above, TB mortality rates plummeted in South Africa from the late 1940s. This decline was brought about by the introduction of effective anti-tuberculosis drugs that saved the lives of thousands of TB patients. However, this impressive achievement disguised the fact that efforts to control TB through the use of chemotherapy and BCG vaccination were only marginally successful in preventing the further spread of the disease. In fact, TB control efforts may have contributed to a real rise in the incidence of TB during the 1950s and early 1960s.

Armed for the first time with a 'silver bullet', in the form of streptomycin (SM) and isoniazid (INH), South African medical authorities launched an all-out attack on TB during the 1950s. Mass x-ray surveys were carried out in both urban and rural areas to identify existing cases, hospital accommodation was increased and educational campaigns developed. By the mid 1950s medical authorities in South Africa, like their counterparts elsewhere, were expressing confidence that they would soon be able to bring TB under control.

A few medical authorities, however, such as the Medical Officer of Health of Cape Town, were less certain and noted that while chemotherapy provided an instrument for saving the lives of TB victims and thus for lowering TB mortality rates, not all cases were being identified. Moreover, many of those who were identified were for one reason or another being only partially treated.[14]

These problems affected all TB control efforts in South Africa, but were much more severe among blacks than among whites. This reflected both the differences in the conditions under which the two groups lived and in the allocation of health resources.

If one compares the accumulation of black cases on TB registers with the accumulation of white cases during the 1950s and 1960s, it is immediately apparent that the two differed not simply in the number of cases recorded, but in the pattern of case accumulation. TB registers include all reported cases that have not been cured. The rate at which the number of cases on a register increases, therefore, reflects both

the rate at which new cases are identified and the rate at which they are cured. A continual accumulation of cases indicates that new cases are being identified faster than existing cases are being cured. In South Africa black TB registers reveal this type of steady accumulation of cases between 1950 and 1960, but white TB registers, by contrast, show an initial increase in cases followed by a leveling off and eventual decline by 1960. Since both black and white populations were subject to active case-finding efforts during this period, the difference in the pattern of accumulation reflects the fact that white cases were being cured at a rate which equalled and often exceeded the rate at which new cases were being identified. New black cases of TB, on the other hand, were accumulating faster than existing services could handle them. This difference in cure rates in turn reflected disparities in access to health services.[51]

In a study conducted in the western Cape, Yach and Bell[51] found that the percentage of patients completing their treatment were 73,2 for blacks, 86,6 for coloureds and 95,6 for whites. They note that these figures are falsely high because information about defaulters is not readily available in compliance surveys. However, the relative difference between the rates of sub-groups remains valid.

Measuring medical services simply by the number of beds available for TB cases (an inadequate measure, but one which health authorities were fond of using), makes the difference in treatment availability clear. Taking 1957 as an example, there were approximately 1 350 new white cases of TB. The accommodation available for these cases in the same year was 1 230 beds. By contrast there were approximately 40 000 new black cases, and the number of beds available nation-wide for all blacks in TB institutions in 1957 was 14 410. In effect there were nearly three times as many black cases per available bed as there were white cases per bed.

The nationalist government, in fact, made considerable efforts to increase the number of beds available for blacks and the number nearly tripled between 1952 and 1957. Yet the number of beds remained inadequate and a massive backlog of patients who could not find accommodation remained.

The situation was in fact worse than it appeared. To begin with, black TB patients frequently required longer stays in hospitals than whites, because their disease tended to be more advanced or serious in nature. For example, in Durban in 1954, whites averaged 6,2 months per stay while blacks averaged 12 months. By 1958 the figures for both groups had been reduced by improvements in the effectiveness of treatment, yet the differential remained, with the average white stay being 3,6 months and the average black stay 5,4 months.[31] This meant that the turnover of patients was much faster for whites than for blacks, making the disparity in the number of beds available for each group even greater.

Secondly, many of the TB beds were in TB centres or settlements, which had been established from public donations and a small provision from the government, by the South African National Tuberculosis Association (SANTA), a private voluntary organization. These settlements were specifically set up to cope with ambulatory and convalescent patients whose disease was of a mild form. They did not treat the more serious cases which so often occurred in the urban areas among blacks. As the Medical Superintendent of the Nessie Knight Hospital in the Transkei wrote, the settlement idea takes:

> ... *no cognizance of the vast majority of Native sufferers who are quite unsuitable for admission to SANTA settlements and whose only hope is accommodation in proper hospitals where they must stay in bed for varying lengthy periods.*[28]

The lack of hospital accommodation for advanced cases prevented many blacks from gaining any treatment until they had infected others.

Lack of hospital accommodation forced the government to begin treating discovered cases on an out-patient basis rather than to wait for accommodation to become available. For a number of reasons out-patient treatment programmes have been largely a failure in South Africa. To begin with, even with out-patient treatment, serious cases still needed to begin treatment within a hospital setting and there were simply not enough beds to treat them.[14] Secondly, local health authorities were overtaxed by the large numbers of cases which needed treatment, and it was impossible to visit, much less keep track of, all the cases on the books. Contact tracing was often inefficient or non-existent. Finally, not all municipalities were willing to bear the cost of providing rations for TB patients receiving treatment, despite the government's offer to cover seven-eighths of this cost.

Some municipalities were clearly more efficient and spent more money than others on TB work. For example, while Durban had 2 000 beds for TB cases and 18 full-time TB officers in 1955, Johannesburg, with twice the population, had only 300 beds and one TB officer.[29] On the other hand, Durban did not initially participate in the government's ration scheme.[31]

Treatment failures

In the absence of adequate health facilities or staff to supervise treatment, responsibility for ensuring that patients received treatment-to-cure was left up to the patients themselves. For a variety of reasons, this often resulted in patients failing to complete their full course of chemotherapy. Recommended treatment with INH and PAS was for 12 months, though it was believed on the mines that a cure could be obtained in milder cases in six to nine months in at least 50 per cent of the cases.[24] Many patients, however, felt considerably improved after two or three months and, if not supervised, began missing treatments. Patients who failed to complete their treatments were labelled 'defaulters', which term implied that it was the patient who was at fault, and white medical authorities often attributed treatment failure to the black's ignorance or 'native mentality'. Yet in South Africa completion of treatment was discouraged by a range of factors. Some of these are common to all out-patient TB treatment programmes, while others are peculiar to the South African political and economic environment of the 1950s, 1960s and 1970s.

Lack of financial resources was perhaps the primary reason why a high percentage of blacks did not complete their treatment. Most blacks who contracted TB and were diagnosed as having the disease lost their jobs, only a few enlightened employers permitting infected workers to continue working while they received treatment. From the start, therefore, TB patients and their families were faced with a financial crisis. While black TB patients were eligible for disability grants, the amount that was provided was both less than that provided for white patients and inadequate for the needs of black families who had no other source of income. In 1965 the disability grant was R3,50 per month plus R1,25 per child. No support was available for spouses. A family of four would thus receive R6 per month. In the same year, the poverty datum line for a family of four in Johannesburg was roughly R53. By contrast, a white tuberculosis patient received R31 for himself, plus R16 for his wife and R9 per child, which for a family of four came to R56 per month.[37]

Not only were disability grants inadequate, but they were administered in a way which discouraged many black workers from obtaining them. The Nationalist policy of separate development, which denied the vast majority of urban workers permanent residence rights within the urban areas, together with a provision which prohibited the payment of pensions or disability grants outside the area in which a worker lawfully and permanently resided, meant that the majority of disabled black workers had to leave the place in which they had been employed and return to a rural homeland in order to obtain these inadequate support payments. For many workers who had not been born in an urban area, but who had worked there on a continuous basis for a number of years, such a move would eliminate their chance of obtaining urban residence status under section 10(b) of the Urban Areas Act. In addition, the chances of obtaining treatment for the disease were, as will be shown below, severely reduced within the rural areas. For both reasons, black TB patients were understandably reluctant to collect the small disability grant that was available to them.

Lacking alternatives, many black bread winners chose to seek new employment as soon as they felt well enough to work, which was frequently long before they were 'cured'. This often meant looking for a new job since their old employer would be aware of their condition and refuse to employ them. While looking for work and, if fortunate enough to find a new job, while working, it was difficult for a patient to continue his or her treatment. Visiting clinics meant loss of pay and sometimes employment. Few clinics operated evenings or Sundays to accommodate employed patients, since TB patients were by definition unemployed.[32, 45]

Prospects for TB patients varied a good deal. In Durban, for example, Dormer was successful in convincing some employers to allow patients who were on treatment but no longer infectious to return to employment. Yet, in 1964 a survey of firms found that only 38 of them provided treatment facilities on the premises so that the worker would not have to lose wages while getting treatment.[32] In Cape Town evening clinics were held during the first week of every month at the central chest clinic in Chapel Street. This was said to benefit the patient who returned to work and almost guarantee against relapse. However, for the black worker in Guguletu or Langa townships, getting to the Chapel Street clinic often represented an expense which discouraged attendance. There were no evening clinics at the Langa or Guguletu clinics during the 1960s.

Those who were unemployed had an additional incentive to quickly seek employment. For the Native Laws Amendment Act required blacks residing in the urban areas to possess an employment contract. Failure to do so placed a TB patient at risk of being repatriated. Prior to 1960 there was no provision for exempting black tuberculotics from this rule and, as Dr A Strating of the Transvaal Peri-Urban Health Board stated, this often caused them to fall foul of the law:

> *Native patients in urban areas receiving home treatment were often arrested by the police on their way to clinics because they were not in possession of a service contract. These Natives often spent several weeks in jail.*[27]

Strating proposed that local authorities prepare a special form stating that the bearer was a tuberculotic and not capable of carrying a service contract. This system, however, placed such cases in a Catch–22 dilemma. For, while the attachment of such a document to patients' identity papers might save them from being arrested or facing repatriation, it also effectively barred them from employment.

While the combination of financial constraints and discriminatory legislation created obstacles for all blacks seeking treatment, migrant workers were at greatest risk of defaulting. Lacking a support network within the urban areas and being ineligible for the payment of disability grants in the urban areas, migrants often had to return to the homelands.

Getting treatment clearly became more difficult during the 1960s as the Nationalists got serious about enforcing the Group Areas Act while also tightening up influx control. The Medical Officer of Health in Port Elizabeth claimed that, as a result of removals under the Group Areas Act, patients were forced to move away from clinics to which they had been going for treatment.[37] In Cape Town, Western found that coloureds who had been removed from Mowbray were on average 5,29 km further from the nearest hospital than they had been before relocation.[50] The movement of coloureds beyond Athlone during the mid-1960s resulted in a decline in coloured TB notifications and an increase in the percentage of clinic first attenders lost to treatment from 1964.[35] A survey of TB patients living in a black residential area of Cape Town found that 50 per cent of those interviewed had experienced difficulty getting treatment, distance from the clinic being noted as an important problem.[44] The Medical Officer of Health for Durban also noted that the removal of blacks from Cato Manor to Kwa-Mashu during the 1960s led to cases being lost to treatment.[33] In more extreme cases, patients attending urban clinics were removed to rural resettlement camps with the same effect. The creation of homelands caused a further reshuffling of people within the rural areas as people were relocated in their 'appropriate' ethnic areas.

This had a similar negative impact on treatment and follow-up.[4, 13]

Additional problems were caused by the transformation of homelands into so-called 'national states', each with its own health service, during the 1970s and early 1980s. There are currently no less than 17 separate authorities responsible for health in South Africa, with minimal coordination among them. This fragmentation has further increased the likelihood of patient default. As members of a medical team working in the Gazankulu 'homeland' located in the eastern Transvaal noted in 1984:

> *Homeland borders and structures limit us and fragment services. Just over half of our patients come from Lebowa; but we may not follow them up at home, visit their families or organize SAC [supervised ambulatory care] for them. We also cannot trace contacts or defaulters, or do case finding in Lebowa.[4]*

Fragmentation also resulted in the use of different drug regimens by neighbouring health authorities. Thus, a patient from Lebowa, who began one regimen in a hospital in Gazankulu, would find another set of drugs being supplied by local health authorities when he or she returned home to complete his or her ambulatory care. This change inhibited the patient's recovery and could contribute to drug resistance.[4]

The problem of coordinating treatment was even greater for blacks living on white farms. A large proportion of the TB patients showing up at Gazankulu hospital came from white farm areas, and similarly, health authorities in Bophuthatswana claimed in 1984 that many of the most severe cases of TB came from the neighbouring white farm areas. In this situation, not only did local health workers lack the authority to follow up and supervise the treatment of the farm workers who came to them for help, but there were no local authorities to take up these responsibilities within the white farming areas.[2, 4]

In short, while patient defaulting from ambulatory treatment programmes has been a common problem of tuberculosis control programmes in Africa, the inequitable distribution of health and social services in South

Africa, combined with the pattern of racial segregation and control enforced by the Nationalist government and the fragmentation of local health services, exacerbated these problems, decreasing the likelihood that black cases would be effectively cured and increasing the number of half-cured chronic cases who were sources of infection to others.

The director of the South African Tuberculosis Research Institute (TBRI) optimistically claimed that medical authorities had treated more than half a million people between 1972 and 1982 and probably rendered 90 per cent of them non-infectious. While this may be an accurate figure, rendering a patient non-infectious is not the same as curing him or her. In fact, most cases are rendered non-infectious after only a few weeks of treatment, but if treatment is stopped at this point or before a cure is achieved, the patient has a good chance of relapsing and becoming infectious once again. The Brown Commission of Inquiry into Health Services estimated in 1986 that nation-wide only 25 per cent of out-patients were effectively treated.[4, 15] In addition relapse rates have been very high. In 1980 it was estimated that 38 per cent of all hospital TB patients represented relapse cases,[17] which finding led the then head of SANTA to conclude that the treatment programme '… had to a considerable degree been a failure'.[7]

The medical team at Gazankulu estimated that in 1980 and 1981 only 38,7 per cent of their admitted patients completed enough treatment. In 1981 the figure was 44,1 per cent. Using shorter regimens and full supervision they were able to increase this to 84 and 86 per cent in 1982 and 1983 respectively. This was viewed as exceptional and required a commitment of staff and resources which were both far in excess of those employed by the average rural health service and in all likelihood not sustainable in Gazankulu, given its limited health budget.

Treatment failure figures disguised a wide divergence between urban and rural health services and it is clear that once a patient was relegated to a rural area, his or her chances of receiving a full course of treatment declined sharply. A comparative study of treatment in several therapeutic settings found that the percentage of patients receiving 75 per cent of their treatments ranged from 50 per cent for Cape Town clinics to 25 per cent for clinics in the Ciskei.[44] Similarly, a follow-up study of 50 cases referred to local clinics for therapy in Natal found that those referred to urban clinics had a compliance rate of 68 per cent, while only 28 per cent of those referred to rural clinics completed their treatment.[51] On the other hand, a follow-up survey of patients receiving treatment in Soweto in 1978 found that only 21 per cent received 80 per cent or more of their prescribed treatments.[39]

It should be noted that the low rates of treatment success recorded for rural areas were roughly similar to those recorded in neighbouring countries, but it must also be recognized that these countries lacked the resources available in South Africa. More importantly, it was only in South Africa that people who could not find jobs were forcibly removed to rural areas where their chances of getting treatment were greatly reduced.

The inability of patients to complete their treatment meant not only that the number of chronic 'half-cured half-ill' cases continued to climb, but also that the number of patients who developed resistance to INH increased, further complicating efforts at TB control. By 1986 50 per cent of the patients treated in many of the rural areas of the country had an acquired resistance to INH.[16]

In the long run, moreover, the recurrent development of patient resistance led to the development of INH- and SM- resistant strains of tubercle bacilli. By 1978, 10 per cent of blacks in treatment in Pretoria had primary resistance to INH, and in 1986 it was estimated that primary resistance was 15 per cent nation-wide.[16] By contrast, in other African countries with well-established TB treatment services, the figure for primary resistance is generally about eight per cent.[40] Resistance to other drugs have also been reported. Primary resistance to rifampicin for example is 1,2 per cent, while secondary resistance occurs in 5,6 per cent of old cases.[21]

While the prospects for cure for blacks who were discovered through various case-finding methods were not good, it is clear that many cases simply were not discovered until they were dead or near death. For example, while notification rates for Johannesburg in the early 1950s hovered around 200/100 000, an x-ray survey of domestic workers concluded that one per cent or 1 000/100 000 had TB. It was estimated that there were 5 000 cases of undetected TB in Johannesburg in 1955.[26] Similarly the Medical Officer of Health for Cape Town noted that:

> *It is astonishing that so many persons with advanced disease, particularly men, can remain unknown, at least to official agencies by avoiding the case-catching net — however wide the mesh — until abject illness or some catastrophe brings them to the notice of the clinics.*[14]

If the situation was bad in the urban areas, it was impossible in the rural reserves. Only a small proportion of the estimated 25 000 cases of active TB in the Transkei were actually seen and treated, and this situation became increasingly worse after 1960. Given inadequate case finding and low patient cure rates, it is highly unlikely that treatment programmes had a significant impact on the prevalence of TB among blacks in South Africa.

The use of BCG

Health authorities in South Africa did not restrict their control efforts to curative measures. They also engaged in preventive work. However, given the limits placed by South Africa's political economy on major structural changes which would alleviate the conditions which gave rise to the disease, preventive work in practice meant medical intervention in the form of BCG campaigns. Like their curative efforts, attempts to prevent the early onset of TB among children through vaccination was only partially effective.

The objective of BCG vaccination is to reduce the incidence of tuberculosis among children, and in particular of severe forms such as tuberculosis meningitis. Worldwide, the use of BCG in third world countries has led to mixed results. In fact, the level of protection afforded by BCG in well-conducted trials has ranged from none to 80 per cent. Numerous factors have contributed to poor protection levels, including low potency of vaccines, sensitization by non-tuberculous mycosensitizing bacteria, the health and nutritional status of the vaccinated population and the fact that heavy or repeated infection may overwhelm immunity derived from BCG.[3] In South Africa, where BCG campaigns began in the early 1960s, the effects of these various factors are difficult to sort out. A study of the effect of BCG on children in the households of known adult TB cases in Pretoria suggested that BCG provided considerable protection for children under four years of age but little protection for children from five to fifteen years old.[6] However, an investigation of TB meningitis cases in Cape Town in 1979–81 found that 45 per cent of the diagnosed cases had had BCG vaccinations.[11] This strongly suggests that high levels of malnutrition among young black children in the country, combined with overcrowding in an environment in which TB is endemic, can overwhelm the protection offered by BCG.

The distribution of BCG coverage, moreover, like that of South African health services as a whole, was highly uneven. In the rural areas where children were increasingly at greatest risk, only a small percentage of children were vaccinated prior to 1970.[8] In Kwazulu, a recent study suggested that only a small percentage (18,4 per cent) of pre-school children had been vaccinated. This figure is based on the appearance of BCG scars. Coovadia notes that BCG does not always leave scars, but concludes that the percentage vaccinated is still unacceptably low. In 1972 only 1,5 per cent of children in the Transkei had BCG scars.[38] BCG coverage was also limited in the many peri-urban slums and squatter camps that surrounded the major cities of the country.[47] Both the limited coverage and the questionable effectiveness of BCG in the face of malnutrition and widespread opportunities for infection make it highly unlikely that BCG campaigns had much effect on the incidence of TB prior to 1970.

BCG coverage increased significantly in the 1970s and 1980s, however. A random survey of 418 pre-school children in rural Ciskei in 1984 found that 68,7 per cent had been vaccinated according to medical records. For children under one year the figure was 87,5 per cent, whereas for five year olds the percentage was only 39,2 per cent.[6] This increase may account for the declining percentage of black children under five years of age among notified cases between 1971 and 1984.[22] On the other hand, this decline may also reflect the large number of black children in this age group who were removed to resettlement camps that were officially outside the statistical boundaries of South Africa during this same period.

CONCLUSION

Although efforts to control TB in South Africa have all but eliminated the disease among the white population, their effectiveness in reducing the toll of TB among blacks is highly questionable. Since the beginning of the century, the overriding concern of government planners for maintaining a system of white privilege and separate development has prevented the creation of an efficient system of health care, while perpetuating the existence of living and working conditions that seriously undermine the health of South African blacks.

Nonetheless, many medical authorities in South Africa appear to be convinced that TB among blacks is declining and that prospects for controlling the disease are bright. Much of this optimism is based on the results of prevalence surveys conducted by the TBRI over the last decade and a half. As has been mentioned earlier, these studies, while impressive in scale, have drawn conclusions about longitudinal changes in black infection and prevalence rates that are highly questionable from a methodological standpoint.[30]

Clearly TB notification rates for blacks have declined since the mid-1960s. Yet this decline need not reflect any change in the underlying incidence of the disease. It may in fact represent the impact of significant cutbacks in TB control efforts, and thus in case-finding efforts. In this regard it is worth noting that in the western Cape, where the collection of health statistics is most complete, both black and coloured TB notification rates are on the rise. The national decline in black TB notifications from the 1960s to the early 1980s was almost certainly also produced by the mass removals that have transferred large numbers of actual and potential cases of TB outside the statistical boundaries of South Africa into 'black homelands', where inadequate medical services prevent the collection of accurate health statistics. In effect, the policy of exclusion that has marked TB control efforts in South Africa since the beginning of the century has continued to operate, sweeping TB under the rug rather than effectively curtailing its spread. As one observer noted when describing the impact of forced removals on TB notifications: 'Logically one could continue this trend and eliminate TB altogether with a few flourishes of a statistical pen'.[38]

REFERENCES

1 Alexander M J, 1921. The problem of tuberculosis in South Africa. *South African Medical Record.* 19, 226–30.

2 Annual Report of the Health Department, Bophuthatswana. 1984.

3 Benatar S R, 1982. Tuberculosis — an overview. *Conference on TB in South Africa: Consumption in the Land of Plenty, University of Cape Town, Cape Town, 2–4 August 1982.*

4 Buch E, Johnson K & Mashabane R, 1984. Can good tuberculosis care be provided in the face of poverty? *Carnegie Conference Paper, No. 198.* Cape Town: University of Cape Town.

5 Burke G & Richardson P, 1978. The profits of death: A comparative study of miner's phthisis in Cornwall and the Transvaal. *Journal of Southern African Studies.* 4, 2, 147–71.

6 Coetzee L & Fourie P B, 1986. Efficacy of BCG vaccination. *South African Journal of Science.* 82, 388–9.

7   Collins T F, 1981. Applied epidemiology and logic in tuberculosis control. *South African Medical Journal.* 59, 566–9.

8   Coovadia H, 1982. Controversies in BCG: BCG in South Africa. *Conference on TB in South Africa: Consumption in the Land of Plenty, University of Cape Town, Cape Town, 2–4 August 1982.*

10 Davies R H, 1979. *Capital State and White Labor in South Africa, 1900–60.* Brighton: Harvester Press

11 Denny J, 1984. *Epidemiology of Tuberculosis Meningitis in the Western Cape, 1979–81.* Cape Town: Carnegie Conference Paper, No. 175.

12 Dubos R & Dubos J, 1953. *The White Plague.* Boston: Little Brown and Company.

13 Dubow, S, 1982. Consumption and underconsumption: the effects of population resettlement on the spread of tuberculosis. *Conference on TB in South Africa: Consumption in the Land of Plenty, University of Cape Town, Cape Town, 2–4 August 1982.*

14 DuPre Le Roux J J, 1957. Report of the Tuberculosis Conference, Johannesburg, 2–4 Dec., 1957.

15 Eighth Interim Report of the Commission of Inquiry into Health Services. Pretoria: Government Printer. 1986.

16 Fourie P B & Knoetze K, 1986. Tuberculosis prevalence and risk of infection in southern Africa. *South African Journal of Science.* 82, 387.

17 Glatthaar E, 1982. Where have we gone wrong — a look at the future? *Conference on TB in South Africa: Consumption in the Land of Plenty, University of Cape Town, Cape Town, 2–4 August 1982.*

18 Grigg E N R, 1958. The arcna of tuberculosis. *American Review of Tuberculous Respiratory Diseases.* 78, 446

19 Johnstone F A, 1976. *Class, Race and Gold.* London: Routledge and Kegan Paul.

20 Katz E N, 1974. White workers' grievances and the industrial color bar. *South African Journal of Economics.* 42, 127–56.

21 Kleeberg H H, 1986. TB bacteriology and the laboratory situation. *South African Journal of Science.* 82, 394.

22 Kustner H C V, 1986. Tuberculosis notifications: an update. *South African Journal of Science.* 82, 386–7.

23 Marks S & Andersson N, (in press). The State, Class and the Allocation of Health Resources. *Social Sciences and Medicine. Special Issue on the Political Economy of Health, in Africa and Latin America.*

24 Martiny, 1954. *Witwatersrand Native Labour Association. Testimony.* Chamber of Mines Archives. Silicosis – TB Dept CTE.

25 Mckeown T, 1979. *The Role of Medicine. Dream, Mirage or Nemesis.* Oxford: Blackwell.

26 News report, 1955. Apathy is allowing TB to kill at random, says expert. *The Star,* Johannesburg. 14th Nov. 1955.

27 News report, 1955. *The Star.* 4th May, 1955.

28 News report, 1956. Doctor says SANTA is unwittingly hindering fight against TB. *The Star.* 19th Nov., 1956.

29 News Reports, 1955–6. *The Star.* 2nd Nov., 1955 and 14th Feb., 1956.

30 Packard R, 1989. *White Plague, Black Labor: Tuberculosis and the Political Economy of Health and Disease in South Africa.* Los Angeles, Berkeley: University of California Press.

31 Report of the City Medical Officer of Health, Durban. 1958.

32 Report of the City Medical Officer of Health, Durban. 1964.

33 Report of the City Medical Officer of Health, Durban. 1965.

34 Report of the Medical Officer of Health, Cape Town. 1961.

35 Reports of the Medical Officer of Health, Cape Town, 1964–75.

36 Report of the Medical Officer of Health, East London. 1931.

37 Report of the Medical Officer of Health, Port Elizabeth. 1965.

38 Sasha W, 1982. Control of tuberculosis in the homelands. *Conference on TB in South Africa: Consumption in the Land of Plenty, University of Cape Town, Cape Town, 2–4 August 1982.*

39 Saunders L D, 1982. An evaluation of the management of TB patients in Soweto. Paper presented to *Conference on Tuberculosis in the Eighties, Pretoria, 1982.*

40 Shennan D H, 1982. Changes in problems of tuberculosis control in Africa between the sixties and eighties. Paper presented to *Conference on Tuberculosis in the Eighties, Pretoria, 1982.*

41 Smit Committee, Union Government, 1942. *Report of the Interdepartmental Committee on the Social Health and Economic Conditions of Urban Natives.* Pretoria: Government Printer.

42 South African Institute of Race Relations. *Surveys of Race Relations, 1953–4* and *1962–7.*

43 Thomson E M & Myrdal S, 1986. The implementation of tuberculosis policy in three areas in South Africa. *South African Medical Journal.* 70, 258–62.

44 Thomson E M & Myrdal S, 1986. Tuberculosis — the patients' perspective. *South African Medical Journal.* 70, 263–4.

45 Thomson L, 1982. State policy with regard to TB Control. *Conference on TB in South Africa: Consumption in the Land of Plenty, University of Cape Town, Cape Town, 2–4 August 1982.*

46 Thorton E H, 1934. Secretary for Public Health, to Provincial Secretaries, TAD, GES 997 401/173, Cape Town, Bloemfontein, Pietermaritzburg, Pretoria. 21 Feb., 1934.

47 Toms I, 1990. Director, University of Cape Town Community Health Clinic, Crossroads. Personal Communication.

48 Tuberculosis Research Committee, 1932. *Tuberculosis in South African Natives with Special Reference to the Disease among Mine Labourers on the Witwatersrand and Johannesburg.* Johannesburg: South African Institute for Medical Research.

49 Van Onselen C, 1982. *Studies in the Social and Economic History of the Witwatersrand, 1886–1914.* Vol. 1. London: Longmans.

50 Western J, 1981. *Outcast Cape Town.* Minneapolis: University of Minnesota Press.

51 Yach D & Bell J, 1986. *Tuberculosis Patient Compliance in the Western Cape.* Unpublished paper.

52 Yeats J R, 1986. Attendance compliance for short course chemotherapy in clinics in Estcourt and surroundings. *South African Medical Journal.* 70, 265–6.

CHAPTER 4

Epidemiology of tuberculosis in South Africa

P M Strebel and J R Seager

INTRODUCTION

Although the causative organism, *Mycobacterium tuberculosis,* was recognized over 100 years ago, tuberculosis programmes are still struggling to control one of the world's most important infectious diseases. Worldwide, the estimated annual incidence of tuberculosis is 8–10 million and about three million people die of the disease each year.[128] In addition to the enormous burden imposed by the disease itself, another one billion persons are believed to be infected, which makes tuberculosis one of the most prevalent infections in the world.[9]

It has been estimated that 6–10 million South Africans are infected with *Mycobacterium tuberculosis,*[57] resulting in approximately 60 000 notified cases[37] and 6 000 registered deaths[131] each year. However, tuberculosis is not uniformly distributed throughout southern Africa, and the purposes of this chapter are to describe the distribution of tuberculosis by person, time and place (descriptive epidemiology); discuss the determinants of tuberculosis (analytic epidemiology); and to review South African studies which have used epidemiological methods to evaluate tuberculosis control strategies.

Epidemiological characteristics of tuberculosis

Tuberculosis is a chronic infectious disease with a complex natural history (Figure 4.1)

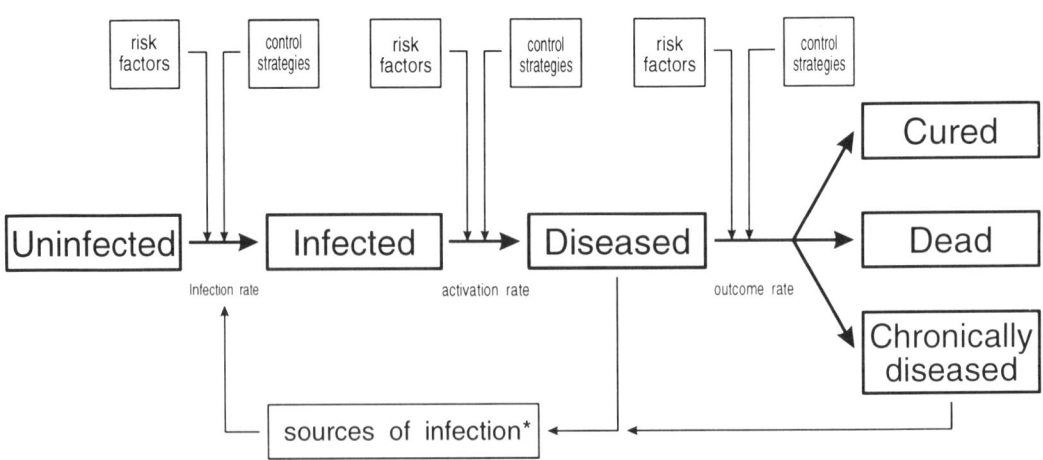

* reinfection of cured or asymptomatic infected persons may also occur

Figure 4.1. Simplified model of the natural history of tuberculosis.

which is characterized by a long and variable incubation period. The interval between infection with *Mycobacterium tuberculosis* and either a demonstrable primary lesion or significant tuberculin reaction is about 4–12 weeks.[7] For the majority of people, infection with *Mycobacterium tuberculosis* results in an immune response without any apparent illness, but there does remain a lifetime risk of 5–15 per cent for progression to overt disease.[30] Occurrence of disease in the previously infected individual may be caused by the reactivation of dormant bacilli in the primary lesion (endogenous disease), or it may be the result of a new challenge caused by reinfection (exogenous disease). The proportions of tuberculous disease attributable to endogenous reactivation and exogenous reinfection are very difficult to determine, but have major implications for prevention.

Transmission of tuberculosis is almost entirely by droplet infection from a source case who is coughing and producing sputum contaminated with *Mycobacterium tuberculosis*. The infectiousness of pulmonary tuberculosis is therefore directly associated with bacillary load in the sputum, cough frequency and environmental factors such as closeness of contact and duration of exposure.[28]

The impact of tuberculosis on a community is best quantified by studying the three phases in the natural history of TB: asymptomatic infection (infection); active disease (disease) and outcomes from TB, which include cure, death, disability or chronic disease.

INFECTION

Definition

Infection with *Mycobacterium tuberculosis* is usually detected by the tuberculin skin test which measures the cell mediated response to mycobacterial antigens. There are various methods of testing (Mantoux, Heaf, Tine and Mono), but most involve the intradermal introduction of a small quantity of a purified protein derivative (PPD) of *Mycobacterium tuberculosis* and then measurement of the size of the resulting induration or swelling after two to seven days,

depending on the type of application. Considerable attention has been given to standardizing both materials and test methods.[125] Unfortunately, the response of an individual to this type of test does not provide an absolute 'positive' or 'negative' result. For example, it is difficult to distinguish infected individuals with small reactions from uninfected individuals who react to the physical trauma of the test.[114] The problem is exacerbated by non-specific reactions to mycobacteria other than tuberculosis (MOTT) and reactions due to BCG vaccination. Both these factors produce reactions which, on average, fall between the normal positive and negative reactions[47, 91] (Figure 4.2). Despite these limitations, the prevalence of infection with *Mycobacterium tuberculosis* in a population can be effectively quantified by studying the distribution of reaction sizes to PPD.

BCG reactions to the Mantoux tuberculin test do not usually produce induration greater than 15 mm, so this amount can be used as a cut-off point for determining the prevalence of infection.[47] However, using a simple cut-off point underestimates the true reactor population since positive reactions are normally distributed around the 15 mm mark, and those below 15 mm overlap the reactions due to BCG. Various formulae using cut-off points ranging from 10 to 15 mm have been devised for estimating the true infected population. In South African populations showing a clear mode around 15 mm, the most consistent results were obtained by adding reactions ≥10 mm to those ≥15 mm and dividing by two.[47]

The tuberculin test provides a valuable research instrument and a useful diagnostic aid. A positive tuberculin skin test indicates a high probability of tuberculous infection, but cannot, in isolation, give any indication of disease status.

Prevalence of infection

Congenital infection is extremely rare[98] and as people pass through life the probability of becoming infected accumulates, resulting in increased prevalence of infection with increasing age. Table 4.1 shows the prevalence of infection at different ages for South African ethnic groups.[47] The prevalence of

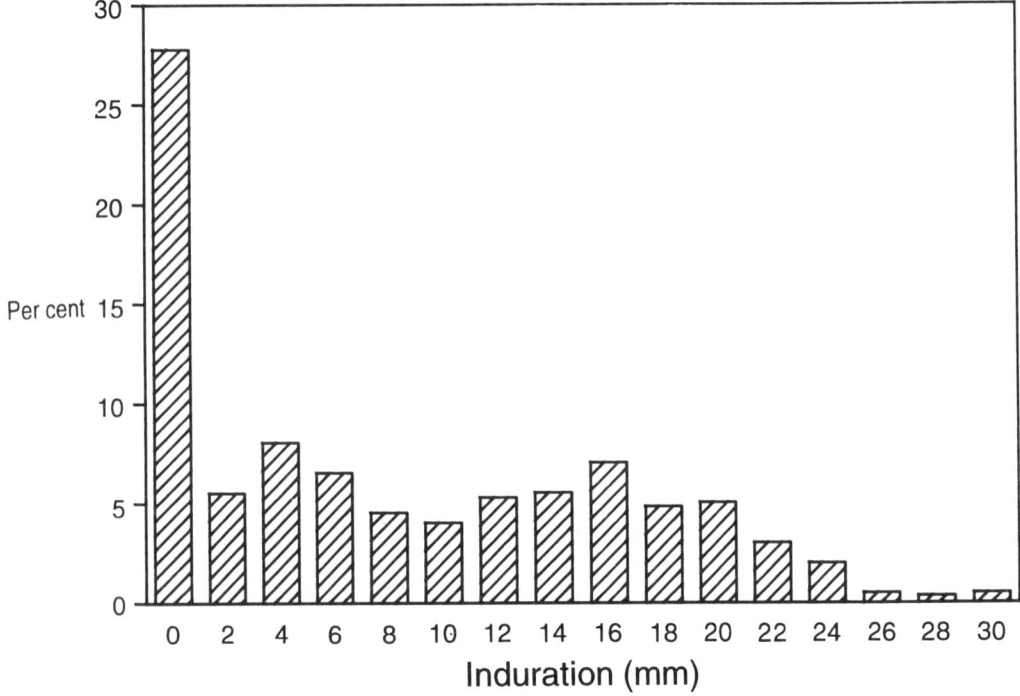

Figure 4.2 (a). Tuberculin hypersensitivity patterns in black children 10–14 years old without BCG scars from Transkei and Ciskei showing the effect of non-specific (MOTT) sensitivity .[47]

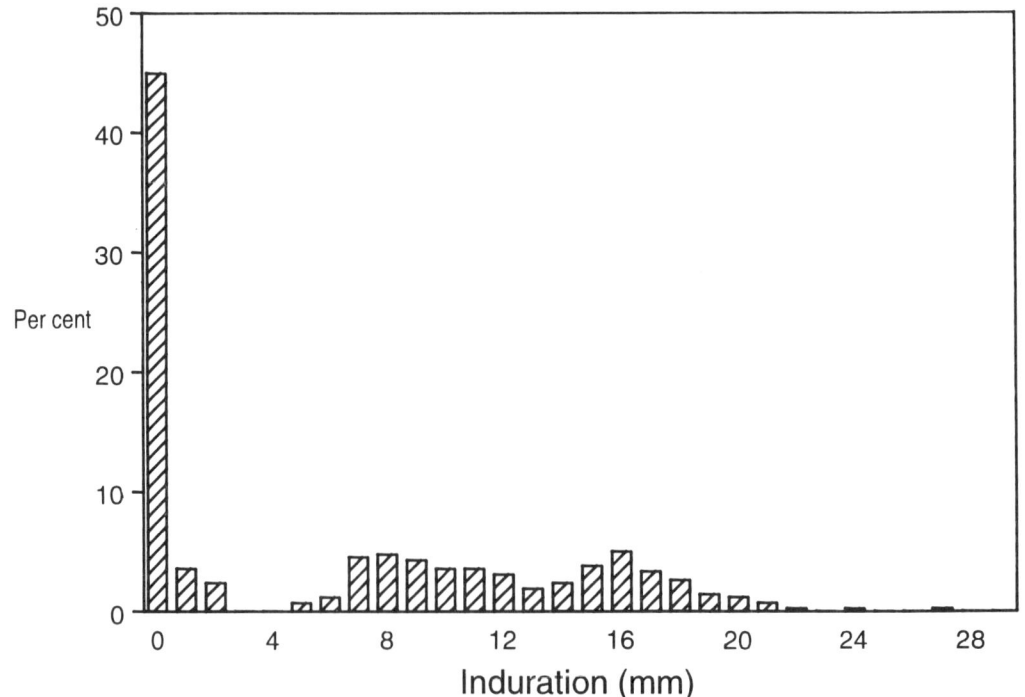

Figure 4.2 (b). Tuberculin hypersensitivity patterns in coloured children aged five to nine years from Cape Town who had been given BCG within the previous 12 months .[92]

infection is higher in lowland regions, which may reflect either historically earlier contact with the disease along the coast, or possibly the climatic factors which facilitate transmission of the bacillus.

Risk of infection

The *annual risk of tuberculous infection* (ARI) is the probability of an individual becoming infected with tubercle bacilli in the course of one year. The ARI can be calculated (using a model developed by Styblo[114]) from surveys of the prevalence of infection in the same population at different times, and it has been used extensively to estimate the risk of infection and trends in risk.[8, 43, 47, 105, 109, 114] The annual risk of infection reflects the extent of transmission of tubercle bacilli in a community. It is one incubation period ahead of disease data and, unlike mortality and notification data, is not dependent on the quality of a routine surveillance system. For these reasons the ARI is the best epidemiological measure of the tuberculosis situation in the community.

By repeating tuberculin skin test surveys the Tuberculosis Research Institute (TBRI) of the Medical Research Council has been able to compare the prevalence of infection for various areas of South Africa and calculate changes in risk of infection (Table 4.2).

Most ethnic groups are experiencing a declining risk of infection, with the possible exception of the coloured population whose population growth rate currently exceeds the decline in risk of infection.[48] There are marked differences in both prevalence and risk of infection between races, urban and rural areas and inland and coastal regions. In general, the highest risks of infection have been observed in blacks living in coastal areas, followed by coloureds and then blacks in inland areas.

Risk factors for infection

There appears to be little gender difference for risk of infection up to the age of 10, but between the ages of 12,5 years and 18,5 years, nine per cent more males than females are infected.[81, 114] This may be the result of greater exposure in males due to social mobility or greater susceptibility after puberty. There are marked differences in the prevalence of infection between ethnic groups (Table 4.1), which are the result of large numbers of active cases of TB among adults in the black and coloured communities living in overcrowded conditions with subsequent transmission to children. Although socio-economic conditions are the major determinant of infection in South Africa, a study in the United States suggests

Table 4.1
The average prevalence rates of tuberculous infection in South Africa (1974–80) according to ethnic group, geographical location and age[47]

Ethnic Group and Geographical Location	Age group 5–9 years Mean Age (yrs)	Pre-valence (%)	No. Tested (N)	Mean Survey Year (19...)*	Age Group 10-14 years Mean Age (yrs)	Pre-valence (%)	No. Tested (N)	Mean Survey Year (19...)*	Age Group 15-19 years Mean Age (yrs)	Pre-valence (%)	No. Tested (N)	Mean Survey year (19...)*
Black												
Highland	7,4	11,4	28 531	76,9	11,7	18,6	8 296	76,9	16,6	31,0	3 732	77,6
Lowland	7,3	21,9	8 555	76,8	11,6	31,7	2 302	76,6	16,7	40,3	1 046	76,8
Urban	7,4	14,0	32 865	76,9	11,6	20,9	7 939	77,2	16,7	33,8	3 830	77,8
Rural	6,9	12,3	4 221	76,9	12,0	22,4	2 659	76,0	16,1	30,1	948	76,0
All regions	7,4	13,9	37 086	76,9	11,7	21,4	10 598	76,9	16,6	33,1	4 778	77,4
Coloured												
Highland	7,1	7,6	8 113	76,8	11,8	14,0	3 534	77,5	16,3	19,5	1 427	77,9
Lowland	6,7	9,6	7 448	77,2	12,2	16,9	3 464	77,6	16,1	20,1	2 120	77,8
All regions	6,9	8,6	15 601	77,0	12,0	15,4	6 998	77,5	16,2	19,9	3 547	77,9
Asian												
Highland	7,0	2,5	4 618	77,5	11,6	5,7	1 680	78,9	16,3	11,1	943	78,9
Lowland	6,2	3,2	2 607	76,9	11,5	4,7	465	78,2	16,0	7,5	380	78,0
All regions	6,7	2,8	7 225	77,3	11,6	5,5	2 145	78,7	16,2	10,1	1 323	78,6
White												
Highland	7,1	0,9	11 683	77,3	12,0	1,6	9 667	77,1	16,1	3,3	5 030	77,7
Lowland	7,1	1,5	5 515	77,0	11,9	3,5	5 124	76,5	16,0	4,6	2 245	76,3
All regions	7,1	1,1	17 198	77,2	12,0	2,3	14 791	76,9	16,1	3,7	7 275	77,3

*In this column the first two figures indicate the year, the third the month e.g. 76,9 – September 1976.

Table 4.2
The risk of tuberculous infection and estimated annual change in risk for South African children aged 5–9 years[51]

Survey Group	Mean Survey Year (19...)†	Mean Age (yrs)	No. Tested+	Prevalence (%)	Risk of Infection 1985 (%)	Annual Change in risk (%)
Indian	76,8	6,7	6 148	2,7		
	81,2	6,9	2 500	1,7	0,1	–11,1
Coloured	76,6	6,9	13 713	8,3		
	81,4	6,9	4 003	7,5	0,9	–2,2
Black (inland)	75,9	7,4	23 224	11,7		
	81,3	7,4	9 855	7,8	0,6	–7,9
Black (coastal)	76,2	7,2	8 262	22,8		
	82,2	7,2	3 788	16,3	1,6	–6,2

* Periods of data collection: 1972–8 and 1979–85.
+ Children without BCG scars only.
† In this column the first two figures indicate the year, the third the month, e.g. 76,8 = August 1976

that differences in host susceptibility may also be involved.[102]

Infection with *Mycobacterium tuberculosis* requires exposure to an infectious source case and the proximity and frequency of that exposure is important as is the severity of the source case.[85] The smear positive case excretes sufficient bacilli for them to be visible in a sputum smear examined by direct microscopy, whereas the case positive on culture excretes so few bacilli that these can only be detected by culturing the organism.[120] Studies[63, 123] have demonstrated that household contacts (and particularly those sharing the same sleeping area as a TB case) have the highest risk of becoming infected, whereas immediate neighbours of source cases have a risk which is only slightly higher than that of the general population.[71, 78]

Most transmission of tuberculosis takes place within households, where the secondary infection and disease rate is relatively low (30 per cent risk of becoming infected and a one to two per cent risk of progression to active disease within one year) when compared with common childhood diseases such as measles and pertussis.[7] Secondary infection rates may, however, become much higher in enclosed environments such as prisons and mental institutions where prolonged, intimate exposure may occur.

Adolescents and young adults appear to be most susceptible to infection.[43, 115] It should be noted that a successful immune response to an initial tuberculous infection may have a protective effect against future disease, but dormant bacilli usually remain within the body and do present a lifetime risk of reactivation.

American data indicate that lower economic status increased the prevalence of infection up to fourfold.[84] Worldwide, risks of infection have been found to be higher in urban areas than in rural areas.[28, 116] There are no published data from southern Africa relating to risk factors for infection except for the broad urban/rural and highland/lowland data presented by Fourie.[47] Other South African data which refer to types of source cases and socio-economic risk factors are dealt with later in this chapter because of their direct influence on control strategies.

DISEASE

The extent of active tuberculous disease (tuberculosis) may be measured in two ways: the prevalence of tuberculosis (number of both new and old cases) which indicates the total disease burden at any point in time; and incidence of tuberculosis (number of new cases over a specified period of time — usually one year) which is a measure of the risk of becoming diseased.

Table 4.3
The bacteriological prevalence of tuberculous disease in the rural black population, South Africa, 1974–84[51]

| | BACTERIOLOGICAL PREVALENCE (%) | | | |
| | MICROSCOPY | | CULTURE | |
	(1974–8)	(1979–84)	(1974–8)	(1979–84)
Treatment history				
present	5,0	2,6	7,4	5,6
absent	1,0	0,6	1,5	1,0
Age				
<50 years	1,0	0,6	1,1	0,9
≥50 years	2,0	1,1	3,6	2,3
Gender				
male	2,4	1,0	3,8	1,9
female	1,0	0,6	1,3	1,0
Geographic area				
coastal	2,0	0,9	4,2	2,1
inland	0,9	0,6	0,9	0,7

Source: Tuberculosis Research Institute of the S A Medical Research Council

Prevalence of disease

The prevalence of tuberculosis is best estimated by conducting population-based surveys of the adult population, using culture and direct smear microscopy of sputum as the basis for determining a case.[107] Smear-positive patients represent the major sources of infection in the community and one unknown smear positive case may, on average, infect about 10 persons with tubercle bacilli during one year. Untreated, an infectious case remains infectious for about two years.[109] The disadvantages of population-based surveys are that they require a large sample size, are costly and need to be repeated to gain an idea of change in prevalence.

Surveys to determine the prevalence of active disease in the rural black population of South Africa were conducted by the TBRI over the period 1974 to 1984[124] (Table 4.3). Approximately 18 000 adults were examined bacteriologically in these surveys and the results were reported for the two periods 1974–8 and 1979–84. Tuberculosis, as indicated by a positive culture, was found

in 1,3 per cent of women and 3,8 per cent of men in 1974–8; and 1,0 per cent of women and 1,9 per cent of men in 1979–84. Comparison of the prevalence of tuberculosis in these two periods suggests a decline of approximately 10 per cent per year.

Bacteriological prevalence of tuberculosis was associated with a history of previous treatment, age, gender and geographic area. Prevalence, as determined by smear and culture positivity, was four to six times higher among persons with a history of previous tuberculosis treatment than amongst untreated persons, which is suggestive of high relapse rates. The higher prevalence in men over 50 years of age is consistent with the age-specific notification rates, which are highest in this age-gender group. Bacteriologic prevalence was between 1,8 and 3,7 times higher in coastal areas when compared to inland areas. Explanation for this difference is largely speculative and may be due to confounding by other variables or may reflect the historical origins of the tuberculosis epidemic in coastal settlements.[81]

In 1984 a tuberculosis prevalence survey was conducted in Ciskei by the TBRI[50] Of the 3 542 persons surveyed, 0,7 per cent were smear positive, 2,2 per cent culture positive, and 15 per cent had parenchymal changes on x-ray (three per cent of which were judged to be of recent origin). These findings indicate that about two out of every 100 adults in rural Ciskei were excreting viable tubercle bacilli at the time of the survey. In Transkei in 1982 the bacteriological prevalence of tuberculosis in adults over the age of 14 years was 2,4 per cent, which was half the proportion found in 1972.[51] In 1987, a survey of 1 039 adult residents of a township in Bophuthatswana produced a case yield of 0,86 per cent by microscopy, 0,96 per cent by culture and 0,58 per cent by radiology.[94] Case yields vary according to the case definition used, with culture (which has both the highest sensitivity and specificity) being the preferred definition for an overall figure.

The prevalence of tuberculosis may also be measured by the number of patients on tuberculosis treatment during a period of time (e.g. one year). This measure of prevalence is of particular relevance in terms of quantifying the health resources spent on tuberculosis treatment. In 1985, patient management data from the TB Control Programme (TBCP) for the seven health regions of South Africa excluding Transkei, Bophuthatswana, Venda and Ciskei were analysed for the first time, revealing a total case load of 93 020 cases and a prevalence of 478 per 100 000 total population.[22] The annual case load increased by six per cent between 1985 and 1988 to an estimated prevalence of 489 per 100 000 total population.[37] Tuberculosis prevalence was highest in the western Cape (955 per 100 000 total population) and lowest in the northern Transvaal (83 per 100 000). Figure 4.3 shows that regions with a high tuberculosis prevalence rate tended to have a low proportion of cases treated

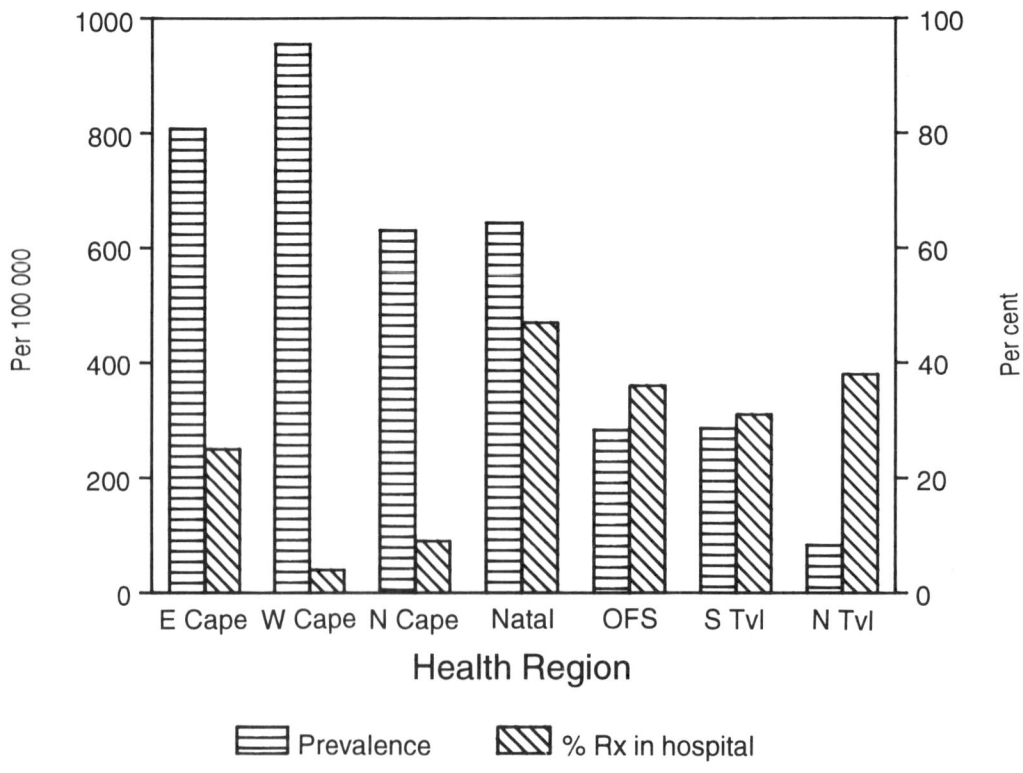

Figure 4.3. Prevalence of tuberculosis and proportion of patients hospitalized by health region in South Africa (excluding Transkei, Bophuthatswana, Venda and Ciskei), 1988.[37]

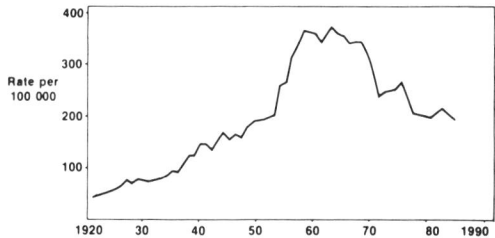

Figure 4.4. Tuberculosis notification rate in South Africa, 1921–85.[130]

in hospital, possibly indicating a shortage of hospital beds for tuberculosis patients in these areas. Data from the TBCP indicate the western Cape to be the health region with the highest tuberculous disease rates. Coastal regions were found to have a higher prevalence than inland regions, a finding similar to the TBRI bacteriological prevalence surveys.

Incidence of disease

In 1988, there were 61 475 tuberculosis cases notified in South Africa (notification rate 172 per 100 000).[37] The notification process is a passive surveillance system which relies on the participation of all medical practitioners to report cases of tuberculosis to their local and regional health offices. For notification purposes a case of tuberculosis is:

> *... a person in whom bacteriological, radiological or histological/cytological evidence of tuberculosis is found, or a pleural effusion which responds to antituberculous therapy, or a child under five years of age with symptoms and a strongly positive tuberculin skin test.*[38]

Despite the limitations of a passive surveillance system, which include variable case detection and reporting practices, notifications offer an ongoing national view of new tuberculosis cases over time.

Figure 4.4 indicates the tuberculosis notification rate in South Africa for the period 1921 to 1985.[130] It suggests that the peak of the tuberculosis epidemic was in the early 1960s when the notification rate was in excess of 350 per 100 000 total population, representing the first major tuberculosis epidemic among the black population in

southern Africa, and actually spanning the greater part of the twentieth century.[24] The sudden increase in tuberculosis notifications in the late 1950s was probably the result of the enhanced case-finding efforts which followed the introduction of effective chemotherapy for tuberculosis.[39] Unlike much of the developed world, South Africa experienced the introduction of effective chemotherapy when tuberculosis was still increasing, and therefore there is the potential for a greater health impact. However, the future course of the epidemic in South Africa is unpredictable and will depend on many factors, including socioeconomic development, the effectiveness of the Tuberculosis Control Programme, and the impact of the AIDS epidemic on tuberculosis.

The coloured population in Cape Town experienced extremely high tuberculosis morbidity and mortality rates in the early part of the twentieth century. Sixty years before the height of the tuberculosis epidemic in South Africa as a whole, tuberculosis mortality among blacks (of whom more than 90 per cent were coloured) living in Cape Town was in excess of one per cent[74] (Figure 4.5). Tuberculosis death rates among whites in Cape Town were in decline by 1903, and were probably similar to rates in Europe where major tuberculosis epidemics occurred in the eighteenth and nineteenth centuries.[60] The timing of the zenith in tuberculosis incidence in the different ethnic groups in South Africa is in keeping with the hypothesis that *Mycobacterium tuberculosis* was brought to the African subcontinent by European settlers, initially took hold in coastal settlements, and subsequently spread inland to involve the majority of the South African population.[81]

Figure 4.6 indicates the tuberculosis notification rate for South Africa by ethnic group for the period 1971 to 1984.[73] Since the early 1970s the tuberculosis notification rate among the coloured population has been increasing. This trend has been especially marked for people living in the western and northern Cape and the Orange Free State.[36] Tuberculosis notification rates in the black population are declining but remain high. In 1987 the ethnic group-specific

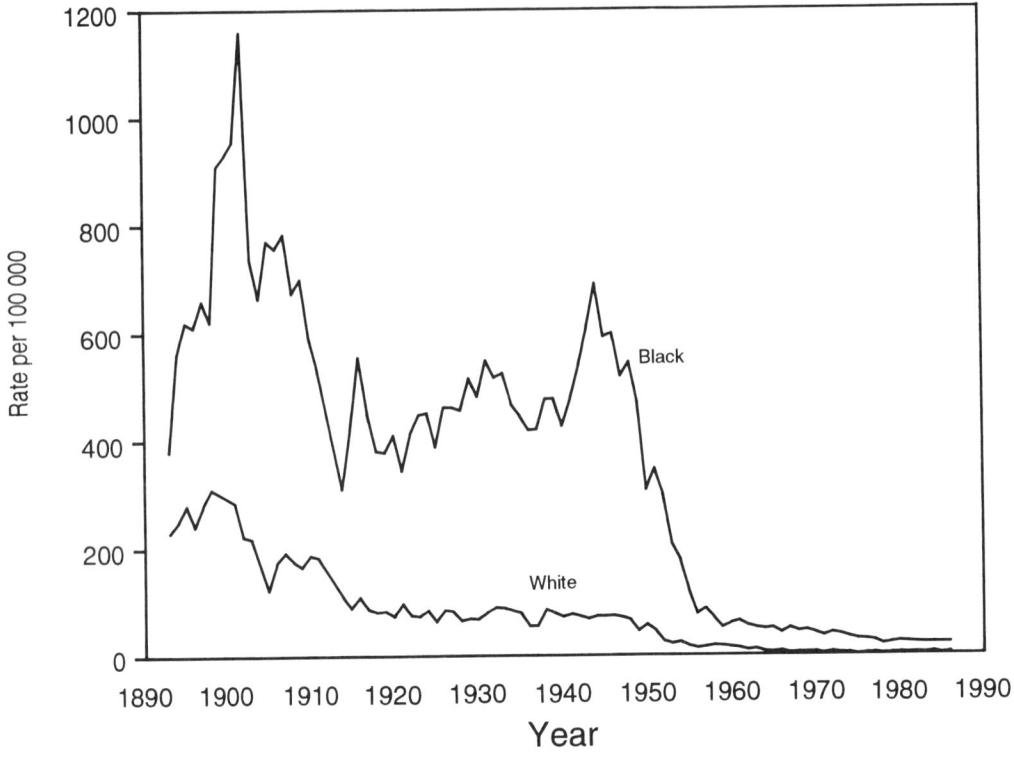

Figure 4.5. Tuberculosis mortality rate (all forms of tuberculosis) by ethnic group for the City of Cape Town 1893–1986.[107]

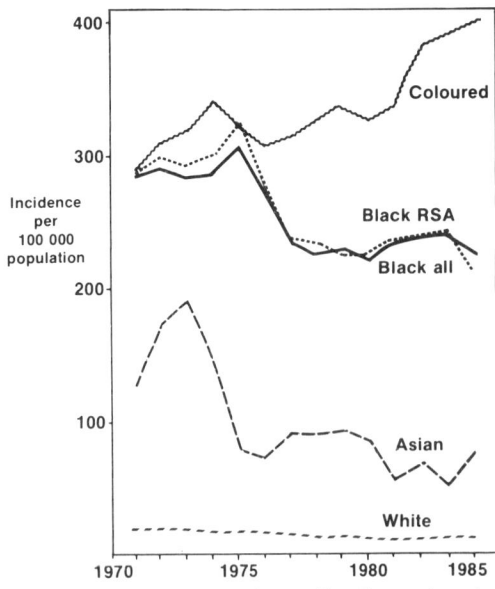

Figure 4.6. Tuberculosis notification rates by ethnic group, South Africa 1971–84.[130]

notification rates were: Indians 60 per 100 000, blacks 194 per 100 000, coloureds 453 per 100 000 and whites 14 per 100 000 total population.[124] Relative to whites, Indians were approximately four times, blacks 14 times and coloureds 32 times more likely to be notified as suffering from tuberculosis.

Although the national tuberculosis notification rate is on the decline, there is evidence that the tuberculosis problem in the western Cape is getting progressively worse. The pulmonary tuberculosis notification rate among coloured people resident in the western Cape in 1987 was higher in rural areas (510 per 100 000 total population) than in urban areas (393 per 100 000 total population) and had increased 106 and 59 per cent respectively since 1971.[107] The tuberculosis problem appears to be as great for blacks living in the western Cape. Using a Human Sciences Research Council sample

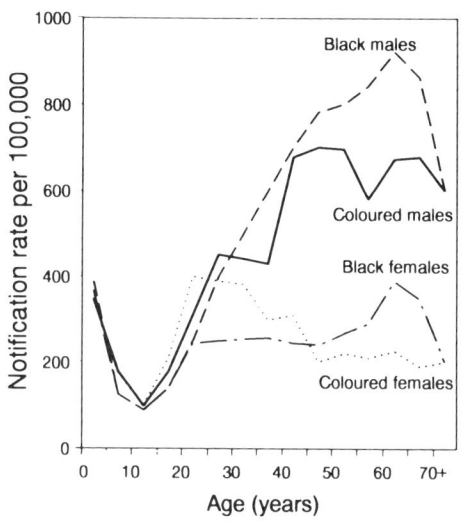
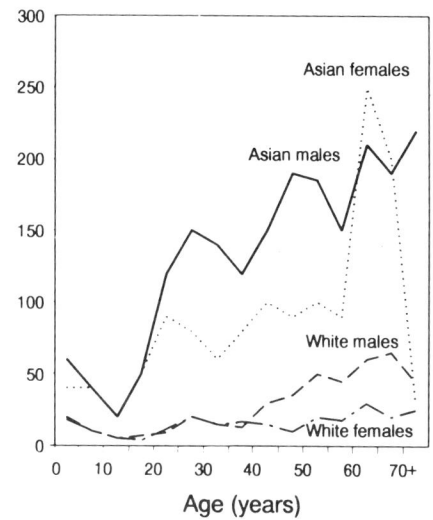

Figure 4.7. Age-ethnic group-gender-specific tuberculosis notification rates, South Africa 1975.[72]

survey of the black population of Cape Town done in 1988, the estimated pulmonary tuberculosis notification rate was 633 per 100 000.[107] At present there is little evidence that the tuberculosis epidemic is affecting whites and Indians resident in the western Cape.

Factors contributing to the worsening tuberculosis epidemic among the coloured and black populations in the western Cape include rapid urbanization with poor housing conditions, overcrowding, poor nutritional status, alcoholism and unemployment, particularly in those areas with the highest tuberculosis case loads.[117] A shortage of nursing staff in western Cape clinics which deal with large numbers of tuberculosis patients has resulted in the inability to perform adequate contact tracing and follow-up of defaulters. In addition the western Cape has the lowest proportion of tuberculosis patients managed in hospital because of a long standing shortage of hospital beds.[75]

Figure 4.7 indicates that tuberculosis notification rates vary markedly according not only to ethnic group, but also to gender and age.[72] In all ethnic groups the tuberculosis notification rates were high in young children (under five years of age), de-

creased to a minimum at age 10–14 years, and then increased into adulthood. This age distribution is characteristic for tuberculosis in many areas of the world[28] and is probably the result of primary disease in young children (who appear to be particularly susceptible to progressive disease following infection in their first two years of life) and secondary disease in adults. In blacks, male and female notification rates were similar up to 20–24 years of age, from which point onwards males had higher rates, peaking at age 55–59 years; a rate approximately twice the female rate for the same age group. In the coloured population the pattern was similar but gender-specific rates peaked earlier than in blacks; for males at 40–45 years and females at 20–25 years. Indian and white gender-specific tuberculosis notification rates were markedly lower (note the different scales in Figure 4.7) but still show an adult male excess with highest rates in those over 60 years of age. These data indicate that coloured and black adult males are the groups at highest risk for tuberculosis. The earlier peak in age-specific tuberculosis notifications in coloureds, a large proportion of whom are resident in the western Cape, is suggestive of an epidemic close to its zenith.

Although tuberculosis may involve diverse organ systems, 93,7 per cent of all notified tuberculosis cases in South Africa excluding Transkei, Bophuthatswana, Venda and Ciskei in 1987 were pulmonary[124] (Table 4.4). Pulmonary tuberculosis in adults is in most instances 'secondary' disease (i.e. the result of endogenous reactivation of a childhood infection), but exogenous reinfection may play an important role in the pathogenesis of adult disease, particularly in areas where transmission is high as it is in South Africa.

The most common extrapulmonary forms of tuberculosis notified in 1987 were primary tuberculosis (clinically determined infection of the lymphatic system; cervical lymph nodes or hilar nodes of the lung) together with more than 100 cases each of tuberculous meningitis, bone and joint tuberculosis, miliary tuberculosis and intestinal tuberculosis. The age group most

affected by the extrapulmonary forms of tuberculosis is children under five years of age. Women of reproductive age and men aged 65 years and older were the groups at highest risk for genito-urinary tuberculosis.[21]

When risk of infection with *Mycobacterium tuberculosis* is high, primary tuberculosis occurs in young children and has a wide spectrum of severity, ranging from an asymptomatic tuberculin skin test conversion to miliary tuberculosis and tuberculous meningitis (TBM). This poses particular problems in clinical diagnosis, as well as in determining a workable case definition for reporting purposes.[104] In 1980, primary tuberculosis was made a notifiable medical condition in South Africa, and 57 per cent of all cases of primary tuberculosis in 1987 were reported from the western Cape.[21] Although diagnostic and reporting practices vary by area, this finding suggests that the

Table 4.4
Notified tuberculosis cases and case fatality ratios by type of tuberculosis in the Republic of South Africa (excluding Transkei, Bophuthatswana, Venda and Ciskei) 1987[124]

TYPE OF TUBERCULOSIS (ICD 9)	NUMBER OF CASES	(%)	NOTIFICATION RATE PER 100 000	CASE-FATALITY RATIO
Pulmonary (011)	50 243	(93,7)	173,6	4,3
Primary (010)	2 079	(3,9)	7,2	0,1
Intestinal (014)	403	(0,8)	1,4	3,2
Central nervous system (013)	242	(0,5)	0,8	27,7
Bones and joints (015)	177	(0,3)	0,6	4,5
Miliary (018)	150	(0,3)	0,5	19,3
Other respiratory (012)	71	(0,1)	0,2	8,5
Genito-urinary (016)	58	(0,1)	0,2	0,0
Other organs	204	(0,4)	0,7	2,9
TOTAL	53 627	(100,1)	185,3	4,3

Source: Directorate of Epidemiology, Department of National Health and Population Development

western Cape is the area with the highest risk of tuberculous infection in South Africa.

The overall completeness of the tuberculosis notification system in South Africa is unknown. Estimates have been made that between a third and a half of all tuberculosis cases go unreported,[69] but few studies using appropriate methodology have measured the extent of under-reporting for tuberculosis. A study of TBM in the western Cape over a nine year period found that 56 per cent of all TBM cases were notified as such and that this proportion was consistent over the period of the study.[35] In this study the annual TBM incidence rate was 7,5 per 100 000 children in the 0–14 year age group. Rates were highest in black and coloured children under two years of age, a finding which was consistent with notification data. A study of the management of children with tuberculosis in Cape Town in 1984 found that 308 out of 331 (93 per cent) of children treated in clinics, and 44 out of 89 (49 per cent) of hospitalized children were notified correctly.[68] Data from the TBCP for the years 1985–8 found the annual tuberculosis notifications to be between 16 and 23 per cent less than the number of new cases placed on treatment.[37] In addition to the problem of under-reporting, some cases notified as tuberculosis may not be true cases. These studies suggest that the notification data should be interpreted with the awareness that they are underestimates of the true incidence of tuberculosis.

A further limitation in the collection and reporting of notification data has been the constantly changing political boundaries in South Africa. As far as possible, notification data for the whole of South Africa have been presented, but where data are only available for the Republic of South Africa with Transkei, Bophuthatswana, Venda and Ciskei excluded, this is indicated in the figure or legends.

Risk factors

It is not sufficient to say that tuberculosis is caused by *Mycobacterium tuberculosis*. The association between poverty and tuberculosis has been recognized for a long time, both in South Africa and internationally.[40, 64, 122] The multifactorial aetiology of tuberculosis, which involves an interplay between agent, host and environment, together with its variable incubation period and duration (both vary from weeks to a lifetime), provide specific challenges in the study of tuberculosis. For these reasons studies of the natural history of and risk factors for tuberculosis have played an important role in the development of modern epidemiology, and tuberculosis has been referred to as 'the bridge to chronic disease epidemiology'.[28, 29] The term 'risk factor' is used here in its broadest sense in that some factors have been strongly associated with risk of disease in infected persons by rigorous analytic studies, while other factors have come to be accepted by inference from numerous clinical observations.

Whereas the risk of infection with *Mycobacterium tuberculosis* is mostly associated with extrinsic factors, such as exposure to an infectious case and overcrowding, the risk factors for the development of disease after infection are largely intrinsic characteristics of the individual.[28] Comstock *et al.*[29] draw an analogy between the distinctly two-stage character of tuberculosis aetiology and the two-hit theory of cancer pathogenesis: infection with tubercle bacilli being the necessary cause, and a breach in cellular immunity the independent sufficient cause. Many factors have been associated with the activation of tuberculosis in infected persons.[28] Certain factors are useful in a clinical setting for identifying persons at high risk of active disease, whereas other factors are amenable to prevention and so have greater public health importance.

Factors NOT amenable to prevention

The risk factors described here may be useful in raising clinical suspicion of tuberculosis in a patient, but they are not amenable to prevention.

Size of the tuberculin reaction

Tuberculin reactions larger than 20 mm are almost always the result of infection with *Mycobacterium tuberculosis*, whereas infections with other mycobacteria cause smaller reactions. Because other mycobacteria seldom cause disease, the risk of subsequent tuberculosis is directly related to the size of reaction.[1, 28]

Time since infection

The risk of disease is highest in the first year after infection, declining over the next seven years (and probably longer).[28] For this reason, recent converters discovered by regular tuberculin skin testing (e.g. in schools) should be referred for medical examination to exclude the presence of active disease.[23]

Age

Follow-up of a group of persons with a newly positive tuberculin skin test has shown that the risk of disease is highest in the early years of life, decreasing sharply to a minimum at 10 years of age, and then increasing again to a peak in early adult life (around 20 years of age), decreasing once more to lower levels during middle age.[31] Ultimately, about 10 per cent of children infected by the tubercle bacillus will develop tuberculous disease during their lifetime.[31] In the early years of life the effects of young age and recent tuberculous infection combine to provide an extremely high risk of disease, which may be disseminated (as in TBM and miliary TB).[28]

Ethnic group

A study in Puerto Rico which involved following up a large number of persons in a BCG vaccination trial showed no major differences in the incidence of tuberculosis between black and white tuberculin reactors.[31] South African data indicate large ethnic differences in the prevalence of tuberculous infection (see Table 4.1), and similar ethnic differences are seen in the incidence (notification rates) of tuberculosis, suggesting that the latter are due mainly to differences in the risk of infection. There are no South African data which indicate that certain ethnic groups have increased genetic susceptibility to activation of latent tuberculous infection.

Gender

Data from the TBRI surveys indicated that adult black African men were roughly twice as likely as women to be tuberculin skin test positive. This male to female ratio was similar for the prevalence of bacteriologically confirmed tuberculosis and for notified tuberculosis rates. Therefore, the higher tuberculosis notification rates seen in males compared to females across all ethnic groups in South Africa (Figure 4.7) appears to be best explained by a higher risk of infection in males.

Rare medical conditions

Table 4.5 summarizes data taken from Rieder *et al*.[85] on a number of medical conditions which have been associated with an increased risk of active tuberculosis among infected persons. Although the measure of association (odds ratio or relative risk) may be large, the rarity of these conditions in South Africa suggests that they may have little public health importance.

Table 4.5
Rare conditions which are risk factors for tuberculosis following infection[85]

| | MEASURE OF ASSOCIATION | |
RISK FACTOR	ODDS RATIO	RELATIVE RISK
Carcinoma of head or neck		16
Haemophilia		9,4
Immunosuppressive treatment		11,9
Haemodialysis		10–15
Diabetes		2,0–3,6
HLA–A11–B15	3,6	
HLA–DR2	1,6	
Gastrectomy		5
Jejuno-ileal bypass		27–63

Factors amenable to prevention

The risk factors for active tuberculosis discussed in this section are both amenable to prevention and prevalent in South Africa, and are therefore of significant public health importance. Interventions aimed at controlling these factors will not only result in a reduction of the risk factor itself (most of which are major health problems in their own right), but will also lower the incidence of tuberculosis (if their association with tuberculosis is causal).

HIV/AIDS

Throughout most of the developing world the prevalence of tuberculous infection in adults is around 30–60 per cent[66] and in many areas of Africa (including parts of South Africa) it reaches 80 per cent.[52] Most of these infections would normally remain quiescent, since the estimated lifetime risk of active disease among infected persons is 10 per cent.[28] A recent study among intravenous drug users in New York City[96] found

the rate of active tuberculosis among tuberculin skin test positive persons to be higher in human immunodeficiency virus (HIV) positive individuals (12/279) than in HIV negative individuals (0/240). The risk of tuberculosis in HIV positive persons was comparable to the risk of disease in infected contacts within the first year after tuberculous infection.[10] A study of women attending an antenatal clinic in Africa found that HIV infection increased the risk of activating latent tuberculous infection 10-fold (M Braun, personal communication).

The historical decline in tuberculosis in the United States has been halted, and part of this phenomenon is thought to be due to the impact of the epidemic spread of HIV to persons with latent tuberculous infection.[85] This effect was first seen in 1985, and by 1987 this had resulted in an estimated excess of 9 226 tuberculosis cases, found particularly in groups with a high prevalence of HIV infection. The potential for synergism between the HIV epidemic

Table 4.6
Summary of studies of the prevalence of HIV infection in tuberculosis patients.

COUNTRY	AGE GROUP	TYPE OF TB	HIV+ (PERCENT)
Burundi[100]	<20	TB	3
	20–40	TB	62
	>40	TB	3
Central African	Adult	TB (all forms)	31
Republic[13]	Child	TB (all forms)	11
	Adult	Lymphatic	64
	Child	Lymphatic	18
	Adult	Extrapulmonary	60
	Child	Extrapulmonary	17
Rwanda[76]	Adult	PTB	31
	Adult	Lymphatic	75
Sierra Leone[3]	—	TB	15
Uganda[97]	—	TB	61
Zaire[20]	Adult	PTB	33
	Adult	Extrapulmonary	48
Zimbabwe[73]	<2	TB	52
	3–15	TB	12
	16–40	TB	43
	>40	TB	17
North America[97]			
New York		TB	42
Florida		TB	31
Seattle		TB	18

and tuberculosis is even greater in many parts of Africa where the overlap of persons infected with both tubercle bacilli and HIV represents a much larger proportion of the population. Indeed, in several African countries with high HIV seroprevalence the reported tuberculosis rates are increasing.[16, 79, 97, 110]

Further evidence for an increased risk of tuberculosis in HIV infected persons comes from the rates of HIV infection found in tuberculosis patients (Table 4.6) which are much higher than those found in the general population. The highest prevalence of HIV infection was found in adult tuberculosis patients, particularly in the sexually active age groups. A study conducted in Zimbabwe found that 52 per cent of tuberculosis patients under two years of age were also HIV positive,[73] a finding which suggested that perinatal infection with HIV may even further increase the risk of active tuberculosis in children exposed to tubercle bacilli in the early years of life. The data in Table 4.6 also suggest that HIV infection is a risk factor for extrapulmonary tuberculosis, as HIV prevalence is often highest in patients with lymphatic or other extrapulmonary tuberculosis.

In the United States, matching of case registries showed that tuberculosis was also diagnosed in more than 10 per cent of AIDS cases in Florida[14] and 5,4 per cent of AIDS cases in Connecticut.[15] In the Florida study the prevalence of tuberculosis in AIDS patients was about 30 per cent in Haitians and about 10 per cent in non-Haitians. These differences were attributed to differences in the underlying prevalence of tuberculous infection in the two groups and suggest that a large proportion of AIDS cases who are infected with *Mycobacterium tuberculosis* will progress to active TB.

Although the HIV/AIDS epidemic in South Africa is apparently less advanced than in many areas in Africa, its potential to promote a major resurgence of tuberculosis is equally great.

Anthropometric status

Weight loss is a common presenting complaint in tuberculosis patients and is generally thought to be a result of the disease process. However, there is also good evidence that being underweight is itself a risk factor for the development of tuberculosis in infected persons.[85] Prospective studies conducted in the United States have found that the incidence of tuberculosis among persons below ideal body weight was 2,2 to 4 times greater than for persons with normal weight for height.[32, 41, 82] A study in Norway found a trend to increasing tuberculosis rates in persons with lower body mass index.[121]

In South Africa the combination of protein-calorie malnutrition and tuberculosis has been observed in clinical settings, but studies which adjust for other contributory factors, and so demonstrate a direct, independent effect of undernutrition on the risk of developing tuberculosis, have not been reported.

Smoking

Tobacco smoking is not a generally accepted risk factor for activating latent tuberculosis. However, a study in Shanghai found tuberculosis incidence was higher (relative risk 2,2) among smokers than among non-smokers after adjustment for age, sex, type of work, history of contact and area of housing.[134] Because of the high prevalence of tobacco smoking among black men (some 60 per cent of black men in Cape Town townships were smokers),[106] even a weak causal association between smoking and tuberculosis could have a major impact on tuberculosis rates.

Alcohol

A case-control study conducted in Mamre in the western Cape found an association between alcohol problems in the household and tuberculosis (odds ratio adjusted for employment status: 2,2, 95 per cent confidence interval 1,3–3,8).[19] A similar association between alcoholism and tuberculosis has been observed in the United States,[56] where alcoholics have been identified as forming a high risk group requiring screening for tuberculous infection and active disease.[17]

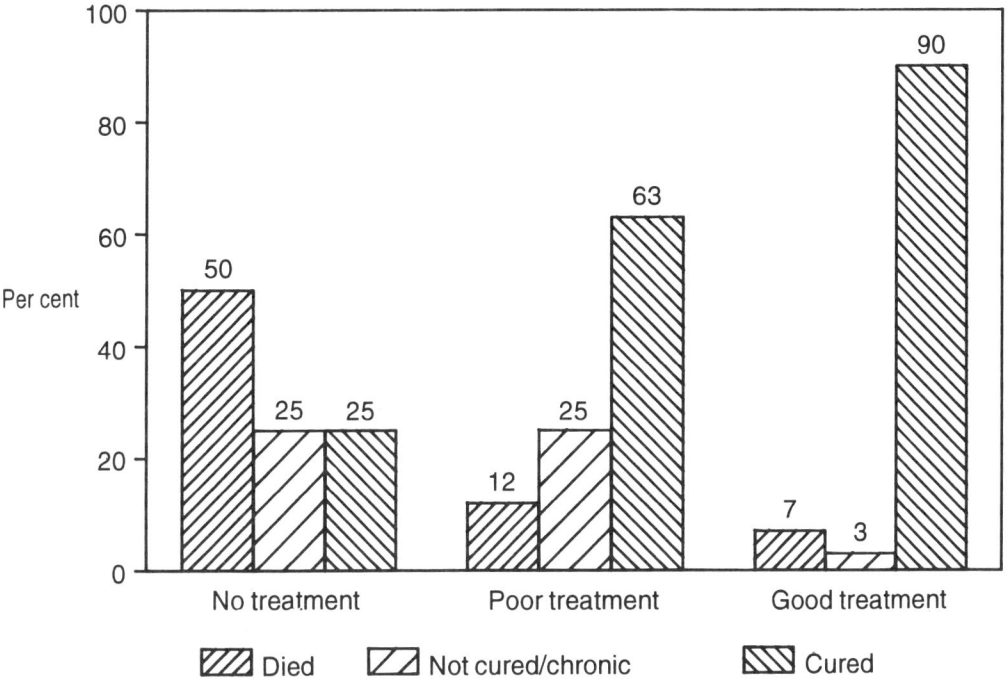

Figure 4.8 (a). Outcomes of tuberculosis with no treatment, poor treatment and good treatment.[62]

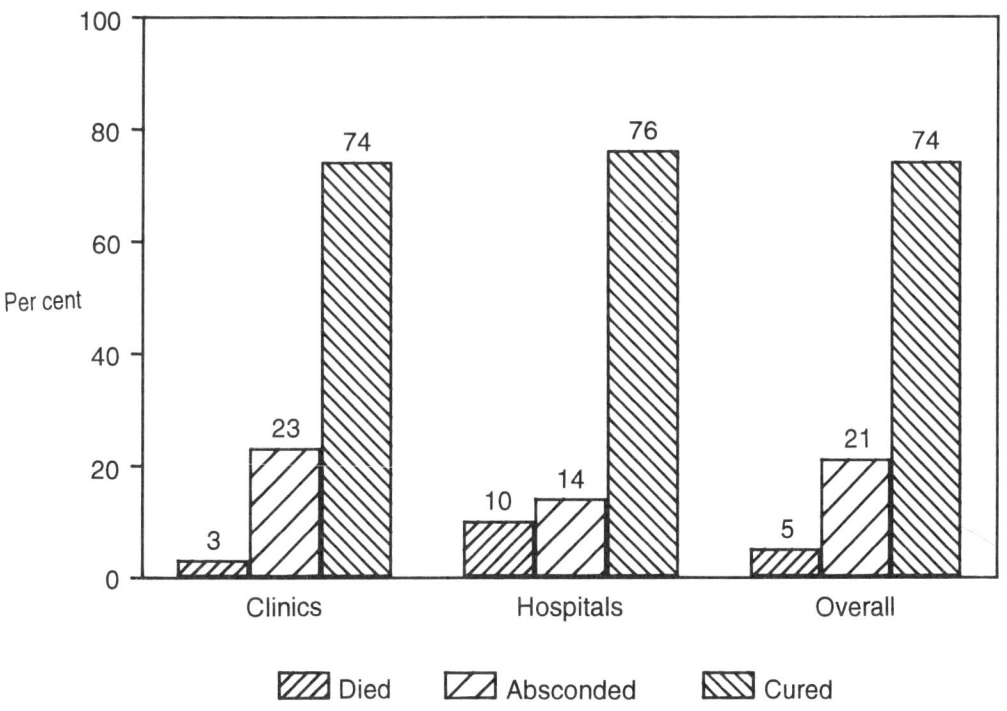

Figure 4.8 (b). Outcomes of tuberculosis in South Africa (excluding Transkei, Bophuthatswana, Venda and Ciskei) as reported in the TB Control Programme 1988.[37]

Silicosis

It has been estimated that the incidence of tuberculosis among miners with silicosis is 30 times greater than among miners without silicosis.[83] It is less clear whether silica dust exposure (in the absence of silicosis) increases a person's risk of activating latent tuberculosis.[99] The large numbers of miners working in dusty environments in South Africa emphasize the potential public health importance of silicosis and silica dust exposure as risk factors for tuberculosis (see Chapter 12).

OUTCOMES OF TUBERCULOSIS

A case of active tuberculosis may have four recognizable outcomes: cure, which implies being bacteriologically sterile and healthy usually as a result of treatment or, more rarely, 'spontaneous' cure; disability which involves bacteriological cure but residual physical, mental or psychological handicap; chronic disease which implies ongoing excretion of tubercle bacilli in symptomatic (rarely asymptomatic) individuals; and death.

Estimates of the fate of patients with bacillary tuberculosis but no treatment have been made by Grzybowski from the results of a number of follow-up studies.[62] Of bacteriologically positive tuberculosis cases, 50 per cent will die, 25 per cent remain sputum positive and 25 per cent attain sputum negative 'cure' after five years of follow-up (Figure 4.8a). With a good treatment programme which involves individualized chemotherapy, the outcome of bacillary patients is markedly improved: approximately 90–93 per cent are cured (rendered sterile); five to seven per cent die and two to three per cent remain chronically sputum positive.[6, 62]

Cure

The TBCP data from the seven health regions of the Republic of South Africa (excluding Transkei, Bophuthatswana, Venda and Ciskei) indicate that, of the 99 251 tuberculosis patients with known outcome in 1988, 74 per cent were cured, five per cent died and 21 per cent absconded (Figure 4.8b).[37] The outcome of

the absconders is unknown — some may have died, while others may have been cured or remained bacillary excretors. The proportion of tuberculosis patients cured has declined steadily from 78 per cent in 1985 to 74 per cent in 1988 and the percentage of absconders has risen from 16 per cent to 21 per cent. The cure rate estimated from the TBCP data is less than the 90 per cent suggested by Grzybowski as being the level attainable by a highly effective tuberculosis control programme. These findings point to an increasing problem of case-holding in South Africa, with the consequences of ongoing transmission of potentially drug resistant tubercle bacilli, continued morbidity and possibly death.

Disability

Relatively few published studies have looked at the disability resulting from tuberculosis in South Africa. This is not because disability from tuberculosis does not occur, but rather because it is overshadowed by the numbers of current tuberculosis cases and deaths. Disability may be minor in an uncomplicated case of pulmonary tuberculosis, or severe as in a case of tuberculous meningitis. A study of 185 TBM patients in the western Cape found that 47 per cent of patients had residual disability ranging from mild mental retardation, epilepsy, deafness or behavioural problems to severe mental retardation with physical abnormalities such as hemiparesis or athetoid movements.[35] In this study 26 per cent of the patients recovered fully and 24 per cent died.

Collins states that the majority of 'cured' patients suffer some degree of permanent disability,[26] and interest in the extent of pulmonary disability has been shown by welfare organizations such as the South African National Tuberculosis Association (SANTA). Attempts at quantitative assessment of lung function in the treated tuberculosis patient are extremely difficult since it proves almost impossible to separate deterioration due to the disease from the effects of age, smoking and other confounders.[92]

Death

Although surveillance of tuberculosis deaths is the least sensitive epidemiologic indicator

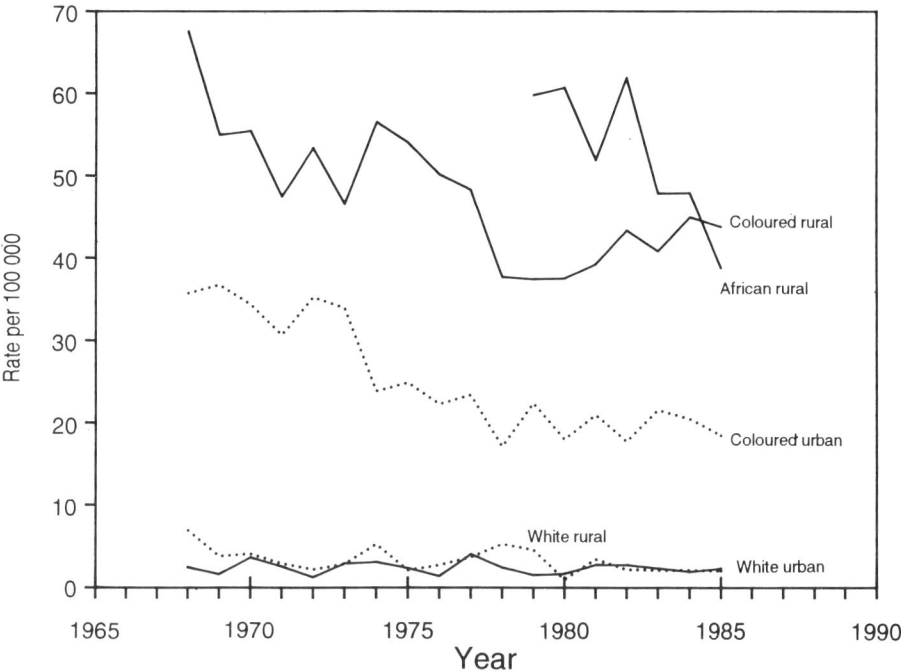

Figure 4.9. Tuberculosis mortality rates for urban and rural areas of the Western Cape Health Region by ethnic group, 1968–85.[107]

of the tuberculosis situation in a community, deaths do represent a preventable outcome and hence are an indication of programme effectiveness.[107] In 1984 there were 5 773 registered tuberculosis deaths in South Africa,[131] mortality being highest in coloured and black adults aged 15-64 years where it is responsible for six to eight per cent of all deaths.[131]

In most areas of South Africa the trend in tuberculosis mortality is thought to be downward,[6] but in the western Cape there is evidence that this trend has levelled off for coloured people and may even have increased slightly in the rural areas of the western Cape (Figure 4.9). As with tuberculous disease there are large ethnic and regional differences with respect to tuberculosis mortality. In the western Cape, calculation of standardized mortality ratios (SMR's), using urban white death rates for 1980–5 as the reference, indicated a 15 times increased risk for a tuberculosis death in the urban coloured population, and 37 and 28 times increased risks for the rural coloured and black populations respectively.[107]

The overall tuberculosis case-fatality ratio (CFR) in South Africa based on notifications (calculated as the number of notified deaths divided by the number of notified cases multiplied by 100) was four per cent in 1988.[131] This estimate is dependent on the assumption of equal bias in the reporting of cases and deaths. A study comparing notified and registered tuberculosis deaths (the latter based on death certificates) found that in 1980, only 28 per cent of registered black deaths were notified. The comparable proportions for whites, coloureds and Indians were 46, 53 and 62 per cent. Using the TBCP data for 1988, the tuberculosis CFR was five per cent.[131] However, as some absconders may have died this is probably a minimum value. Interpreting these data together with other reports in the literature suggests that the overall tuberculosis CFR in South Africa is probably between four and eight per cent.

Tuberculosis CFR's vary widely according to the organ system involved and the age of the patient (Table 4.4), the highest CFR's being found in TBM (27,7 per cent) and miliary tuberculosis (19,3 per cent). An active surveillance project for TBM in the western Cape found a CFR of 23,8 per cent which is similar to the CFR for TBM based on notifications.

Risk factors for a poor outcome

Factors affecting the outcome of patients with active tuberculosis include age, type of disease, stage at diagnosis, and compliance with therapy.[6, 65] The effect of age and type of disease on CFR's have already been discussed.

Poor prognosis is associated with advanced stage of tuberculous disease at diagnosis, and this is a reflection of poor access to curative health services, ineffective case-finding strategies and a need for improved health education. That these latter factors are important in the South African setting was indicated in a study of TBM in the western Cape in which it was found that children from rural areas were diagnosed at a later stage of the disease and more of them died (31 per cent as opposed to 17 per cent).[35]

CONTROL STRATEGIES

The dynamics of the tuberculosis epidemic are complex and it is often impossible to separate the many determinants of the epidemic's progress from the efforts to control the disease.

Case-finding and contact tracing

The infectious case (sputum smear positive) is the priority for case-finding operations,[55] but most routine case-finding programmes do not specifically focus on this aspect. Data from the published reports of the Medical Officers of Health of the larger South African municipalities allow reasonable estimates of the efficiency of different case-finding methods to be made.[88, 90] Figure 4.10 shows the routine case yields from the four main sources of cases — mass x-ray campaigns; screening of so-called 'risk groups'; contacts of known tuberculosis cases; and

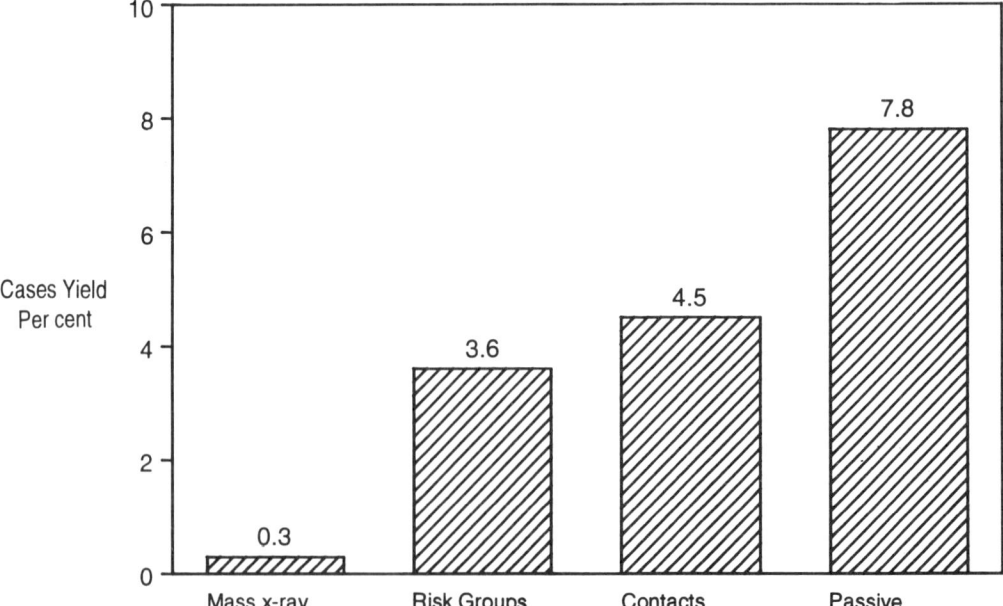

See text for explanation of categories.

Figure 4.10. Case yields (cases found/persons screened x 100) from tuberculosis screening in the larger South African cities 1980–3.[88]

people found by passive case-finding (i.e. where the patient voluntarily seeks treatment). The case yield is defined as the ratio of cases identified to persons screened and is expressed as a percentage. Mass x-ray refers to people who were screened at pre-employment checks but did not undergo any selection on health grounds. This indiscriminate approach produces a very low case yield and reflects the 'healthy worker effect', with a tuberculosis prevalence lower than the national average. Higher yields will be found initially in some industrial settings,[77] but in repeated mass x-ray campaigns in the same area the yield rapidly decreases to approach the national average. Selective screening of the unemployed and hostel residents increases the case yield to 3,6 per cent, and contacts of known tuberculosis cases produce a yield of 4,5 per cent. The highest yield (7,8 per cent) comes from passive case-finding (Figure 4.10).

Indiscriminate mass x-ray is a poor method for finding cases as only about a quarter of x-ray positive tuberculosis cases are infectious.[49] A case yield of 0,25 per cent by mass x-ray represents one case

found in every 400 x-rays taken, and the yield of the priority infectious cases could be as low as one in 1 600. Clearly this is a very expensive way of finding cases.

At the other extreme, passive case-finding produces quite a high case yield but is the hardest to influence directly. Passive case-finding depends upon the individual's awareness of signs and symptoms of tuberculosis, a willingness to attend for screening, and the availability of health services. Although a high yield can be expected, there is the risk that the disease may be in an advanced stage before a patient becomes sufficiently motivated to attend a clinic of his or her own accord.

In case-finding research, 'patient's delay' is used to refer to the delay between the onset of the disease and the patient seeking medical attention, and 'doctor's delay' (more accurately health service delay) is the delay between the patient first presenting at a medical facility and the start of treatment. Both these delays can be long and, although there are no accurate figures for South Africa, the average patient's delay is likely to be more than three months[4] —

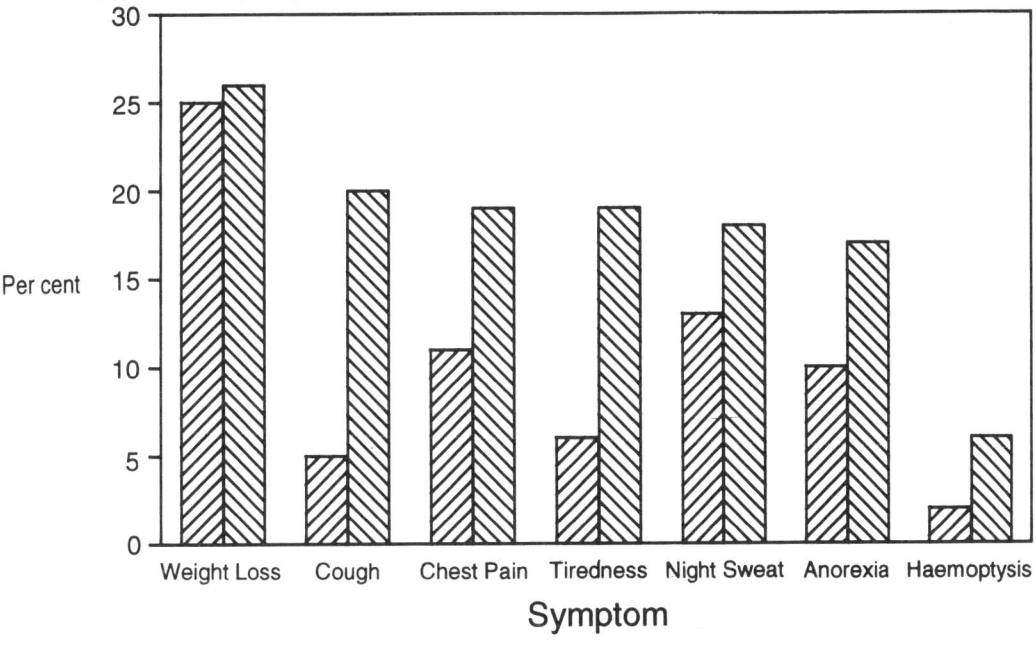

Figure 4.11. Symptom recognition and perception of 'illness' by 165 rural blacks attending a free tuberculosis check up facility in Transkei.[90]

three months during which contacts will be exposed to a potentially infectious source. There have been reports of doctor's delays in excess of 12 months in some areas (R F Ingle, personal communication) but this is probably the exception rather than the rule.

Health education of both patients and service providers is the most obvious way to reduce both types of delay. There is still ignorance regarding tuberculosis among medical practitioners, who fail to comply with recommended practice[132] and among the general population who do not know the common signs and symptoms of the disease.[90, 103]

Figure 4.11 shows the symptoms reported by 165 rural blacks attending a village screening point in Transkei which offered free check-ups for TB according to whether or not the client considered him- or herself to be 'ill'. Almost equal numbers in both groups said that they had experienced a loss in weight, so, for this population weight loss would not be sufficient motivation for attending the clinic. Night sweats were also almost as common in the 'not ill' group as the 'ill' group, but the most common sign of tuberculosis — a productive cough of long duration — was

recognized as being a sign of illness. From this rather small sample it appears that a cough and tiredness are most likely to be considered as signs of illness. Overall, 39 per cent of the people who said they were not ill had at least one of the classical signs of tuberculosis. In an urban sample the percentage decreased to 24 per cent, but this is still high enough to have serious consequences for passive case-finding. Clearly there is a need to increase people's awareness of the importance of the signs and symptoms of tuberculosis if passive case-finding is to increase.

Prevalence surveys provide data which can be used to determine the potential efficacy of various contact tracing procedures within families under optimal conditions. The TBRI has data collected over 11 years from random samples from the relatively high prevalence areas of KwaZulu, Transkei, Ciskei, Lesotho and the border region of the eastern Cape (Table 4.7).[90]

For these surveys five categories of index cases were selected: children under 15 years of age with Mantoux reactions ≥14 mm; children under five years with Mantoux reactions ≥14 mm; culture positive

Table 4.7

Case yields (cases found/persons screened x 100) for contact tracing from various types of index cases under optimized conditions[90]

INDEX CASE		NO. SCREENED		CASES FOUND				CASE YIELD (PER CENT)		
TYPE	AGE	INDEX	CONTACTS	MX+ CHILD	C+ ADULT	S+ ADULT	C+S+ ADULT	TOTAL	PER FAMILY	PER CONTACT
Child										
Mx+	<15 yr	176	1 093	16	6	0	8	30	17,0	2,7
Mx+	<5 yr	129	648	16	5	0	5	26	20,2	4,0
Healthy	<15 yr	100	758	1	1	0	0	2	2,0	0,3
Adult										
C+	>15 yr	87	442	20	1	0	0	21	24,1	4,8
S+	>15 yr	26	124	2	0	0	0	2	7,7	1,6
C+S+	>15 yr	68	411	17	1	1	0	19	27,9	4,6
Healthy	>15 yr	100	722	1	0	0	1	2	2,0	0,3

Mx+   Mantoux reaction ±14 mm
C+   Culture positive
S+   Direct microscopy. Smear positive
C+S+   Culture and smear positive

adults; adults positive by both culture and smear; and adults positive by smear only. The control groups were healthy adults negative by all tests except Mantoux, and healthy children who had Mantoux reactions less than 10 mm. The total case yield ranged from 1,6 per cent for the contacts of smear positive adults to 4,8 per cent for the contacts of culture positive adults. The low yield from contacts of smear positive adults is surprising and suggests that there were some false positive smears in these data as the smear positive individual is generally more infectious than one who is positive only on culture. The yield of adult cases from contacts of existing adult cases was low, but the adult case yield was much higher among contacts of Mantoux positive children. This is an important difference because the priority infectious cases are generally adults, so it seems that contact tracing from children will have the greatest epidemiological impact. Clearly the child case also needs attention but the epidemic is mainly propagated by adults. The case yield from the healthy control group was 0,3 per cent which is marginally higher than is normally achieved by mass x-ray and

confirms that mass x-ray campaigns appear to select people who may be healthier than average.

The case yield per contact of a proven case averages out at around four per cent, but case yields per family can be as high as 28 per cent. In other words, contact tracing from confirmed TB cases or infected children in high prevalence areas will find another case in every fourth or fifth household. Thus contacts are not only a definite risk group, but the yields from contact tracing are high enough to warrant special attention.

Another risk group that might be considered for special case-finding efforts consists of people from poor socio-economic conditions. Stories of squatter areas that are 'full of TB' are common among tuberculosis workers, and yet there are few statistics to support these claims. Of the various socio-economic indicators, overcrowding is the most strongly related to the transmission of infection. There is a strong tendency to assume that squatter or slum housing will automatically be overcrowded, but in a developing community near Pretoria the mean crowding index for slums was 2,56

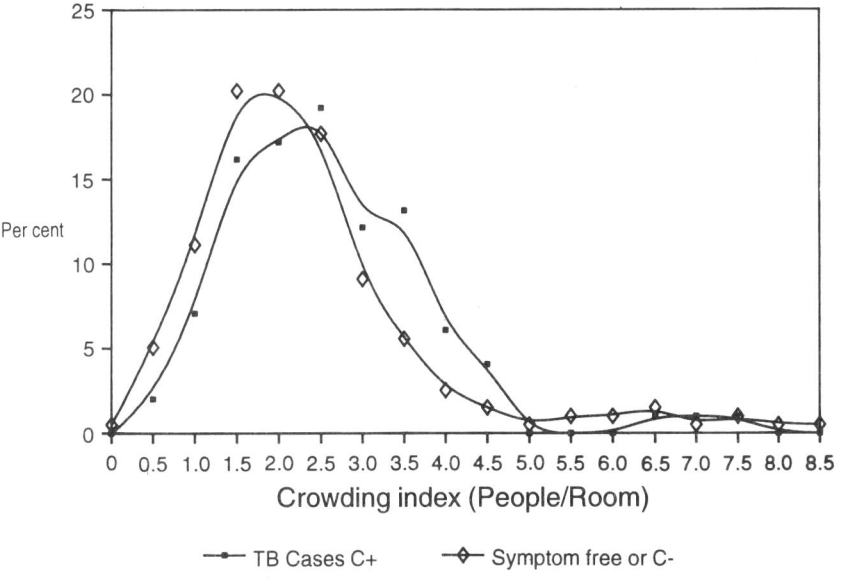

C+ culture positive, C- culture negative

Figure 4.12. Smoothed frequency distributions of crowding indices for tuberculosis cases (culture positive) and persons without active tuberculosis.[94]

people/room (*just* overcrowded according to the Slums Act); for traditional huts 2,33 and for township houses 2,37. These values were not significantly different. The mean crowding index for luxury houses was significantly lower at 1,93.[94]

In the same study, of 1 039 adults questioned, 441 or 42 per cent had at least one symptom of tuberculosis and were eligible for sputum examination. Twenty-five per cent of respondents admitted a cough of more than two weeks duration and 7,4 per cent of these proved to be tuberculosis cases; only one per cent of respondents had bloodstained sputum and 6,7 per cent of these were tuberculotics. The people with a cough yielded 95 per cent of the cases whereas those with bloodstained sputum only amounted to five per cent of the total. So, for case-finding purposes, a productive cough of long duration (more than two weeks) is the best indicator of tuberculosis. Blood stained sputum, while obviously needing investigation, is such a rare symptom that it is of little use for population-based screening programmes.

Studies in Transkei[11] and Mamre (western Cape)[19] failed to show any association between overcrowding and tuberculosis. However, in the Pretoria study mentioned above, when the frequency distributions of crowding indices for tuberculosis cases were compared with people proven to be free from active tuberculosis, there were more tuberculosis cases in the overcrowded homes (Figure 4.12). Unfortunately, the two distributions overlap almost completely, making case-finding efforts based on overcrowding alone impractical.

Case-holding

Once the diagnosis of tuberculosis has been made, the major determinant of outcome is the ability of the health service to 'hold the patient to cure'. Case-holding can be discussed under two headings: patient compliance; and compliance by the health service with tuberculosis policy.

Patient compliance

The most appropriate way to measure patient compliance with tuberculosis therapy is to use a cohort (or follow-up) study which involves enroling a representative sample of newly diagnosed tuberculosis patients and following them up at regular intervals until after the treatment has ended in order to determine their outcome.[133] Compliance with tuberculosis treatment was studied in 560 patients in Soweto in 1978.[87] At follow-up after one year, only 159 (or 28 per cent) had received 80 per cent or more of their required treatment. The compliance was better for hospitalized patients (42 per cent) than for non-hospitalized patients (20 per cent). At least 17 per cent of patients over 10 years of age had tubercle bacilli in their sputa on microscopy more than four months after therapy had been started.

A cohort study of 374 patients placed on daily supervised outpatient treatment in the Hewu district of Ciskei found that 75 per cent of patients had received more than 80 per cent of their prescribed doses.[33] The results from Hewu indicate the extent to which case-holding can be improved by active follow-up of patients. A cross-sectional study of tuberculosis compliance in the western Cape in 1984 indicated that 82,5 per cent of patients had completed more than 75 per cent of their expected treatment by the day of the survey.[5] However, cross-sectional studies tend to overestimate the compliance as patients removed from the treatment register at the time of the study (as a result of death or defaulting) may be excluded.

Together these studies indicate that patient compliance varies widely according to the setting, and they suggest that case-holding for a prolonged period of anti-tuberculous chemotherapy can be improved by making the clinic service more responsive to the patients' needs with mechanisms for follow-up and supervision of treatment.

Compliance with tuberculosis policy

Surveillance of tuberculosis management practices is an important tool for improving national control programme standards.[53, 54, 55] At issue here is the compliance of practitioners and local authorities with the national TBCP guidelines for diagnosis, treatment and follow-up.

A study of Local Authority compliance with tuberculosis policy in the western Cape found that there was a lack of clear definitions in the policy guidelines as to what constitutes patient compliance, defaulting and treatment failure.[5] In addition, the notification criteria for children and management of children with tuberculosis showed a lack of uniformity between local authorities. Some of the problems faced by local authorities when carrying out tuberculosis policy guidelines included a lack of hospital beds for tuberculosis patients, lack of patient transport, alcohol abuse, lack of cooperation of employers, unemployment, and low socio-economic status of the patients.[5]

A useful measure of the effectiveness of a tuberculosis control effort is the proportion of 'new' cases with tuberculosis presenting at a health service who have a history of

prior tuberculosis treatment. These patients fall into two groups: those who did not complete the required number of doses (defaulters) and those who completed treatment but then relapsed (relapses). A study of 95 patients presenting with sputum positive tuberculosis at a hospital in the Thaba Nchu district of Bophuthatswana found that 35,8 per cent had been previously treated for tuberculosis. Reasons for relapse in these patients were that 50 per cent had had inadequate outpatient treatment after hospitalization, 25 per cent had absconded from treatment, and 25 per cent had multiple admissions with haphazard drug regimens. Only one patient was a treatment failure.[59] A study of the rates of relapse in 150 hospitalized tuberculosis patients in the Johannesburg/Pretoria area in 1985 found that 26 per cent had had previous treatment and six per cent were judged to be

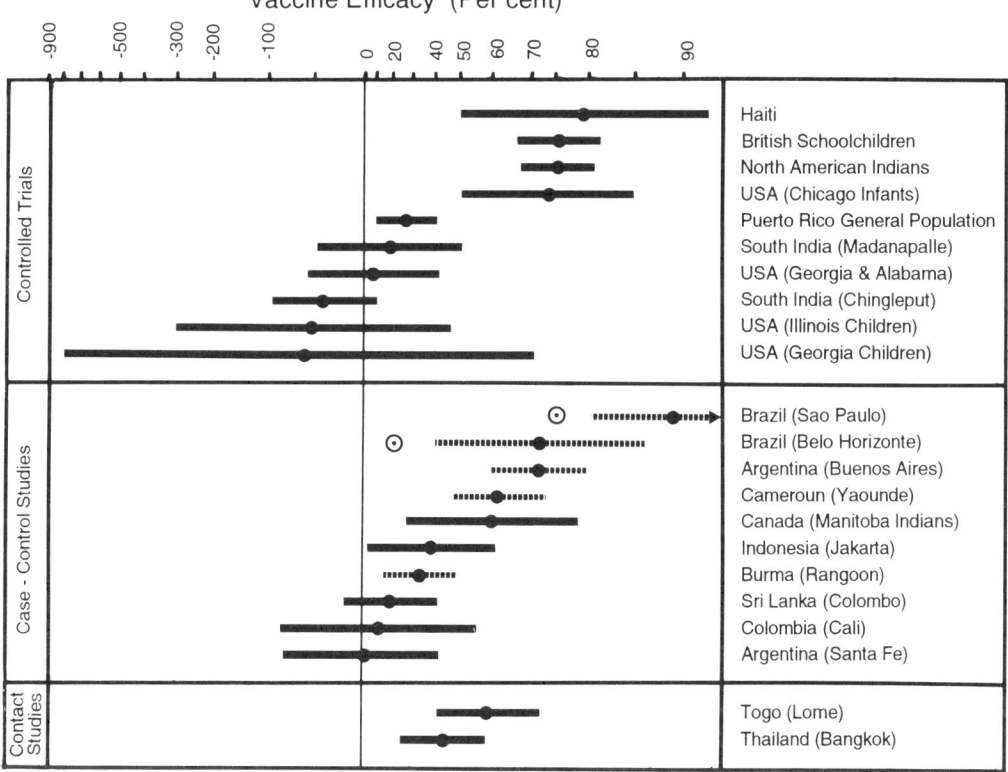

Figure 4.13. Summary of estimates of the efficacy of BCG vaccines against tuberculosis. (Source: Fine P E M, 1989. The BCG story, lesson from the past and implications for the future. Review of Infectious Diseases. (Suppl. 2) 353-9.

treatment failures.[44] These studies point to the need for improved case-holding rather than to a problem with drug resistance.

Drug resistance

Programme effectiveness is a product not only of compliance with the regimen but also of the efficacy of the drugs used. A major reason for treatment failure in a compliant patient (i.e. the failure to render a tuberculosis patient sterile, or a relapse in a fully treated person within 12 months of therapy having been completed) is drug resistance. Analysis of over 22 000 sputum cultures collected throughout South Africa between 1965 and 1978 revealed INH resistant organisms in 17,5 per cent of cultures and streptomycin-resistant organisms in 15,8 per cent.[6] The TBRI has monitored drug resistance to INH since the mid-1960s by studying patients on antituberculous chemotherapy. Approximately one third had had previous tuberculosis treatment. In 1986 INH resistance was found in 11 per cent of new cases and 24 per cent of old cases.[70] Comparing the 1986 data with the earlier estimates suggests no worsening of the drug resistance situation, but data from the TBCP for 1988 does indicate an increasing problem of patients absconding, which would tend to promote drug resistance.

BCG (bacille Calmette-Guérin)

Tuberculosis is one of the six target diseases specified under the World Health Organization's (WHO) Expanded Programme on Immunization (EPI), and in South Africa BCG vaccination was compulsory for all newborn children between 1973 and 1989. BCG vaccination was removed from the statute book in 1989, but not from the EPI programme, as a result of recognizing the futility of legislation which is virtually impossible to enforce.

The efficacy of BCG vaccination was called into question after the publication of results of a large trial in South India, which indicated very little protective effect.[67] Over the years various trials of BCG vaccine efficacy around the world have continued to produce variable results (Figure 4.13).[46] These results suggest, however, not so

much that BCG may be ineffective but, rather, that variability existed in the vaccines used, the populations studied and the methodologies which were employed. Evaluating vaccine efficacy is complicated by the extremely widespread use of BCG which is given routinely in virtually all countries of the world except the United States, Iceland and the Netherlands.[126] Also, the impact of BCG is difficult to evaluate since most BCG programmes were introduced at the same time as other social, economic and (particularly) case-finding and chemotherapy interventions.

Recent South African studies indicated a 65 per cent protective effect attributable to BCG against active disease for children under five years of age in an urban setting[18] and 58 per cent in a rural population.[48] Other studies have reported that vaccinated children develop tuberculosis in a milder form,[58] and that vaccination gives a protective effect against serious forms of tuberculosis which lasts for about five years.[12] The latter two observations have not been confirmed in large controlled trials of BCG vaccine. The assumption that BCG must be ineffective merely because many children developing TB meningitis have been vaccinated is erroneous. If there was 100 per cent vaccine coverage with an 80 per cent effective vaccine, *all* cases would arise in vaccinated children.

Styblo & Meijer[112] pointed out that BCG vaccination at birth does not have much impact on the transmission of infection as the protective effect lasts for 10–15 years at the most[109] and children rarely spread infection. Also, more than 95 per cent of children with tuberculosis and 75 per cent of primary clinical tuberculosis cases aged 15–29 are smear negative.[111] This does not, however, preclude BCG vaccination since there is some evidence that BCG protects children from the most severe forms of TB (TBM and miliary TB).

Recently the routine use of BCG for newborns has been questioned in view of rising HIV prevalence and the potential risk of disseminated BCG disease in immunocompromised infants. The most recent WHO guidelines recommend BCG vaccination for newborn infants, even when the mother is

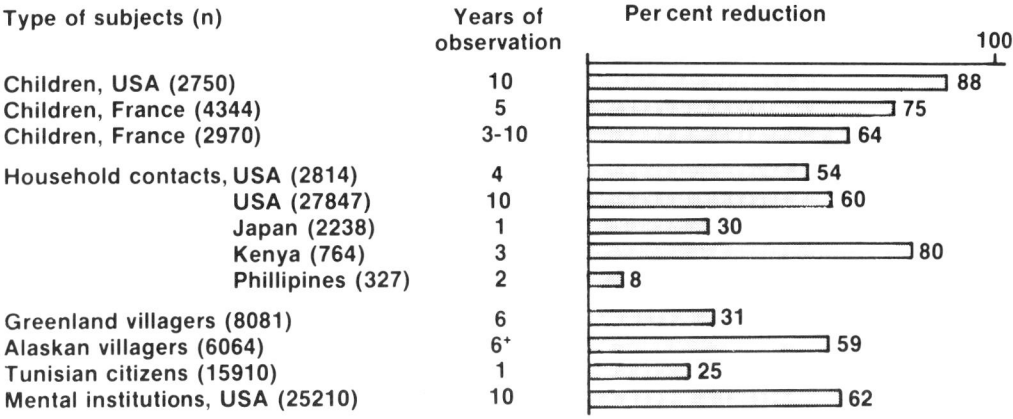

Type of subjects (n)	Years of observation	Per cent reduction
Children, USA (2750)	10	88
Children, France (4344)	5	75
Children, France (2970)	3-10	64
Household contacts, USA (2814)	4	54
USA (27847)	10	60
Japan (2238)	1	30
Kenya (764)	3	80
Phillipines (327)	2	8
Greenland villagers (8081)	6	31
Alaskan villagers (6064)	6+	59
Tunisian citizens (15910)	1	25
Mental institutions, USA (25210)	10	62

+Reduction persisted up to 19 years

Figure 4.14. Summary of the results of controlled trials of isoniazid in preventing tuberculosis.[27]

suspected of being infected with HIV.[129] BCG should, however, be withheld from individuals with *symptomatic* HIV-infection.[127]

Chemoprophylaxis

Thirteen INH chemoprophylaxis trials were conducted in seven countries during the 1950s and 1960s, and included some 100 000 participants.[45] The majority of these trials showed a reduction of at least 50 per cent in the number of tuberculosis cases in the treated group (Figure 4.14). Trials showing smaller protective effects were either said to have had inadequate sample sizes or, in the case of the Greenland trial, used inadequate doses of INH.

The conclusion from these studies is that prophylactic treatment of primary tuberculosis can reduce the bacillary burden and thereby decrease the likelihood of reactivation. The beneficial effect of prophylaxis has been shown to last for up to 20 years in the United States and is presumed to be for the lifetime of the individual.[42]

In the South African setting, prophylaxis can only be realistically considered for children, since the prevalence of infection in adults is generally too high for routine prophylaxis to be feasible. There are two important questions regarding the feasibility of prophylaxis — (i) can the infected child be reliably identified? and (ii) once treated, will the child be susceptible to reinfection?

Identification of infection

There are problems with both sensitivity and specificity of the tuberculin skin test. Eleven per cent of infected schoolchildren will be falsely classified as uninfected as a result of various host factors that cause a reaction of less than 15 mm, and 10 per cent of uninfected school entrants will show a positive reaction due to BCG given at birth.[93] By the age of 11 the 'false' positive rate increases to 25 per cent because of BCG given on school entry. Whilst careful interpretation of tuberculin reactions to find appropriate cut-off points is useful at the population level, there will inevitably be at least 10 per cent misclassification at the individual level due to the overlap of the upper limit of BCG reactions and the lower limit of tuberculosis reactions. In a mass chemoprophylaxis programme there is the risk that a high proportion of infected

Table 4.8
Potential effects of misclassification in allocating 10 000 5–15 year old children for prophylactic treatment on the basis of Mantoux test results[93]

	INFECTED		
	Yes	No	
MANTOUX ≥15 mm	1 350	150	1 500
MANTOUX <15 mm	935	7 565	8 500
	2 285	7 715	10 000

1 350/2 285 (59 per cent) of the infected children are CORRECTLY IDENTIFIED by the Mantoux test.
935/2 285 (41 per cent) of the infected children are MISSED by the Mantoux test (false negatives).
150/7 715 (2 per cent) of the uninfected children would be INCORRECTLY IDENTIFIED as infected and GIVEN TREATMENT UNNECESSARILY (false positives).

children (41 per cent) will be missed because of the poor sensitivity of the skin test (Table 4.8).

Exogenous reinfection

There has been considerable debate over the years as to whether adult tuberculosis is the result of the reactivation of a childhood infection or the result of recent infection. Some argue that reinfection is rare,[25, 62, 100] whereas others claim it is common, particularly in high prevalence areas.[108, 119] Locally, the TBRI has demonstrated that INH-resistant infections are equally common in the elderly as in the young.[70] Many of these older people would have been infected before the introduction of INH, so at least some of their present infections must be due to reinfection. This debate has produced two opposing schools of thought as to whether prophylaxis will ultimately have a significant impact on the course of the epidemic.[34, 98, 109]

In the United States the results of the various prophylaxis trials have been taken as being a strong indication for widespread implementation of prophylactic treatment for all recent tuberculin converters. However, hepatotoxicity of INH for persons over 35 years may be a problem.[27, 118] As a result, the American Thoracic Society and the Centers for Disease Control formally recommended an INH prophylaxis programme for household contacts, newly infected persons and tuberculin skin test reactors under 35 years of age.[2]

There is certainly a wealth of evidence to show that prophylaxis prevents disease, but the major argument against a general campaign in a high prevalence area like South Africa is the heavy demand for limited resources which might be better utilized for case-finding, case-holding and treatment. Despite this it can be argued that the risks of adverse effects from chemoprophylaxis in young people are minimal and are outweighed by the possibility of preventing some cases of tuberculosis. The South African National Tuberculosis Association has been providing prophylactic treatment for large numbers of schoolchildren over the past few years, and this intervention is currently being evaluated in a randomized controlled trial run by the Centre for Epidemiological Research of the Medical Research Council (MRC).

Effects of HIV on the control programme

Active TB has been seen to occur earlier in the natural history of HIV infection than other opportunistic infections (such as *Pneumocystis carinii* pneumonia and

Mycobacterium avium complex) which are commonly part of the clinical manifestations of AIDS.[66] Consequently many people will present first to a tuberculosis facility and might have their HIV infection overlooked if a high index of suspicion for HIV is not maintained.

In addition, it has been suggested that tuberculosis may accelerate the progression of HIV infection to AIDS.[128] The implications of this for infection control are considerable, especially in those areas where streptomycin injections are still given with reusable syringes and where the Heaf gun is routinely used for initial screening. Disposable equipment and suitable sterilizing agents are available but both cost and supply will present problems in many developing countries.

Established diagnostic procedures may have to be reviewed as many HIV positive patients will be anergic, thus rendering the tuberculin skin test less useful as an initial screening device. Recent guidelines from the United States suggest accepting a 5 mm Mantoux reaction as positive in the HIV-infected individual and continuing preventive therapy for 12 months.[17] Much work still needs to be done to determine appropriate guidelines for the diagnosis and management of tuberculosis in HIV-infected persons.

ACKNOWLEDGEMENTS

The authors wish to thank Professor G W Comstock and Dr H L Rieder for helpful input to this chapter and to Drs D Yach and C Metcalf for suggestions which contributed to earlier drafts.

REFERENCES

1 Almeida F & Almeida J M, 1964. Relation between degree of tuberculin sensitivity and prevalence of tuberculosis. *Bulletin of the World Health Organization.* 30, 519–28.

2 American Thoracic Society and Centers for Disease Control, 1986. Treatment of tuberculosis and tuberculosis infection in adults and children. *American Review of Respiratory Diseases.* 4(2), 355–63.

3 Andrew K, 1989. Prevalence of HIV I and II seropositivity in groups of healthy individuals and patients in Sierra Leone. *Paper presented at IEA African Regional Conference, Harare, August 1989.*

4 Aoki M, Mori T & Shimao T, 1982. Studies of factors influencing patients', doctors' and total delay of tuberculosis case-detection in Japan. *Paper presented at 25th World Conference on TB and Respiratory Disease, Buenos Aires, 1982.*

5 Bell J & Yach D, 1988. Tuberculosis patient compliance in the western Cape. *South African Medical Journal.* 73, 31–3.

6 Benatar S R, 1982. Tuberculosis in the 1980s with particular reference to South Africa. *South African Medical Journal.* 62, 359–64

7 Benenson A S (ed.), 1985. *Control of Communicable Diseases in Man.* 14th ed.

8 Bleiker M A & Styblo K, 1978. The annual tuberculosis infection rate and its trend in developing countries. *Bulletin of the International Union Against Tuberculosis.* 53, 295–307.

9 Bloch A B, Rieder H L, Kelly G D, Cauthen G M, Hayden C H & Snider D E, 1989. The epidemiology of tuberculosis in the United States. Implications for diagnosis and treatment. *Clinics in Chest Medicine.* 10(3), 297–313.

10 Braun M M, Truman B I, Maguire B *et al.*, 1989. Increasing incidence of tuberculosis in a prison population — association with HIV infection. *Journal of the American Medical Association.* 261, 393–7.

11 Burney P G & Sittampalam Y, 1984. The social parameters of tuberculous infection among children in the Transkei. *Tropical Geographical Medicine.* 36(1), 37–43.

12 Cartwright J D. BCG vaccination of the newborn. *South African Medical Journal.* 54, 65–67.

13 Cathebras P, Vohito J A, Yete M L *et al.*, 1988. Tuberculose et infection par le virus de l'immunodeficience humaine en Republique Centrafricaine. *Medecine tropicale.* 48(4), 401–7.

14 Centers for Disease Control, 1986. Tuberculosis and acquired immunodeficiency syndrome — Florida. *MMWR.* 35, 587–90.

15 Centers for Disease Control, 1987. Tuberculosis and AIDS – Connecticut. *MMWR.* 36, 133–5.

16 Centers for Disease Control, 1989. Advisory committee for elimination of tuberculosis. Tuberculosis and human immunodeficiency virus infection. *MMWR.* 38, 236–50.

17 Centers for Disease Control, 1990. Screening for tuberculosis and tuberculous infection in high-risk populations and the use of preventive therapy for tuberculous infection in the United States. Recommendations of the Advisory Committee for Elimination of Tuberculosis. *MMWR.* 39 (No. RR–8), 1–12.

18 Coetzee L, Fourie P B, & Viljoen M J, 1986. A simple model for establishing the association between BCG scar status and the risk of tuberculosis in child contacts of adult tuberculotics. *Curationis.* 9(1), 25–9.

19 Coetzee N, Yach D & Joubert G, 1988. Crowding and alcohol abuse as risk factors for tuberculosis in the Mamre population, results of a case-control study. *South African Medical Journal.* 74, 352–4.

20 Colebunders R L, Ryder R W, Nzilambi N *et al.,* 1989. HIV infection in patients with tuberculosis in Kinshasa, Zaire. *American Review of Respiratory Disease.* 139(5), 1082–5.

21 Collie A, 1987. Extrapulmonary tuberculosis in the Republic of South Africa with special reference to the western Cape health region. *Epidemiological Comments.* 14(9), 2–20.

22 Collie A & Küstner H G V, 1989. The Tuberculosis Control Programme, 1985–6. *South African Medical Journal.* 76, 676–80.

23 Collins T F B, 1981. Applied epidemiology and logic in tuberculosis control. *South African Medical Journal.* 59, 566–9.

24 Collins T F B, 1982. The history of southern Africa's first tuberculosis epidemic. *South African Medical Journal.* 62, 780–8.

25 Collins T F B, 1984. Will SANTA'S new project succeed? *SANTA News.* 23 (11), 4–5.

26 Collins T F B, 1990. Ultra-short course preventive treatment for children. *SANTA News.* Jan. 1990, 5–6.

27 Comstock G W, 1981. Evaluating preventive therapy: The need for more data. *Annals of International Medicine.* 94, 817–9.

28 Comstock G W, 1982. Epidemiology of tuberculosis. *American Review of Respiratory Diseases.* 125, 8–15.

29 Comstock G W, 1986. Tuberculosis — a bridge to chronic disease epidemiology. *American Journal of Epidemiology.* 124, 1–16.

30 Comstock G W & Edwards P Q, 1979. The competing risks of tuberculosis and hepatitis for adult tuberculin reactors. *American Review of Respiratory Diseases.* 3, 573–7.

31 Comstock G W, Livesay V T & Woolport S F, 1974. The prognosis of a positive tuberculin reaction in childhood and adolescence. *American Journal of Epidemiology.* 99(2), 131–8.

32 Comstock G W & Palmer C E, 1966. Longterm results of BCG vaccination in the southern United States. *American Review of Respiratory Diseases.* 93, 171–83.

33 Conradie H H, 1983. Evaluation of compliance to tuberculosis outpatient treatment in the Hewu district of Ciskei, 1983–6. *TBRI Symposium on Tuberculosis in Southern Africa, May 1987.*

34 Crawford J T, Eisenach K D & Bates J H, 1989. Diagnosis of tuberculosis, present and future. *Seminars in Respiratory Infections.* 4(3), 171–81.

35 Deeny J E, Walker M J, Kibel M A, Molteno C D & Arens L J, 1985. Tuberculous meningitis in children in the western Cape. *South African Medical Journal.* 68, 75–8.

36 Department of National Health & Population Development, 1984. A rise of tuberculosis among coloureds. *Epidemiological Comments.* 11(5), 1–43.

37 Department of National Health & Population Development, 1990. Tuberculosis Control Programme — 1988. *Epidemiological Comments.* 17(1), 3–13.

38 Director General of Health, 1982. *Guide to the Use of Tuberculosis and Immunization Statistics Forms.* Circular 22 of 1982. Pretoria: Department of National Health and Population Development.

39 Dormer B A, 1952. Procedures in the control of tuberculosis. *South African Medical Journal.* 93–6.

40 Dormer B A & Wiles F J, 1946. Tuberculosis in the Bantu. *South African Medical Journal.* 262–5.

41 Edwards L B, Livesay V T & Acquaviva F A, 1971. Height, weight, tuberculous infection and tuberculous disease. *Archives of Environmental Health.* 22, 106–12.

42 Farer L S, 1982. Chemoprophylaxis. *American Review of Respiratory Diseases.* 125 (3 part 2), 102.

43 Fayers P M & Barnett G C, 1975. TSRU Report No 3. The risk of tuberculous infection in Saskatchewan. *Bulletin of the International Union Against Tuberculosis.* 62–9.

44 Felten M K & Kahler R, 1987. Estimated rates of 'relapse' and 'failure' in tuberculosis hospitals. *TBRI Symposium Against Tuberculosis in Southern Africa, May 1987.*

45 Ferebee S H, 1970. Controlled trials in tuberculosis, a general review. *Advances in Tuberculosis Research.* 17, 28–106.

46 Fine P E M, 1989. The BCG story, lessons from the past and implications for the future. *Reviews of Infectious Diseases.* (Suppl. 2) 353–9.

47 Fourie P B, 1983. The prevalence and annual rate of tuberculosis infection in South Africa. *Tubercle.* 64, 181–92.

48 Fourie P B, 1989. BCG vaccination and the EPI. *South African Medical Journal.* 72, 323–6.

49 Fourie P B, Gatner E M S, Glatthaar E & Kleeberg H H, 1980. Follow-up TB prevalence survey of the Transkei. *Tubercle.* 61, 71–9.

50 Fourie P B & Knoetze K, 1984. Random sample survey of tuberculosis prevalence in Ciskei, 1984. *Tuberculosis Research Institute Report 8512.*

51 Fourie P B & Knoetze K, 1986. Tuberculosis prevalence and risk of infection in southern Africa. *South African Journal of Science.* 82, 387.

52 Fourie P B & Zeelie S, 1984. *Third Survey of TB Prevalence in Transkei 1982.* TBRI Epidemiology Section (unpublished).

53 Fox W, 1983. Compliance of patients and physicians, experience and lessons from tuberculosis — I. *British Medical Journal.* 287, 33–5.

54 Fox W, 1983. Compliance of patients and physicians, experience and lessons from tuberculosis — II. *British Medical Journal.* 287, 101–5.

55 Fox W, 1988. Tuberculosis case-finding and treatment programmes in the developing countries. *British Medical Bulletin.* 44(3) 717–37.

56 Friedman L N, Sullivan G M, Bevilagua R P & Loscos R, 1987. Tuberculosis screening in alcoholics and drug addicts. *American Review of Respiratory Diseases.* 136, 1188–92.

57 Glatthaar E, 1982. Tuberculosis control in South Africa — 'Where have we gone wrong?' and 'A look at the future.' *South African Medical Journal.* 62, 36–41.

58 Greefhuyzen J & Freidman I, 1973. Tuberculosis notwithstanding BCG vaccination. *South African Medical Journal.* 49, 1706–8.

59 Griffiths M L, Makgothi M M & Nordesjo G, 1981. Tuberculosis management in a rural community — factors in failure. *South African Medical Journal.* 59, 14–6.

60 Grigg E R N, 1958. The arcana of tuberculosis – with a brief epidemiologic history of the disease in the USA. Parts I and II. *American Review of Tuberculosis.* 78, 151–72.

61 Gryzbowski S, 1980. Epidemiology of tuberculosis and the role of BCG. *Clinical Chest Medicine.* 1, 175–87.

62 Grzybowski S, 1983. Tuberculosis, A look at the world situation. *Chest.* 84, 756–61.

63 Grzybowski S, Barnett G D & Styblo K, 1975. Contacts of active pulmonary tuberculosis. *Bulletin of the International Union Against Tuberculosis.* 50, 90–106.

64 Hinman A R, Judd J M, Kolnik J P & Daitch P B, 1976. Changing risks in tuberculosis. *American Journal of Epidemiology.* 103, 486–97.

65 Hoerwitz O, 1973. Disease, cure and death, epidemiologic and clinical parameters for chronic diseases illustrated by a model-tuberculosis. *American Journal of Epidemiology.* 97, 148–59.

66 Hopewell P, 1989. Tuberculosis and human immunodeficiency virus infection. *Seminars in Respiratory Infections* 4(2), 111–22.

67 Indian Council of Medical Research, 1980. Tuberculosis prevention trial, Madras, trial of BCG vaccines in South India for tuberculosis prevention. *Indian Journal of Medical Research.* 72, suppl., 1–74.

68 Jacobs M, Coetzee G J, Fisher S, Yach D & Kibel M, 1987. Management of children with tuberculosis in a local authority of Cape Town. *Second TBRI Symposium on Tuberculosis in Southern Africa, Cape Town, 1987.*

69 Kleeberg H H, 1982. The dynamics of tuberculosis in South Africa and the impact of the control programme. *South African Medical Journal.* 62, 22–3.

70 Kleeberg H H, 1986. TB bacteriology and the laboratory situation. *South African Journal of Science.* 82, 394–5.

71 Kumar R, Saran M, Verma B L & Srivastava R N, 1984. Pulmonary tuberculosis among contacts of patients with tuberculosis in an urban Indian population. *Journal of Epidemiology and Community Health.* 38, 253–8.

72 Küstner H G V, 1979. Trends in four major communicable diseases. *South African Medical Journal.* 55, 460–73.

73 Legg W, Mahari M, Houston S *et al.*, 1989. Association of tuberculosis and HIV infection in

Zimbabwe. *Paper presented at IEA African Regional Conference, Harare, August 1989.*

74 Medical Officer of Health of the City of Cape Town, 1903. *Annual Report.*

75 Medical Officer of Health of the City of Cape Town, 1986. *Annual Report.*

76 Mets T, Ngedenahayo P, van de Perre P & Mutwewingabo A, 1989. HIV infection and tuberculosis in central Africa. *New England Journal of Medicine.* 321(8), 542–3.

77 Myers J E, 1986. Tuberculosis screening in industry. *South African Medical Journal.* 70, 251–2.

78 Nair S S, Ramnathrao G & Chandrashekar P, 1971. Distribution of tuberculosis infection and disease in clusters of rural households. *Indian Journal of Tuberculosis.* 18, 3–9.

79 Nkowane B, 1989. Epidemiology and control of AIDS in Africa. *Paper presented at IEA African Regional Conference, Harare, August 1989.*

80 Nyboe J, 1957. Interpretation of tuberculosis infection age curves. *Bulletin of the World Health Organization.* 17, 319–39.

81 Packard R M, 1989. *White Plague, Black Labor. Tuberculosis and the Political Economy of Health and Disease in South Africa.* Berkeley: University of California Press.

82 Palmer C E, Jablon S & Edwards Q, 1957. Tuberculosis morbidity of young men in relation to tuberculin sensitivity and body build. *American Review of Tuberculosis.* 76, 517–39.

83 Paul R, 1961. Silicosis in northern Rhodesia copper miners. *Archives of Environmental Health.* 2, 96–109.

84 Reichman L B & O'Day R, 1978. Tuberculous infection in a large urban population. *American Review of Respiratory Diseases.* 117, 705–12.

85 Rieder H L, Cauthen G M, Comstock G W & Snider D E, 1989. Epidemiology of tuberculosis in the United States. *Epidemiological Review.* 11, 79–98.

86 Rieder H L, Cauthen G M, Kelly G D, Bloch A B & Snider D E, 1989. Tuberculosis in the United States. *Journal of the American Medical Association.* 262, 385–9.

87 Saunders L D, Irwig L M, Wilson T D, Kahn A & Groeneveld H, 1984. Tuberculosis management in Soweto. *South African Medical Journal.* 66, 330–42.

88 Seager J R, 1984. X-ray case-finding in tuberculosis. *Tuberculosis Research Institute Bulletin.* 5(1), 9–13.

89 Seager J R, 1986. Health education in TB hospitals. *South African Journal of Science.* 82, 388–9.

90 Seager J R, 1986. Is active case-finding an effective TB control measure? *South African Journal of Science.* 82, 389.

91 Seager J R, 1989. *Project Screen Ravensmead.* Cape Town: CERSA, Medical Research Council (unpublished).

92 Seager J R, Felten M K, Collins T F B & Kerr J, 1987. Screening of successfully treated tuberculosis patients for signs of chronic respiratory failure. *Paper presented at the 2nd TBRI Symposium on Tuberculosis in Southern Africa, Cape Town, 1987.*

93 Seager J R, Fourie P B, Kleeberg H H & Felten M K, 1985. Is preventive treatment of schoolchildren worthwhile? *SANTA News.* 24 (4), 4–5.

94 Seager J R, Schoeman J H, Wilkinson I S & Westaway M S, 1987. An attempt to optimize tuberculosis case finding by identifying high risk socio-economic groups. *Second TBRI Symposium on Tuberculosis in Southern Africa, Cape Town, 1987.*

95 Seager J R, Strebel P M & Joubert G, 1990. *A Century of Tuberculosis Control in South Africa: the Epidemic Continues.* Ninth Epidemiological Conference, East London.

96 Selwyn P A, Hartel D, Lewis V A *et al.*, 1989. A prospective study of the risk of tuberculosis among intravenous drug users with human immunodeficiency virus infection. *New England Journal of Medicine.* 320, 545–50.

97 Slutkin G, Leowski J & Mann J, 1989. Tuberculosis and AIDS. The effects of the AIDS epidemic on the tuberculosis problem and tuberculosis programmes. *Bulletin of the International Union Against Tuberculosis.* 63(2), 21–4.

98 Smith M H D & Teele D W, 1989. Perinatal tuberculosis. In: Remington J S & Klein J O (eds): *Infectious Diseases of the Fetus and Newborn Infant.* 3rd ed. Philadelphia: W B Saunders & Co.

99 Snider D E Jr, 1978. The relationship between tuberculosis and silicosis. *American Review of Respiratory Diseases.* 118, 455–60.

100 Standaert B, Niragira F, Kadenda P & Piot P, 1989. The association of tuberculosis and HIV infection in Burundi. *AIDS Research into Human Retroviruses.* 5(2), 247–51.

101 Stead W W, 1967. Pathogenesis of a first episode of chronic pulmonary tuberculosis in man, recrudescence of the residuals of the primary infection or exogenous reinfection. *American Review of Respiratory Diseases.* 95, 729–45.

102 Stead W W, Senner J W, Reddick W T & Lofgren J P, 1990. Racial differences in susceptibility to infection by Mycobacterium tuberculosis. *New England Journal of Medicine.* 322 (7), 422–7.

103 Steyn M, 1988. *Evaluering van die Tuberkulose Motiverings – Voorligtingsprogram onder Swartes in Geselekteerde Gebiede.* Pretoria: Human Sciences Research Council, Pretoria.

104 Stolz A P, Donald P R, Strebel P M & Talent J M T, 1990. Criteria for the notification of childhood tuberculosis in a high-incidence area of the western Cape Province. *South African Medical Journal.* 77, 385–6.

105 Stott H, Patel A, Sutherland I, Thorup I, Smith P G, Kent P W & Rykushin T P, 1973. The risk of tuberculosis infection in Uganda, derived from findings of national tuberculin surveys in 1958 and 1970. *Tubercle.* 54, 1–22.

106 Strebel P M, Kuhn L & Yach D, 1989. Smoking practices in the black township population of Cape Town. *South African Medical Journal.* 75, 428–31.

107 Styblo K, 1976. Surveillance of tuberculosis. *International Journal of Epidemiology.* 5, 63–8.

108 Styblo K, 1978. Epidemiology of tuberculosis. *Bulletin of the International Union Against Tuberculosis.* 53, 141–52.

109 Styblo K, 1980. Recent advances in epidemiological research in tuberculosis. *Advances in Tuberculosis Research.* 20, 1–63.

110 Styblo K, 1989. The potential impact of AIDS on the tuberculosis situation in developed and developing countries. *Bulletin of the International Union Against Tuberculosis.* 63 (2), 25–8.

111 Styblo K, 1989. Overview and epidemiologic assessment of the current global tuberculosis situation with an emphasis on control in developing countries. *Review of Infectious Diseases.* 11, suppl. 2, 339–46.

112 Styblo K & Meijer J, 1976. Impact of BCG vaccination programmes in children and young adults on the tuberculosis problem. *Tubercle.* 57, 17–43.

113 Styblo K, Meijer J & Sutherland I, 1969. TSRU report no. 1 — the transmission of tubercle bacilli. Its trend in a human population. *Bulletin of the International Union on Tuberculosis.* 42, 5–104.

114 Sutherland I, 1976. Recent studies in the epidemiology of tuberculosis, based on the risk of being infected with tubercle bacilli. *Advances in Tuberculosis Research.* 19, 1–63.

115 Sutherland I & Fayers P M, 1975. The association of the risk of tuberculous infection with age. *Bulletin of the International Union Against Tuberculosis.* 50, 70–81.

116 Sutherland I, Styblo K, Sampalik M & Bleiker M A, 1971. Annual risk of tuberculous infection in 14 countries derived from the results of tuberculin surveys in 1948–1952. *Bulletin of the International Union of Tuberculosis.* 45, 75–114.

117 *Symposium on Tuberculosis in the Western Cape Regional Services Council Area, April 22, 1988.*

118 Taylor W C, Aronson M D & Delbanco T L, 1981. Should young adults with a positive tuberculin test take isoniazid? *Annals of International Medicine.* 94, 808–13.

119 Ten Dam H G & Pio A, 1982. Pathogenesis of tuberculosis and effectiveness of BCG vaccination. *Tubercle.* 63, 225–33.

120 Toman K, 1979. *Tuberculosis Case-finding and Chemotherapy.* Geneva: World Health Organization.

121 Tverdal A, 1986. Body mass index and incidence of tuberculosis. *European Journal of Respiratory Diseases.* 69, 355–62.

122 Union of South Africa, 1914. *Report of the Tuberculosis Commission of 1914.* Cape Town: Cape Times.

123 Van Geuns H A, Meijer J & Styblo K, 1975. Results of contact examination in Rotterdam 1967–69. *Bulletin of the International Union Against Tuberculosis.* 50, 107–21.

124 Weyer K & Fourie P B, 1989. Die epidemiologie van tuberkulose in Suider-Afrika. *Continuing Medical Education.* 7, 239–47.

125 World Health Organization, 1963. The WHO standard tuberculin test. *WHO/TB Technical Guide No 3.* Geneva, World Health Organization.

126 World Health Organization, 1980. BCG vaccination policies. *WHO Technical Report Series.* 652, 1–17.

127 World Health Organization, 1987. Statement from consultation on human immunodeficiency virus (HIV) and routine childhood immunisation. *Weekly Epidemiological Record.* 62, 297–9.

128 World Health Organization/IUATLD, 1989. Tuberculosis and AIDS. Statement on AIDS and tuberculosis. *Bulletin of the International Union Against Tuberculosis.* 64(1), 8–11.

129 World Health Organization/UNICEF, 1989. Statement on early immunization for HIV-infected children. *Weekly Epidemiological Record.* 64, 48–9.

130 Wulfsohn M, Küstner H G V, 1985. Epidemiology of tuberculosis. *Epidemiological Comments.* 12(9), 1–19.

131 Yach D, 1987. Tuberculosis deaths in South Africa (1980). *South African Medical Journal.* 72, 149–51.

132 Yach D, Hoffmann M & van Herzeele, A, 1988. Compliance of local authorities in the western Cape to the national regimen. *South African Medical Journal.* 73, 33–5.

133 Youngelson S M, 1988. Measuring patient compliance in the treatment of pulmonary tuberculosis in Cape Town — pitfalls in study design. *South African Medical Journal.* 73, 28–30.

134 Yu G, Hsieh C, Peng J, 1989. Risk factors associated with the prevalence of pulmonary tuberculosis among sanitary workers in Shanghai. *Tubercle.* 69, 105–12.

CHAPTER 5

Tuberculosis in children

H M Coovadia

DIFFERENCES BETWEEN TUBERCULOSIS IN RICH AND POOR COUNTRIES

Researchers have pointed out the similarities between tuberculosis in present-day developing countries and the disease in nineteenth century Europe — similarities in prevalence patterns, clinical disease, hypersensitivity phenomena and association with malnutrition.[19] This is not surprising given the likeness in social conditions.

Clinically, the onset of the primary complex usually goes unnoticed, although acute pneumonic signs have occasionally been noted to herald this initial infection. These overt manifestations were said to have been more frequent in the United States in the early part of this century,[16] but this is probably due to the fact that minor signs were more thoroughly examined there than to any real difference in disease.

The size of the primary lesion is bigger in tropical countries, while progression of the primary lesions in the lung parenchyma and regional lymph nodes to caseation necrosis is more likely to occur among disadvantaged children; the degree of caseation, cavitation, and extent of segmental lung lesions being more pronounced in the latter than in better-off children. This is a predictable outcome given the larger exposure of children in developing countries to the immunosuppressive effects of malnutrition and other infectious diseases. These diseases lead to a failure of immunological containment of the primary lesion. For the same reasons, multiple lesions are more common, and quiescent foci of tuberculosis are more often reactivated among poor children than those in industrialized temperate countries. It must be remembered, however, that in any situation, reactivation TB is rare in children.

Tuberculin tests, as an index of underlying TB, are less often helpful in developing countries because of secondary immunodeficiencies. Skin sensitivity is more reliable and positive in developed countries.

Hypersensitivity phenomena are relatively uncommon in developing countries, but paradoxically phlyctenular conjunctivitis is said to occur frequently in industrialized countries and also where protein-energy-malnutrition (PEM) is common. It is not an association which has been particularly prominent in the author's experience in Durban, nor is erythema nodosum seen there with any regularity, but phlyctens were seen in ten per cent of untreated cases in the United States in the first half of this century.[16] Hypersensitivity reactions causing effusions from serous surfaces (pleura, peritoneum) are said to be more frequent in developed countries, but these complications may also occur as a result of invasive infection. Probably for these reasons such effusions are not uncommon in South African blacks.

The severest forms of tuberculosis, such as meningitis and cerebral tuberculomata, are rare in the developed world but much more likely to arise as complications in poorer countries. The same applies to peritoneal effusion due to TB abdomen, pericarditis, and clinically evident involvement of the liver and spleen. Choroidal tubercles have been detected with varying degrees of frequency in Europe and the United States. However, they are extremely rare in South Africa and careful fundoscopic searches have failed to reveal tubercles even in cases of miliary tuberculosis. Lymph node enlargement is greater in developing countries. Upper cervical lymphadenopathy may be part of the primary complex, lesions in the mouth accounting for this nodal involvement having been detected more often in the United States when TB was prevalent than at other times.[16] In tropical countries Addison's disease is frequently due to TB among adults, but this is rarely the case in temperate zones. It goes without saying that TB is often an accompaniment of PEM, especially kwashiorkor and marasmus, in South Africa.

In summary, the combination of early primary infection due to overcrowding and poverty and the immunodeficiencies caused by malnutrition and repeated childhood infections increases exposure and decreases both protective host responses to TB and hypersensitivity reactions. These factors account for the differences noted above between tuberculosis in rich and poor countries.

DIFFERENCES BETWEEN CHILD-HOOD AND ADULT TUBERCULOSIS

There are easily noticeable differences in clinical features between children and adults with tuberculosis, and there are a number of reasons for these differences. In children the disease is usually the result of first contact with *Mycobacterium tuberculosis* when the immunological apparatus is naive and unprimed; in adults, TB is most often due to the reactivation of a previously dormant infection which is confronted by immune cells prepared to react by prior sensitization to the microbe. The mechanisms for resistance are relatively less well developed in pre-school children, especially in infants, and there are more opportunities for greater exposure to larger burdens of the infecting organism at this age. This leads to more serious disease than in adulthood. Feeding practices by infected parents may also expose young babies to the dangers of inhaling or swallowing expectorated material. The transition from dormancy to reactivation is initiated by certain immuno-suppressive diseases, chief of which are PEM and measles. These are pre-eminently diseases of infancy and childhood, and therefore they have great importance as aggravating factors during this period.

The natural history of untreated tuberculosis results in some organs being affected soon after infection (lungs, lymph nodes) while others do not become involved until months to years later (kidneys, adrenals). It follows that the latter are less likely to appear in childhood. The maturation of certain tissues such as the breast and uterus renders them vulnerable to disease only after puberty.

For the above reasons blood spread leading to severe disease such as TB meningitis, disseminated TB and miliary TB is more frequently seen in paediatric patients than in adults. Tuberculin tests become positive after a period of temporary suppression, and pulmonary, lymph node and meningeal TB become evident after measles; latent lesions flare up when children develop kwashiorkor or marasmus. A positive tuberculin skin test in pre-school children in the absence of any other evidence of TB often requires isoniazid acid hydrazide (INH) prophylaxis because of the likelihood of malnutrition or infection precipitating overt disease. In adults the chances of such aggravating factors acting are less, but not nil.

In addition to the above, there are other clinical presentations which characterize the disease in childhood. Children have enlarged lymph glands more frequently than do adults, and these often attain larger dimensions. Even when adults develop primary pulmonary TB, the ensuing hilar lymph node growth is less pronounced. Tuberculosis of the tonsils is uncommon at any age but is sometimes seen in adults with pulmonary TB; similarly, infection of the larynx is occasionally noted in adolescents with progressive primary TB. Primary middle ear disease is mostly restricted to infancy, at which time babies are infected during feeding by a mother with TB. Pulmonary lesions are usually apical or sub-apical in adults and adolescents, whereas pneumonia most often occurs in all segments, but particularly in the periphery and in the lower lobes, of the lungs in children. Pleural effusions are infrequent under the age of six years. Bronchial extensions are secondary to lymphadenitis in the young, whereas they are due to leakage of material from cavitating parenchymal lesions in the older age groups. Luminal obstruction of the bronchioles is usually caused through erosion of the bronchial wall by neighbouring glands, but external compression of bronchioles by enlarging glands may rarely also take place in the very young. Genital tuberculosis is usually post-pubertal, salpingitis and uterine TB being evident after puberty. Epididymitis is seen as an isolated lesion in younger boys but occurs as part of an epididymo-orchitis in older boys. Rectal TB and fistula-in-ano are diseases of adults, as is the rare involvement of the myocardium.

Dissimilar immunological behaviour is the reason for children experiencing exudative reactions while older age groups suffer fibrotic lesions — healing of parenchymal and nodal lesions is often by calcification in the former and by fibrosis in the latter.

EVOLUTION OF UNTREATED PRIMARY TUBERCULOSIS[18, 23]

The sequence of events that may occur after an initial infection with *Mycobacterium tuberculosis* which is left untreated is given in Figure 5.1. It reveals the gradual but relentless unfolding of clinical disease with time, some organs such as the lungs being affected early, whilst others like the bones, kidneys and skin are not involved until after a few years.

Figure 5.1. Evolution of untreated primary tuberculosis in children (adapted from references 18, 23)

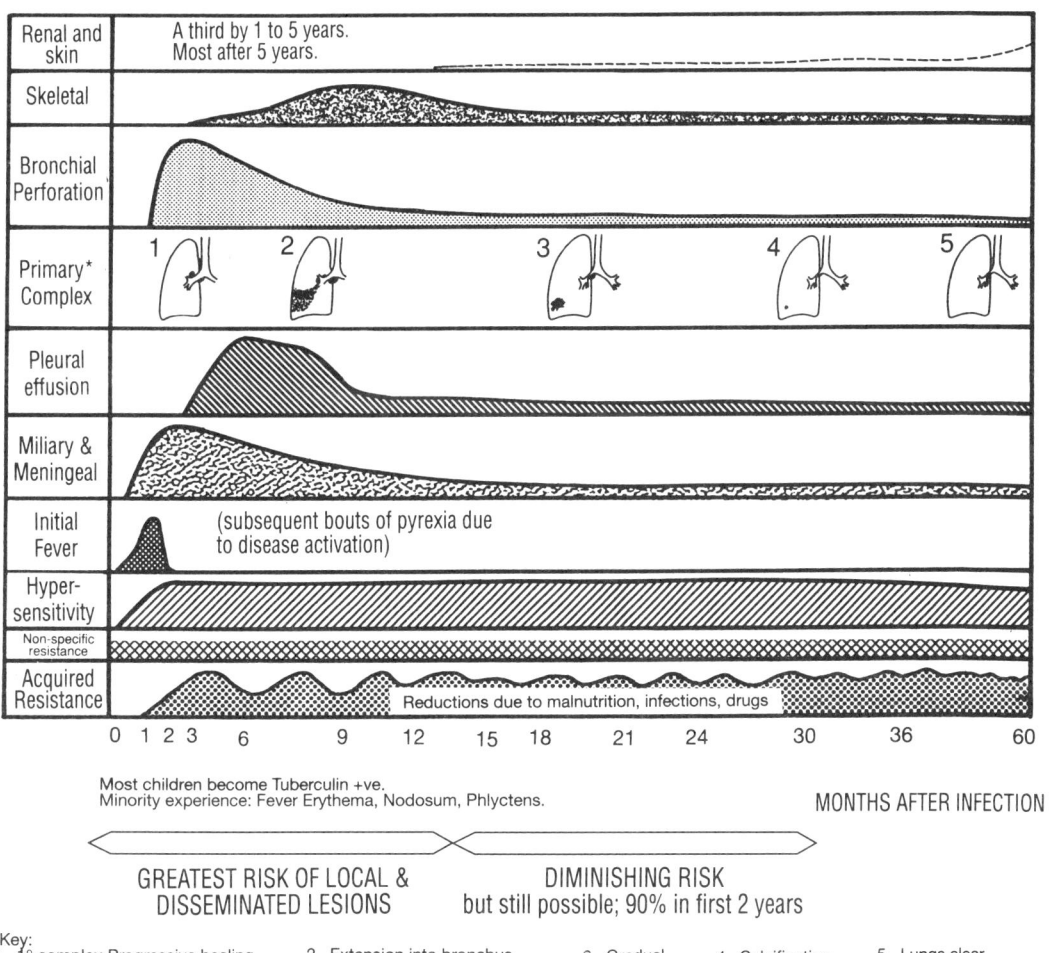

*Key:
1. 1° complex. Progressive healing most cases. Spread from nodes. Ghon focus rarely leads to effusion, cavity, "coin" shadow.
2. Extension into bronchus from node causing consolidation etc.
3. Gradual healing.
4. Calcification may occur.
5. Lungs clear. Calcified lesion reabsorbed.

CONGENITAL TUBERCULOSIS[20,24]

Congenital tuberculosis must be considered when circumstances suggest that infection has passed from a mother to her foetus or newborn baby. Beitzke (1935)[3] had suggested that the minimum requirements for this diagnosis were a demonstrated TB lesion, a primary in the liver, or tubercles in the foetus and uterus after exclusion of all extra-uterine sources of infection. However, these criteria are not useful in the practical situation.

The hormonal and immunological adjustments of pregnancy may lead to reactivation of TB in the mother, which may take many forms — pulmonary, genital, haematogenous, etc. However, the rate of transfer of TB to the foetus is low, even when there is infection of the placenta. Congenital tuberculosis was seen in less than one per thousand cases of TB in the pre-chemotherapeutic era.[16] Abortions or still-births may occur, depending on whether infection is early or late in pregnancy.

Infection may be transmitted by one of three mechanisms: haematogenous spread, through amniotic fluid, or during birth. Bacteraemia in the mother, endometritis or placentitis, result in the spread of organisms through the umbilical vein and ductus venosus. In this case the primary is always in the liver after which there may be dissemination to other organs. Infected amniotic material may be inhaled, swallowed or become lodged at sites such as the ear, this occurring in utero or during birth. The primary focus can be in the lungs with hilar and mediastinal adenopathy, in the oropharynx and abdomen, or in tissues such as the external ear. During birth, amniotic fluid or genital tract infection passes to the baby in a similar manner. Airborne or direct transmission may occur after birth from an infected adult, usually the mother.

There is very little host reaction to *Mycobacterium tuberculosis* in the foetus or newborn, with the result that bacillary growth is high and caseation is marked. Lymphocytes and epithelioid cells are sparse and giant cells uncommon.

Infected babies are usually well at birth with signs gradually developing within a few weeks — the delay in overt disease may be as long as five months. Wasting may be a prominent feature, and the liver is usually enlarged with moderate derangement of liver functions. At least one case has been observed with exuberant lymphadenopathy in the porta hepatis causing obstructive jaundice. In this type of case the differential diagnosis must include the causes of the neonatal hepatitis syndrome or biliary atresia. Pulmonary infection presents with respiratory distress and adventitious sounds in the chest. Large glands in the hilum may cause unilateral partial obstruction to the airways resulting in clinical features mimicking those of congenital lobar emphysema; there is respiratory distress and diminished air entry on the affected side of the chest with the typical radiographic findings of hypertranslucency on the affected side and shift of mediastinum to the opposite lung. Severe congenital disease may present with pallor, lymphadenopathy, skin lesions and meningitis. A subumbilical lymph gland (which usually disappears by eight weeks of age) may enlarge. A white seropurulent ear discharge with pre-auricular lymphadenopathy together with a few enlarged upper cervical glands represents a primary congenital complex in the ear; this may occur as an isolated finding without systemic signs. Occasionally the disease runs a rapidly downhill course resembling acute bacterial septicaemias; this is associated with poor granuloma formation and extensive multiplication of bacilli.

In addition to the conventional investigations for TB, it is useful to seek out the disease in the mother, to examine the placenta for macroscopic and histological lesions in suspicious cases, to culture placental and amniotic fluid material, and occasionally to perform a liver biopsy in the neonate.

INH, rifampicin and ethionamide are given for congenital TB. Response may be slow, with healing by calcification. Prophylactic INH is used for asymptomatic babies born of infected mothers; BCG should be administered under these conditions. The alternative is to give prophylactic INH for six weeks and then to perform a tuberculin test on the baby; if the test is negative, BCG can be given and INH discontinued.

RESPIRATORY SYSTEM

Primary complex

The incubation period of between two and eight weeks is not revealed by overt clinical features; it is a time of silent bacterial growth, occult haematogenous dissemination of a few bacilli to distant body sites and the gradual emergence of sensitization to mycobacterial antigens. The tissues seeded in this early spread, such as the spleen, liver, lymph glands, skin and apices of the lung, may show clinically evident signs at a later stage (8 to 14 weeks after onset of infection). The apices of the lung may subsequently demonstrate calcified lesions arising from such early spread (Simon's foci).

The primary complex is usually asymptomatic, but a short-lasting pyrexia and erythema nodosum have been noted among a proportion of well-nourished pre-school children. The lung is the site of the primary complex in the vast majority of tuberculous infections, with lymphadenitis being the hallmark; extrapulmonary primary infection is uncommon. Autopsy data from work done by Ghon and Kuedlich is quoted as showing the lungs as a portal of entry in 95,93 per cent of children with TB; the bowel in 1,14 per cent; skin in 0,14 per cent; tonsils, nose and middle ear 0,09 per cent each; and eye and parotid 0,05 per cent each.[23] The majority of primary infections are initiated by a single focus. The primary complex resolves in most instances, but the lesion which fails to clear causes pulmonary disease. There may be an acute pneumonic onset with respiratory distress followed by quiescence with an absence of symptoms and signs. This is succeeded by increasing lassitude, low grade fever, loss of weight and an insidious deterioration in health. The probability of finding x-ray evidence of a primary complex decreases with age and malnutrition (in the latter, the disease is usually widespread before detection). Most under-five year olds with TB show radiographic changes of a primary complex, and there may be more than one parenchymal lesion. The primary complex affects the right lung more than the left and slowly resolves over many months with appropriate therapy. Resolution may take about six months in the young and twice this period in older children, but it is sooner when rifampicin is used because the drug acts on both continuously multiplying and intermittently active organisms. The end result on treatment is a fibrous scar or almost complete clearing whereas, without treatment, natural resolution leads to healing by calcification. The differential diagnosis rests on consideration of hilar adenopathy with parenchymal lesions. The tuberculin test which becomes positive aids diagnosis.

Intrapulmonary extension (parenchymal, bronchial)

The clinical manifestations of intrapulmonary extension are numerous, encompassing the entire range of physical signs arising from pulmonary disease. They include features of obstructive airways (brassy cough, stridor, wheeze, decreased air entry), emphysema, collapse, bronchopneumonia, consolidation and pleurisy. Fever, cough and loss of weight of two to three months' duration are the usual presenting symptoms. Weight loss, however, precedes the other symptoms. Haemoptysis is unusual and night sweats are rare.

There is local extension of the lesions with increasing lung destruction and regional lymph node enlargement. The major direction of spread of bacilli is from the primary focus in the parenchyma to the hilar lymph nodes; very few mycobacteria remain in the Ghon focus. Therefore local and extrapulmonary progression of infection occurs as a result of leakage of caseous lymph node contents and not from parenchymal lesions.

In rare instances, bacilli remain in significant numbers within the parenchymal lesion of the primary complex. This is analogous to adult onset TB, and has been mainly noted in older children. The lung focus may become smaller and calcify or enlarge and cavitate. Caseous material from such cavities spills into the bronchi and spreads throughout the lungfields; it may also impinge on the pleura and cause pleural disease. The parenchymal lesion is seen as a round focus on chest x-rays. Other diseases to be excluded are staphylococcal and *Haemophilus influenzae* pneumonia, foreign bodies and congenital cysts.

In the vast majority of cases dissemination is from the lymph node; erosion of the wall of the bronchus by an adjacent node results in caseous material being coughed up or inhaled distal to the point of erosion. Segmental lung lesions after the primary complex occur mostly within three months and within a year in 90 per cent of cases.[16] Bronchopneumonic lesions can be segmental, lobar or involve the entire lung. The consequences are consolidation and/or collapse of the lung. Swollen glands may:

- compress the airways causing a brassy cough, stridor or wheeze;
- produce a ball-valve effect resulting in obstructive emphysema;
- occlude airways and cause collapse or consolidation of a lobe (e.g. right middle lobe). As the airways in infants and children are quite flexible, obstruction is rarely by external compression — it is usually caused by erosion;
- interfere with venous return and cause oedema of the hand and arm or a superior mediastinal compression syndrome; vigorous coughing may force glands into the thoracic inlet and obstruct respiration; these glands may be palpated by inserting the fingers behind the manubrium;
- burst into the mediastinum and point in the supraclavicular fossa;
- perforate into the bronchus, discharging caseous material into the peripheral lung causing bronchopneumonia;
- erode into a blood vessel (e.g. the aorta);
- rupture into the pericardial sac;
- result in a pleural effusion;
- compress the left recurrent laryngeal or phrenic nerve, causing hoarseness or elevation of the left hemidiaphragm respectively; or
- press on the oesophagus causing dysphagia; an oesophageal diverticulum may be produced, and rupture can lead to a broncho-oesophageal fistula.

The physical signs depend on the complications listed above. One point needs to be stressed: extensive bilateral broncho-pneumonia may present with mild pyrexia, marked respiratory distress, and few if any adventitious sounds. Mediastinal glands, pleural effusion and calcification are more common in older children; cavitation in younger children.

Pleurisy

A child may present with the physical signs of pleural thickening or effusion; an aspirate reveals blood or a yellow fluid with a reduced glucose content but which is rich in proteins, macrophages and neutrophils. The fluid may be fibrinous and clot. Dissemination to serosal surfaces takes place early on, within three to six months of infection. Pleural tuberculosis is more common in the older child (over six years of age) than in infants, extension occurring from a subpleural focus and occasionally through blood. The right side is affected more often than the left. The visceral and parietal layers of pleura become adherent.

The onset of pleural disease may be insidious, with fever, malaise, and marked pleuritic pain occurring in the context of hypersensitivity phenomena, especially erythema nodosum. This happens when the pleura is the target of allergic reactions. In many children there is no pleuritic pain, and skin tests are negative. It is therefore often difficult to deduce whether pleurisy is allergic or infective in nature. Effusions in interlobar spaces can be detected on chest radiographs. Spontaneous pneumothorax has been recorded as a complication of TB lung disease. When steroids are used in addition to anti-TB drugs the effusions clear in a few weeks.

POST PRIMARY SPREAD

Post primary spread produces miliary TB and meningitis within a year of infection, and bone, joint and kidney lesions some years later. Spread to the lymph glands is common. In addition to local and bronchogenic extension in the lungs there is haematogenous dissemination, due to erosion of a blood vessel by the lymph glands in the primary complex. Bacilli are released into the blood at repeated intervals and this, with seeding into distant tissues may be followed either by slow progression of infection or latency at sites such as the liver, spleen, skin, lymph nodes, bones, joints or kidneys, with subsequent reactivation. Complications can develop one after another if treatment is not instituted. This is disseminated tuberculosis.

A sudden shower of bacilli into a blood vessel with concomitant disease is acute miliary TB, which formed 5,5 per cent of all TB cases among children seen in the King Edward VIII Hospital, Durban. It is the most serious form of tuberculosis.

MILIARY TUBERCULOSIS

The main features of miliary tuberculosis are:

- sudden shower of heavy bacillary load into blood vessel;
- risk higher in under-five year olds;
- usually within six months of infection;
- incidence reduced by BCG;
- spreads from caseating lymph node in lung;
- spread from lung focus causes generalized dissemination; spread from abdominal focus is initially to the liver;
- dissemination leads to innumerable tiny lesions in lungs, meninges, choroid (rare in black children), skin, liver, spleen, and kidney;
- tubercles are usually of similar size;
- child is acutely ill, fever, loss of weight, few or no signs in chest, hepato-splenomegaly, lymph nodes enlarge, may be signs of meningitis (in about 25 per cent of cases);
- chest x-ray: 'snowstorm' — tubercles greater than 1 mm;
- tuberculin test can be negative;
- tubercles on chest x-ray resolve in 6 to 13 weeks of treatment;
- in pre-chemotherapeutic days, all died of meningitis within three months of diagnosis.

The older literature spoke of the rare complication of 'chronic miliary' which followed an acute attack and during which the tubercles seen on chest radiographs were larger and appeared more dense.[16]

REACTIVATION TUBERCULOSIS

An older child or adolescent who presents with a vague illness, cough, fever and weight loss, and who has an opacity or cavity in the apical or subapical zones on chest radiograph, may have reactivation of a previously quiescent focus of TB. This adult-onset type disease accounts for only a small minority of childhood TB. It is more likely if the first infection occurred after the age of seven years, the disease breaking through many months to years after this primary infection. The initial sensitization usually restricts the lesion to the lungs so that extra-pulmonary dissemination is limited. Within the lungs, extension is through bronchogenic or lymphatic spread. Healing on

Table 5.1
Types and frequency of radiological changes seen in pulmonary tuberculosis

	SOUTH AFRICA		NIGERIA[1]
	DURBAN*	JOHANNESBURG[9]	
Mediastinal glands	42%	43%	54%
Pleural effusion	13%	10%	11%
Calcification	2%	8%	2%
Parenchymal lesions:			73%
Segmental lesions	80%	90%	
Cavities	5%	14%	
Miliary	8%	9%	
Primary complex	Unavailable	7%	

* 281 black children seen at the King Edward VIII Hospital, Durban, 1980–6

treatment is by fibrosis, leaving a scar of prior disease. It is often extremely difficult to distinguish the progressive form of TB that follows the primary complex from reactivation disease.

The type and frequency of radiological changes seen in pulmonary TB in black children in South Africa[9] and Nigeria[1] are given in Table 5.1. Lesions occur more often on the right and are usually of multiple types. In the South African study[9] the sites of segmental lesions in order of frequency were: right lower lobe, left lower lobe, left upper lobe, right middle lobe, left lingula.

CORRELATION BETWEEN CLINICAL AND IMMUNO-LOGICAL FEATURES OF TUBERCULOSIS[15]

In common with other chronic bacterial infections (such as leprosy), tuberculosis presents with a range of different clinical entities which are accompanied by a specific pattern of immune responses. At one end there is aggressive cellular immunity with few bacilli in granuloma and restricted clinical manifestations ('reactive' TB); at the opposite pole there is deficient cellular immunity with a high bacterial load and disseminated disease ('unreactive TB'). Antibodies and circulating immune complexes correlate inversely with cellular immunity. As shifts occur from one polar form to the other (due to treatment or the natural history of the disease), the varying concentrations of antigen and antibody give rise to immune complexes which produce hypersensitivity phenomena such as fever, arthritis, pleurisy, erythema nodosum and phlyctenular conjunctivitis (Table 5.2).

During chemotherapy a number of unspecified local immunological reactions are produced by antigen-specific cells sequestered in selected sites. These may result in enlargement of cerebral tuberculomata, an increase in lymph node size and acute respiratory distress.

Table 5.2
The spectrum of human tuberculosis[15]

		REACTIVE	INTERMEDIATE REACTIVE	INTERMEDIATE UNREACTIVE	UNREACTIVE
Clinical:	Pulmonary lesions	Localized small lung lesions	Small and large lung lesions, cavitation	Small and large lung lesions, cavitation	Miliary
	Dissemination	Localized	Localized	Diffuse	Widespread
	Other features		lymph-adenopathy Serositis	lymph-adenopathy Fistulae	
Immunological					
	Cellular immunity:				
	In vivo test:				
	Tuberculin skin test	++++	+±	±	0
	In vitro test:				
	Leucocyte migration inhibition	++++	++	±	0
	Humoral immunity				
	Antibodies to PPD	±	++±	+++±	++++
	Immune complexes	0	+	+++	++++
Bacillary load (in sputum, tissues)		0	±	+++±	++++
Histological changes in lymph node					
	B dependent zones	±	±	++++	±
	T dependent zones	++++	++±	±	0
Response to treatment		Excellent	Good	Modest	Poor

Table 5.3
Clinical types of tuberculosis in black children*

Pulmonary	99,0%
Other respiratory (e.g. pleurisy)	2,5%
Meninges	14,8%
Gastrointestinal (including abdomen)	8,0%
Bones and joints	3,1%
Genito-urinary tract	0,3%
Lymph nodes	44,0%
Miliary	5,5%
Pericardium	0,3%
Erythema nodosum	0,1%
Eyes	1,2%
Ear, nose and throat	1,2%
Endocrine	1,5%

* As found in 328 black children at the King Edward VIII Hospital, Durban, 1985

Table 5.4
Common symptoms in 328 black children with tuberculosis*

Cough	63%
Fever	40%
Vomiting	31%
Diarrhoea	20%
Anorexia	20%
Weight loss	15%
Weakness	10%
Night sweats	9%
Headache	8%
Convulsions	7%

* As seen at the King Edward VIII Hospital, Durban, 1985

Table 5.5
Common physical signs in 328 black children with tuberculosis*

Lymph node enlargement	46%
Hepatomegaly	56%
Respiratory distress	25%
Splenomegaly	13%
Clubbing	4%
Phlyctens	2%

* As seen at the King Edward VIII Hospital, Durban, 1985

Table 5.3 shows the clinical types of tuberculosis found in 328 black children at the King Edward VIII Hospital, Durban.

The types of TB seen in Durban are similar to those reported from other parts of the third world[1, 11, 17] Pulmonary infection usually accounts for more than 80 to 90 per cent of all cases of childhood tuberculosis. The common symptoms and signs seen in hospitalized cases of tuberculosis are given in Tables 5.4 and 5.5. The common causes of death from TB in Durban are shown in Table 5.6.

LYMPH GLANDS

In tuberculosis these are frequently involved at any site in the body as part of the drainage to nodes from a primary focus. These glandular enlargements have been alluded to in the descriptions of disease of different organs, and are involved early on during the tuberculous process. In this section cervical lymphadenopathy is considered. Peripheral lymphadenopathy, which was mainly cervical, has accounted for 21 per cent of hospitalized cases of TB in Durban. The sites of lymph node enlargement seen in Durban are given in Table 5.7

Miller[18] believes that cervical nodes are usually the regional component of a primary complex, while others hold the view that they may result from blood or lymphatic spread. The classical tubercle granulomata in the nodes cause caseation necrosis, periadenitis, adherence to adjacent nodes and skin, and breaks through the skin resulting in sinuses. Those with matted nodes are often tuberculin positive. In other cases, enlargement of one group of nodes extends to other nodes along the lymphatic chain without adherence to the skin or to each other. The first affected node is usually larger than nodes that are subsequently involved. The younger the child, the larger the nodes. Affected nodes may soften and form abscesses which track, may calcify and become hard; may regress; or may lie dormant for years and then become active once again. It follows that the consistency and adherence of tuberculous lymph nodes varies according to the stage of the disease.

Cervical lymph nodes are more commonly enlarged than any other group. A child with TB cervical nodes may appear surprisingly well; illness often accompanies extension to other sites. Anterior cervical nodes are more often felt than posterior cervical nodes. Submental and submandibular nodes are rarely enlarged; they drain the gums and periodontal tissues. Supraclavicular lymph nodes (detected in 21 per cent of cases of pulmonary TB in Nigeria[1]) are always indicative of some serious underlying disease and are usually unilateral; they accompany mediastinal adenopathy and are evidence of pleural, pulmonary or abdominal disease. A lymph node in the anterior midline of the neck may be mistaken for a thyroglossal cyst.

The neck is the most common site of nodal tuberculosis for a number of reasons: glands may be the regional component of a primary focus, the neck is rich in lymphatics; and repeated upper respiratory tract infections may reactivate previously seeded bacilli.

Fever, malaise, weight loss and *generalized* lymph node enlargement may some-times be seen during the course of lymphatic and blood-borne dissemination.

The other diseases to be considered in the differential diagnosis are chronic fungal, viral and bacterial infections, lymphomas, connective tissue disorders, histiocytosis X, and chronic sinus histiocytosis.

LIVER AND SPLEEN

Liver

The liver as a site of infection is to congenital tuberculosis what the lungs are to childhood and adult disease. Primary TB of the liver is uncommon; in Durban it accounted for only 0,2 per cent of childhood TB, while in a study of hospitalized black patients in Johannesburg it accounted for only 1,34 per cent of all cases of hepatic TB.[6] Primary inoculation may occur via *the lungs* (through the blood), *the gut* (through the biliary system, or from enteric lymph nodes or intestinal mucosa via blood or lymph), *glands in the porta hepatis* (through erosion

Table 5.6
Mortality in tuberculosis in 643 black children at the King Edward VIII Hospital, Durban, 1980–6

Overall	64%
• Miliary	32%*
• Meninges	19%
• Pulmonary	4%
• Gastrointestinal	4%

* Percentage of overall mortality

Table 5.7
Sites of lymph node enlargement in 143 black children with tuberculosis at the King Edward VIII Hospital, Durban

Overall	44%
Pulmonary	26%*
Cervical	21%
Axillary	8%
Submandibular	5%
Generalized	4%
Supraclavicular	3%
Abdominal	3%

* Percentage of 328 cases

of blood vessels, hepatic artery, bile radicle) and *across the diaphragm* (through lymph or blood spread after failure to lodge or establish infection in the lungs). In rare cases the *percutaneous route* may be the channel for primary hepatic TB. More often, mycobacteria get to the liver as part of miliary or disseminated infection; the latter may be blood borne or spread from intestinal and abdominal lesions. Miliary tubercles may be found in the liver even when absent on radiographs of the lungs. Rarely, miliary spread may originate from a primary in the liver. The intrahepatic granulomas which usually affect portal tracts may coalesce and block small bile ducts, form a single tuberculoma and calcify. It has been suggested that hepatic granuloma are analagous to skin reactions to mycobacterial antigens, as hepatomegaly occurs more often in those who are tuberculin skin test positive. Tuberculous glands may obstruct the porta hepatis, and non-specific histological changes, such as focal necrosis, fatty degeneration and periportal inflammation, are also seen.

Hepatomegaly in tuberculous disease is more often seen in the third world than in Europe, and it may be prominent enough to warrant the construction of a differential diagnosis around hepatomegaly or it may be an insignificant finding in a multiplicity of physical signs. In an Indian study the liver was enlarged clinically in seven per cent of children with TB though histological changes were more frequent, 46 per cent.[22] In the King Edward VIII Hospital in Durban the liver was clinically enlarged in 51% of 328 cases of tuberculosis.

In clinical practice the liver may be enlarged due to granuloma, to reticulo-endothelial reaction and to the ensuing malnutrition. There is associated abdominal pain, fever and weight loss. Obstructive jaundice is seen in rare instances. During miliary spread, an acute hepatitis picture with jaundice and liver failure is said to occur when cell mediated immune reactions are blunted and there is gross caseation with an excessive overgrowth of mycobacteria in the tuberculous lesions. Jaundice may also be due to granulomatous involvement of the liver parenchyma during disseminated or primary tuberculosis of the liver. An isolated tuberculoma may be found as a circumscribed hepatic nodule, and calcified nodules may be seen incidentally on abdomen radiographs.

Liver function tests, especially gamma glutaryl transferase and alkaline phosphatase, may occasionally be abnormal. In obscure clinical problems, liver biopsy may be adopted for diagnosis of TB. Hepatic radio-isotope scan is not always useful as it fails to distinguish the disease from other causes of diffuse involvement, abscesses and malignancy.

Spleen

Spread of the infection to the spleen occurs in a similar manner to that in the liver. Accordingly, splenomegaly may be due to granuloma (from miliary, disseminating or abdominal TB) or to reticulo-endothelial responses to chronic infection. Splenomegaly is usually gradual in onset and accompanied by hepatomegaly. An acutely enlarging spleen in the absence of a big liver, occurring in a markedly ill-looking child, is due to leakage of infected lymph node contents into the splenic artery — often there is an associated severe iron-deficiency anaemia in such children. Calcifications may be discovered incidentally on abdomen radiographs; these are small, round, of similar size and regular, in contrast to the irregular calcified areas following trauma or haemorrhage. Reactivation of a previously quiescent focus may account for a palpable spleen in older children and adolescents. The spleen was palpable in 13 per cent of the cases of TB seen in Durban.

ABDOMINAL AND GASTRO-INTESTINAL TUBERCULOSIS

This is an uncommon complication of tuberculosis in South Africa — in Cape Town the overall incidence of TB per thousand population was 176 times greater than that for abdominal TB,[13] while in Durban it accounted for eight per cent of hospital admissions. Most large referral hospitals in the third world would admit about five to six such patients per year. This complication appears to be more common in some parts of Africa, such as in Nigeria where it accounted for 29 per cent of all cases of childhood TB seen at the University College Hospital, Ibadan (where about 20 cases were seen annually).[12] The spread from the primary infection to the abdomen usually takes months, but calcification of nodes rarely occurs under one year.

Abdominal tuberculosis may arise in the following ways:

- secondary spread due to swallowed bacilli coughed up from pulmonary lesions (more than 95 per cent have associated pulmonary TB);
- primary infection from cow's milk. This is rare in South Africa; even when unpasteurized milk was being regularly consumed, bovine TB did not often cause abdominal disease;
- extension from pelvic disease (e.g. salpingitis) which occurs after puberty.

The infection spreads along the following pathway: bacilli are coughed up from lungs, swallowed, trapped in Peyer's Patches or infiltrate mucosa, there is ulceration of mucosa along the length of the bowel, extension of the infection to serosa and draining mesenteric lymph nodes, spread to other lymph nodes along the lymphatic chain, periadenitis and leakage of caseous material from nodes, adherence to visceral peritoneum, low grade sticky peritonitis and encroachment of the bowel lumen. The exudate from the peritoneum may be plastic, watery or haemorrhagic and the surface of the peritoneum may be studded with miliary tubercles or with granulomas undergoing caseation. The viscera become matted together and the infected omentum may be rolled up towards the epigastrium, assuming a sausage-like shape that lies across the abdomen.

The clinical features are due to systemic responses, lymph node enlargement with or without pressure on adjoining tissues, exudate formation and gastrointestinal involvement. The dominance of any one of these pathological processes enabled the Cape Town group to classify the clinical presentation in 59 children with abdominal TB as shown in Table 5.8. Their main symptoms and signs are given in Tables 5.9 and 5.10.

There may be gross ascites or only moderate distension with thickened adherent bowel, swollen omentum and glandular masses producing a doughy feel. Deep palpation reveals masses due to enlarged glands in the right iliac fossa, centrally or along both sides of the spine. Adenopathy can lead to compression of the inferior vena cava and oedema of the lower limbs (this was found in two per cent of abdominal TB cases in Nigeria).[12] Obstruction of intestinal lymphatics can cause steatorrhoea and chylous ascites. In rare cases strangulation of lymphatic channels produces a chylous ascites with considerable abdominal distension, a severe complication which causes relentless wasting and inanition, and which responds poorly to antituberculous therapy. Acute or subacute intestinal obstruction may be caused by stenosis or kinks in the bowel or by external pressure from glands.

Ulcers in the bowel are usually silent, may produce asymptomatic bleeding, and occasionally an erosive gut ulcer can cause frank blood in the stools. Tuberculous enteritis usually involves the terminal ileum, colon, duodenum and rectum. Occasionally interluminal fistulae or an umbilical fistula is produced — chronic fistula-in-ano is rare in children but more often seen in adults. Acute appendicitis-like forms of TB may rarely be detected. Tuberculomas of the caecum present as an intra-abdominal tumour. Granulomas of the oesophagus are most often silent, but in rare cases the scarring from these lesions, or pressure from mediastinal lymph nodes, can lead to luminal narrowing and cause difficulty in swallowing.

Table 5.8
Clinical categories of abdominal tuberculosis*

1. Exudative form	Ascites	49%
2. Nodal form	Palpable nodes	38%
3. Enteric form	Gastrointestinal tract disease	13%

* As seen in 59 children in Cape Town[13]

**Table 5.9
Frequency of symptoms in children
with abdominal tuberculosis***

Weight loss	78%
Cough	52%
Abdominal pain	44%
Vomiting	44%
Diarrhoea	31%
Sweating	36%
Blood in stools	5%
Haematemesis	2%

* As seen in 59 children in Cape Town

**Table 5.10
Frequency of signs in children with
abdominal tuberculosis***

Abdominal distension	92%
Masses	56%
Hepatomegaly	51%
Extra-abdominal adenopathy	47%
Ascites	44%
Splenomegaly	14%

* As seen in 59 children in Cape Town

The differential diagnosis includes lymphoma for abdominal masses, and other causes of intestinal obstruction, ascites and blood in the stools. Supportive evidence for TB is usually obtained from a positive tuberculin test and from chest and abdomen radiographs; the last-mentioned may reveal ascites, calcification or intestinal obstruction. Lymph node biopsy, bacteriology and laparoscopy may be required for confirmation. Ascitic fluid is clear and yellow or haemorrhagic, with lymphocytes, macrophages, increased proteins and adenine deaminase levels, and decreased sugar content. AFB are infrequently detected by culture from ascitic fluid.

Mortality in the early part of this century was about 25 per cent but is now roughly 10 per cent. Post-mortem findings in such cases[12] are given in Table 5.11. Response to currently available anti-TB therapy is generally good, steroids being employed by some workers for severe cases. Most patients are cured within 12 months of treatment, some within 18 months and a minority only by 24 months.

BLOOD AND BONE MARROW

It is uncommon for the blood changes in tuberculosis to be so profound as to attract clinical attention. Studies in black children have failed to demonstrate any consistent pattern, except that due to chronic infection. On the other hand, virtually every known haematological abnormality has been associated with this infection. Cameron[5] has proposed a useful classification of the possible blood changes in TB

based mainly on the degree of dissemination and the extent of anergy.

Restricted disease

In restricted disease with intact cell mediated immunity the features are usually those common to any chronic bacterial infection:

red cells:
  microcytic normochromic anaemia (iron deficiency)
  normocytic hypochromic anaemia, macrocytic anaemia (folate deficiency);
white cells:
  polymorphonuclear leucocytosis, neutropenia;
platelets :
  thrombocytosis, thrombocytopenia.

Tuberculosis affecting the small bowel or bone marrow can lead to vitamin B12 megaloblastic anaemia and a leucoerythroblastic reaction respectively. Toxic depression of the bone marrow causes hypoplastic anaemia. Severe anorexia and wasting are associated with decreased intake of iron and folate, thereby producing microcytic, hypochromic and megaloblastic anaemias.

Disseminated tuberculosis

Disseminated TB appears to overwhelm immune systems occasionally and cause anergy. In such situations, the blood changes appear to be more dramatic, although they also include the above abnormalities. Monocytosis, leukaemoid reactions (myeloid, lymphatic, monocytic), hypoplasia (aplastic anaemia, pancytopenia,

Table 5.11
Post-mortem findings in 28 cases of abdominal tuberculosis[12]

	PERCENTAGE OF TOTAL	
Lymph nodes:		100%
Mesenteric	75	
Peripancreatic	46	
Portahepatic	43	
Subdiaphragmatic	7	
Ileocaecal	4	
Retroperitoneal	4	
Viscera:		70%
Spleen	68	
Liver	46	
Kidney	39	
Pancreas	7	
Adrenals	14	
Gastrointestinal tract:		25%
Ileum	21	
Jejunum	4	
Peritoneum	21	

agranulocytosis, thrombocytopenia), proliferative reactions (leucoerythroblastic anaemia, myelofibrosis) and haemolytic anaemia have all been known to occur. Pancytopenia and myeloid leukaemoid abnormalities are the more common among these extreme reactions. Polycythaemia and thrombocytosis have been documented on rare occasions.

It must be borne in mind that abnormal blood results in patients with this disease may be due to the administration of antituberculous therapy. A very large number of haematological disorders, encompassing the range of findings noted above, caused by the infection itself can follow use of these drugs in conventional doses.

EYES

Coughing or sneezing by an adult with TB near a child can result in primary infection of the conjunctiva. This may be asymptomatic. Overt disease causes conjunctivitis, lacrymation, swelling and reddening of the eyelids and sclera. Eversion of the lid reveals hypertrophied granulation tissue with small yellow areas. There is no pain and onset of symptoms is gradual. The pre-

auricular, and occasionally, the tonsillar lymph nodes enlarge. Trachoma, foreign body and viral conjunctivitis need to be excluded.

Phlyctens, which can be seen at any stage of the disease, are part of the hypersensitivity phenomena of TB, and therefore bacilli are not grown from these lesions; they also indicate active disease. These reactions are seen in about 15 per cent of cases of pulmonary TB of childhood in Nigeria,[1] and in two per cent of cases seen in Durban. In earlier studies from the United States they were noted more often in association with TB of the tonsils, adenoids and middle ear, and accompanied a positive tuberculin test.[16] They are frequently recurrent and occur in crops. The patient complains of intense irritation, pain, lacrymation and photophobia in one or both eyes. Phlyctens are small grey jelly-like nodules at the limbus; running up to each spot is a small leash of injected conjunctival vessels. Phlyctens may migrate onto the cornea dragging a leash of blood vessels along with them. The nodules usually disappear in about a week, but on rare occasions they can ulcerate and involve the cornea in a severe phlyctenulokeratitis, leaving corneal opacities on healing. The pre-auricular lymph node is not enlarged. They must be distinguished from a foreign body, herpes simplex and vernal conjunctivitis. The lack of blood vessel encroachment of the cornea in vernal conjunctivitis helps to distinguish it from phlyctens. Local treatment includes hydrocortisone (one per cent) and atropine (0.25 per cent) drops.

Severe keratitis can lead to scarring and impaired vision.

The lacrymal gland is usually infected through bacteraemic spread; it is only rarely a primary infection. The sac and duct are involved, resulting in epiphora; it can leave scars and spread to the skin around the eye.

Iritis and uveitis cause oedema of the eyelids and conjunctivitis. The anterior chamber of the eye becomes clouded and nodules are seen on the pupillary edge of the iris.

Retinal haemorrhages with unaffected vision can be seen in the extremely rare instances of retinal TB.

Choroidal tubercles are exceedingly rare in black children in South Africa, even with miliary or meningitic disease. Their prevalence rates in the industrialized countries, during the period when tuberculosis was common, varied considerably: in primary TB a figure of six per cent prevalence has been noted, in TB meningitis about 10 per cent and in miliary disease the upper limit was about 70 per cent.[18] Tubercles are yellow circular bodies with a diffuse edge, seen along arteries near the disc, and are said to disappear in six weeks of treatment. There may be a single large tubercle, but usually they are multiple. Without treatment the edge becomes sharper, the central part fades to white, and black pigment appears at the periphery; therefore the result after about three months is a white scar with a black edge.

Flame shaped and coloured lesions on ophthalmoscopic examination indicate choroiditis. These are usually asymptomatic, but they may leave a scar with resultant impairment of vision.

EARS, MASTOIDS

Infection reaches the middle ear either by contiguous spread from the oropharynx through the eustachian tube or by blood-borne bacteria. Extension from the oropharynx usually occurs after the primary focus has already been established either in the mouth or throat or elsewhere in the body. Infection may sometimes be passed from a parent to the young infant whilst feeding, and this also happens when the mother (or father) coughs or sneezes. In this latter instance the tubercle bacilli may be driven through the eustachian tube into the middle ear where they will form a primary focus. Neonates who aspirate infected amniotic fluid also develop a primary focus in the middle ear. Mastoids are most often infected as a direct complication of middle ear disease. Blood-transported material may reach the middle ear or mastoids; from the latter there may develop osteitis and subperiosteal cold abscesses and spread to the middle ear.

In a primary infection of the middle ear there is chronic painless otorrhoea and enlargement of the lymph node between the mastoid and angle of the mandible. More often the following sequence takes place: the ear drum loses its shine, the blood vessels on it dilate, and it becomes thick and swollen so that the normal contours and landmarks disappear. A number of tubercles are seen on the membrane; these liquefy resulting in numerous perforations (especially in the lower half of the ear drum), which coalesce. Tubercles may also be seen in the mucosa of the middle ear cleft.

Through the perforations emerges a pale pink granulation with a watery discharge. Secondary bacterial infection causes it to become purulent. There is an insidious onset of conductive deafness which often goes unnoticed in the very young. Tuberculous inflammation produces greater compression than does purulent disease, and therefore a lower motor neurone facial nerve palsy is not uncommon, especially in those under two years of age.

The chief complications are secondary bacterial infection, osteitis, cold abscesses and meningitis. Spread of infection to the labyrinth is more common after TB than acute otitis media, though symptoms are rare.

What assists in distinguishing TB from other bacterial infections of the middle ear and mastoid is the absence of pain and fever. The diagnosis is made by finding TB bacilli in the discharge or on biopsy of the granulation tissue in the ear. Treatment includes anti-TB treatment, regular toilet of the ear and surgical removal of bony sequestra from the mastoid.

Clues to the diagnosis of tuberculous otomastoiditis include:
- predisposing factors;
- TB in other organs;
- multiple small eardrum perforations;
- large central perforation or total destruction of the drum;
- pale granulation with watery discharge from the ear;
- lower motor neurone facial palsy in a child under two years of age.

OROPHARYNX

Infection at the focus of a dental extraction or mucosal injury leads to a painless ulcer in the dental sulcus, buccal mucosa or on the gums; the submandibular and tonsillar glands become swollen. This oral lesion and regional upper cervical lymphadenopathy represents the primary complex. The initial mucous membrane lesion appears to be less often detected in Africa and India than in Europe.

A primary complex of the tonsils and the tonsillar nodes develops after contact with infected material. The latter may be transmitted through food, drink and utensils, such as spoons; tuberculous material may also be carried on contaminated fingers or through saliva. The feeding of babies by affected parents predisposes the young to tonsillar infection; the practice of pre-masticating infant food can facilitate the passage of tubercle germs. When milk was unpasteurized, it occasionally caused oropharyngeal TB. Bloodspread from a primary in the lungs is rare in children, though more common in adults. Clinically the tonsils are asymmetrically enlarged and red, the crypts become obscured, small yellow nodules appear and shallow grey ulcers are seen on the tonsils and the pillars of the fauces. Cervical adenitis is present.

Adenoids are infected in a similar manner to tonsils; the result is a profuse and excoriating nasal discharge. Phlyctens are alleged to be closely associated with TB of the adenoids, tonsils and middle ear.[16]

Salivary glands are rarely infected; there is chronic enlargement of submaxillary or parotid glands. Miliary tubercles may be seen on the posterior pharynx and tonsillar fauces, and are painful. Tuberculous laryngitis occurs in adolescents, usually during progressive primary disease. Occasionally, infection takes place through bacteraemia, causing hoarseness and pain on coughing or swallowing.

KIDNEYS, URINARY TRACT

This is a later complication of TB, after four to seven years of the primary lesion, and is therefore a disease of adolescents and adults. It accounts for less than one per cent of childhood disease. Spread is always blood-borne, though it has been suggested that because kidney disease is often associated with TB of the spine and pleura, it may be through the lymphatics.[4] Tubercle bacilli can be recovered from the urine in miliary disease without involving the kidney or urinary tract.

Tubercles are seen on the surface of the kidneys or deeper in the cortex but rarely in the pelvis. An encapsulated abscess forms between the cortex and pyramids, and may discharge into the urine, resolve and heal by calcification, or leave a ragged wall cavity with persistent discharge of bacilli. The lesions may, however, progress and cause destruction of the kidney. On rare occasions when infection proceeds to the pelvis, ureters and bladder, there can be ureteric narrowing and hydronephrosis. Before the days of drug treatment 50 per cent of children were dead within five years of the onset of kidney disease.[18]

Chronic sterile pyuria may be detected on routine investigation; mild haematuria and proteinuria may also be present. Groin pain is sometimes a symptom of this problem, and, in the later stages, when there is cystitis, frequency and dysuria occur and there is painless haematuria.

The diagnosis is made by culture of tubercle bacilli from early morning samples of urine and radio-imaging of the kidney which reveals calcification, deformed calyces, cavities, filling defects, destruction of the kidneys or hydronephrosis following on ureteric stenosis. Cystoscopy may reveal ulcers and fibrosis.

The differential diagnosis includes chronic pyelonephritis and other causes of haematuria such as bladder infections and glomerulonephritis. Therapeutic surgery is used in advanced cases in addition to routine anti-TB therapy.

GENITAL TRACT, BREAST

The long interval between primary infection and genital disease results in the latter being rare in childhood, especially in this age of effective drug therapy.

Boys

Primary TB of the penis with bilateral inguinal lymphadenopathy used to be seen after circumcision by an infected operator. Without adequate therapy, roughly half of the babies so infected died of disseminated disease.[16] Epididymitis and orchitis are often associated with renal TB or are secondary to blood spread. Involvement of the epididymis is insidious in onset, usually painless and bilateral with hard and irregular cords. The knotted cord can adhere to the skin, soften and rupture. In young boys this occurs as an isolated infection without spread to the testes. Orchitis, rare before puberty, accompanies epididymitis as a single lesion in older boys. It causes dragging pain, swelling of the scrotum and enlargement of the testicle; sinuses may develop. These infections are followed by sterility in an appreciable number of cases, with bilateral disease being worse for this complication than unilateral disease.

The other conditions to be considered in the diagnosis are hydrocele, torsion of the testis, epididymo-orchitis caused by sexually transmitted diseases and *Escherichia coli*, orchitis due to mumps and *E. coli*, and seminoma.

Prostatic spread is associated with advanced renal TB or epididymo-orchitis. It is usually silent and detected as a nodular mass on rectal examination.

Girls

Primary infection of the vulva and vagina gives rise to inguinal adenitis, while re-infection at these sites results in a local ulcer without regional nodal enlargement. This is recorded where female circumcision is practised or where there is contamination of a small wound in this area. It results in dysuria and an ulcer.

Before puberty, the Fallopian tubes and uterus may be the sites of miliary disease. After puberty, these organs are infected through the blood, or rarely, from TB of the abdomen. Salpingitis is more frequent than uterine TB, and spread to the latter usually is a consequence of tubal infection. In adolescents pelvic inflammatory disease may be caused by TB.

There is abdominal distension and pain in both lower quadrants; amenorrhoea, scanty or irregular menstruation can occur. A mass which is either central or extending to the iliac fossae may be felt in the pelvis or arising from it. Some cases have free fluid in the abdomen. Pelvic examination reveals adnexal masses, and sterility is a frequent complication even with appropriate chemotherapy.

The ovaries are affected by miliary tubercles, blood dissemination or spread from salpingitis. Usually the result is a peri-oophoritis rather than an infection of the ovaries. It is silent.

Breast involvement occurs after puberty as a painless lump which may adhere to the skin, soften and form sinuses or discharge through the lacteal ducts.

SECRETORY AND ENDOCRINE GLANDS

These glands are involved through blood-borne or contiguous spread. So, for example, the salivary gland is infected via TB of the mandible, the testis from the epididymis, the ovaries from the Fallopian tube, and the pancreas from parapancreatic nodes. Lacrymal, salivary and mammary glands can be the site of primary infection. Infection usually occurs late in the course of established TB. Tubercles may be seen on the surface of glands such as the thyroid, pancreas and adrenals (blood or miliary spread) or within the substance of the gland (as, for example, leakage of caseous material from an adjacent lymph node into the pancreas). Isolated cases of TB of the pituitary, pineal and thymus have been recorded.

Clinical manifestations are uncommon (except for genital tuberculosis). The thyroids and parotids may enlarge painlessly. Decreased function such as hypothyroidism or diabetes insipidus is exceedingly rare. The adrenals are usually silently infected in childhood, but TB of the adrenals can be detected at post-mortem in children who had no detectable clinical disease during life. This is because Addison's disease appears 6 to 15 years after bilateral infection, and peaks at 30 years.

TUBERCULOSIS AND IMMUNO-DEFICIENCY STATES

It is to be expected that an infection such as tuberculosis, which is so closely linked to immune mechanisms for both its arousal from dormancy and its expression, will be more frequent and severe in conditions of immunological impairment. Clinical features in TB depend on immunopathology and it is therefore not surprising that signs and symptoms of active disease are often blunted in immunodeficient states. As primary immunodeficiencies are less commonly identified in the third world, the associations which have been detected with TB usually relate to secondary immunodeficiencies. Selected examples given below illustrate these associations.

Protein-energy-malnutrition and TB are social diseases *par excellence*, deeply rooted in impoverishment. The overcrowded and unhygienic conditions which are the social substrate of malnutrition also predispose to the spread of *Mycobacterium tuberculosis*, and *exposure* to this infection is therefore higher. The loss of integrity of mucous membranes, skin and protective tissue facilitates establishment of *infection*. The immunodeficiency of kwashiorkor and marasmus prevents the maintenance of the dormant state of the infection, with the result that there is an escape, *activation* and proliferation of the mycobacteria. The inability of cellular and humoral immune mechanisms to restrict the infection leads to *dissemination* and *severe* disease.

Apathy and loss of appetite are frequent in PEM and will not in themselves awaken suspicions about associated TB. Fever may be absent and lymph node enlargement minimal, despite extensive underlying infection. No adventitious sounds may be heard in the chest, although rapid breathing and recession are seen when there is pneumonia. In southern Africa, the older child with kwashiorkor is at very high risk of also having TB. The anergic state results in negative tuberculin tests, which may take about a month to become positive on nutritional rehabilitation. Accordingly, if TB is suspected, it is advisable to wait for this period before repeating the tuberculin test.

There is no added risk in using live vaccines (including BCG) in PEM, and conventional drug treatment is adequate.

It must be remembered that the other side of the coin is that kwashiorkor or marasmus may be precipitated by TB in a sub-optimally nourished child. Weight loss is an invariable feature of TB.

Severe measles produces profound, extensive and protracted impairment of most limbs of the immune response, and for the same reasons as PEM, there is an association between measles and TB.

Ever since von Pirquet noted that the tuberculin reaction became negative during measles infection, there have been numerous attempts to link causally the development of TB and the depression of skin reactivity to PPD. Implicit in this is the belief that delayed hypersensitivity and immunity are one and the same thing in TB. Although closely related, it would appear that these two facets of the allergic response to the tubercle bacillus are not identical. This, together with the varying degrees of severity of measles may account for some contradictory evidence in this regard.

There are many studies of large groups of children in whom an attack of measles preceded the development of TB, all of which studies suggested that measles both activated and aggravated TB. Two large measles epidemics in the virgin populations of southern and western Greenland in 1951 and 1962 added further support to the association between measles and TB.

In the 1962 epidemic in Greenland a control group without measles was available for comparison.[2] Of 34 000 persons, 10 722 contracted measles whereas the remainder (being immune as a result of previous epidemics) did not. It was found that in adults (more than 20 years of age) in this population, the incidence of TB was significantly higher in those who had suffered from measles than in those who had not.[14] This evidence suggested that persons who had had measles were predisposed to the development of TB. Starr and Berkovich (1965)[25] found that measles had a detrimental effect on patients already on treatment for TB. Flick,[8] in a review of the literature, quotes a number of studies from which he draws the opposite conclusion, i.e. that measles may have a beneficial effect on existing TB. The author's experience is that measles is generally damaging to children and in particular predisposes them to TB.

The strong impression is that, at least in black children, a severe attack of measles not infrequently leads to pulmonary TB. The radiological evidence of measles pneumonia persists, and gradually merges into what turns out to be tuberculosis. The prolonged anergic state after measles renders interpretation of a negative tuberculin test particularly difficult, but the evolution of the pneumonia and repeated skin tests may be helpful in establishing a diagnosis.

Information is accumulating on unusual manifestations of TB in human immunodeficiency virus (HIV) infection, but most of this evidence has been documented in adults and adolescents.[10, 21] The picture in children is still unclear.

In perinatal HIV infection, BCG can be used at birth or soon thereafter, as clinical deterioration is usually delayed for a few months. There is a risk of BCG disseminat-ing; in the third world, however, the risks of this must be weighed against the potential benefits of protection. It has been recommended that where the risks of TB are high, prophylactic INH be employed in AIDS. Treatment for established disease should include three to four drugs for longer periods; this should not be under nine months. Maintenance therapy may be required thereafter. Short course chemotherapy should be avoided.

The data from adults suggests that TB is detected in excess of the expected frequency in patients with systemic lupus erythematosus (SLE).[7] Advanced pulmonary involvement and miliary spread are common. The severity and mortality from tuberculosis correlate with the severity of SLE and the use of steroid therapy for this disease.

REFERENCES

The material for this chapter has been drawn from a number of different sources: personal experience, analysis of tuberculosis at King Edward VIII Hospital, Durban, standard texts and key papers in the literature. The books by Miller F J W and Lincoln E M, Sewell E M have been particularly useful. References are provided only for those points which require clarification.

1 Aderele W I, 1979. Pulmonary tuberculosis in childhood: an analysis of 263 cases seen at Ibadan, Nigeria. *Tropical and Geographical Medicine.* 31, 41–51.
2 Bech V, 1965. The measles epidemic in Greenland in 1962. *Archives des Virusforsch.* 16, 53–64.
3 Beitzke H, 1935. Über die angeborene Tuberkulose Infektion. *Ergeb ges Tuberk Forsch.* 7, 1–30.
4 Burke H, 1954. A new approach to the pathogenesis of extrapulmonary tuberculosis. *British Journal of Tuberculosis.* 48, 3.
5 Cameron S J, 1974. Tuberculosis and the blood — a special relationship? *Tubercle.* 55, 55–72.
6 Essop A R, Moosa M R, Segal I, Posen J, 1983. Primary tuberculosis of the liver — a case report. *Tubercle.* 64, 291–3.
7 Feng P H & Tan T H, 1982. Tuberculosis in patients with systemic lupus erythematosus. *Annals of Rheumatic Diseases.* 41, 11–4.
8 Flick J A, 1976. Editorial: Does measles really predispose to tuberculosis? *American Review of Respiratory Diseases.* 114, 257–65.
9 Freiman I, Geefhuysen J & Solomon A, 1975. Radiological presentation of pulmonary tuberculosis in children. *South African Medical Journal.* 49; 1703–6.
10 Goldman K P, 1987. Editorial: AIDS and tuberculosis. *British Medical Journal.* 295, 511–2.
11 Hatcher L H, 1963. A study of primary tuberculosis in 100 Korean children. *Tubercle.* 44, 355–9.
12 Johnson A O K & Aderele W I, 1979. Abdominal tuberculosis in childhood. *Journal of Tropical Medicine and Hygiene.* 82, 47–52.
13 Johnson C A C, Hill I D & Bowie M D, 1987. Abdominal tuberculosis in children: a survey of cases at the Red Cross War Memorial Children's Hospital, 1976–1985. *South African Medical Journal.* 72, 20–2.
14 Lange P K, 1970. Morbilli and tuberculosis in Greenland. *Scandinavian Journal of Respiratory Diseases.* 51, 256–60.
15 Lenzini L, Rottoli P & Rottoli L, 1977. The spectrum of human tuberculosis. *Clinical and Experimental Immunology.* 27, 230–7.

16 Lincoln E M & Sewell E M, 1963. *Tuberculosis in Children.* New York: Mcgraw Hill Book Company, Inc.

17 Lloyd A V C, 1969. Review article: Tuberculosis in childhood *East African Medical Journal.* 46, 481–8.

18 Miller F J W, 1982. *Tuberculosis in Children: Evolution, Epidemiology, Treatment, Prevention.* Edinburgh: Churchill Livingstone.

19 Morley D, 1973. *Tuberculosis: Paediatric Priorities in the Developing World.* Great Britain: Butterworths.

20 Nemir R L & O'Hare D, 1985. Congenital tuberculosis. Review and diagnostic guidelines. *American Journal of Diseases of Childhood.* 139, 284–7.

21 Pinching A J, 1987. The acquired immune deficiency syndrome: with special reference to tuberculosis. *Tubercle.* 68, 65–7.

22 Ramachandran R S, 1971. Some aspects of tuberculosis in children: 3 000 cases. *Mediscope.* 14 (5).

23 Smith M H D & Marquis J R, 1981. Tuberculosis and other mycobacterial infections. In: Feigin R D & Cherry J D (eds): *Textbook of Pediatric Infectious Diseases,* vol. 1. Philadelphia: Saunders Company.

24 Snider D E & Bloch A B, 1984. Congenital tuberculosis. *Tubercle.* 65, 81–2.

25 Starr S & Berkovich S, 1965. The effect of measles, gamma globulin modified measles, and attenuated measles vaccine on the course of treated tuberculosis in children. *Pediatrics.* 35, 97–102.

CHAPTER 6

Tuberculosis in adults

S R Benatar

Mycobacterium tuberculosis is a hardy organism capable of surviving in all climatic conditions, and it is therefore found worldwide and in all peoples. The disease it causes has plagued mankind for many centuries (see Chapter 1). Tuberculous lesions have been found in the vertebrae of neolithic man in Europe and in Egyptian mummies dating back to 3700 BCE. Hippocrates described the symptoms of an illness he called 'phthisis' (meaning 'to waste away'), and he recognized nodules in the lung as being features of the disease. The Latin name 'tubercula' for such nodules led to the introduction in 1834 of the term tuberculosis for the clinical and pathological description of the disease.[13]

Tuberculosis, as the 'great white plague' in Europe from the seventeenth to the nineteenth centuries, accounted for 20 per cent of all deaths. In Britain tuberculosis reached its peak in the late eighteenth century, at which time the annual death rate from tuberculosis was approximately 500 per 100 000 population per year. This had fallen to 200 per 100 000 population by 1882 when Robert Koch discovered the tubercle bacillus, and to 50 per 100 000 just before anti-tuberculosis drugs came into general use in the 1940s and subsequently down to approximately five per 100 000 per year.[18]

Despite major advances in our understanding of the disease and the development of new, potent anti-tuberculosis drugs, it remains a problem worldwide and especially in developing countries. It is estimated that of three million deaths every year throughout the world from tuberculosis, 75 per cent are in the developing world. The AIDS epidemic and its association with tuberculosis have given a re-emphasis to this disease, both in the developed and developing worlds.

PATHOGENESIS

Tuberculosis is transmitted by the airborne spread of one to three bacilli of *Mycobacterium tuberculosis* suspended in droplet nuclei 1–5 μm in diameter — produced during coughing or speaking by persons with active (open) pulmonary tuberculosis. However, the relatively low infectivity rate requires fairly prolonged and close contact for high levels of transmission. Approximately one-third of close contacts of tuberculous patients are found to have evidence of infection (positive tuberculin skin test).

Inhalation of droplets into the mid and lower zones of the lung results in the development of a small area of bronchopneumonia. Antigen-activated macrophages sensitize T-lymphocytes which accumulate at the site of infection and release a range of lymphokines. In the weeks preceding the development of natural acquired immunity the organisms proliferate, drain into regional lymph nodes and subsequently proceed through the lymphatic system into the systemic circulation which then distributes them to many organs throughout the body. The inflammatory reaction generated and maintained by activated macrophage and T-lymphocyte secretion of a range of cytokines leads to natural acquired immunity which both defends the host against proliferating organisms and damages tissues through the cytotoxic and other effects of the mediators of inflammation (see Chapter 14). The small area of bronchopneumonia with its regional lymphadenopathy constitutes the primary complex, and subsequent calcification of this complex is common.

This, usually asymptomatic, sequence of events is associated with the development of acquired immunity to *M. tuberculosis* which results in the death of most of the bacteria in the primary focus and other sites throughout the body. However, a few bacilli remain alive and dormant following the primary infection (particularly in areas of high PO2 such as the apex of the lung, cortex of the kidneys, and vertebrae). This primary infection confers partial immunity to subsequent re-infection by inhaled bacilli. The development of immunity is associated with development of a positive hypersensitivity skin reaction to tuberculin within four to six weeks of infection. Although natural acquired immunity and the positive hypersensitivity reaction develop simultaneously they are mediated by independent clones of lymphocytes.

It is estimated that approximately 5 to 15 per cent of patients infected by the tubercle bacillus will ultimately develop tuberculous disease, and it is possible that a greater percentage may do so in the very adverse circumstances found in some developing countries. The untreated, but infected, person carries the risk of developing tuberculosis for a lifetime and reactivation can occur at any stage after the primary infection, although the risk is greatest in the first two years. Factors determining who will develop tuberculous disease are complex and include the interaction of a variety of host characteristics, the virulence of the infecting strain and environmental influences. Although there is some evidence for genetic susceptibility to tuberculosis, such as the excess risk observed in monozygotic as compared with dizygotic twins and in blood relations as compared with non-relations living in the same close contact,[7] extraneous factors, such as malnutrition, overcrowding, silicosis, malignant disease or the use of immunosuppressive drugs, are all much more important in determining the progression of infection to disease and in causing later reactivation.

EPIDEMIOLOGY

Tuberculosis is not uniformly distributed throughout the world or through different population groups in individual countries. It is therefore necessary to have a surveillance programme to monitor tuberculosis trends in defined areas so that effective programmes for control of the disease can be designed and the efficacy of these assessed.

There are four methods of surveillance to monitor tuberculosis trends:

- the mortality rate;
- the incidence of disease (the notification rate);
- prevalence surveys; and
- estimates of the annual risk of infection.

The mortality rate was a useful indicator of trends in the pre-chemotherapeutic era of high mortality, but, with the current much lower rates, it is an inadequate measure.

The second method of monitoring tuberculosis — the recording of the incidence of disease — suffers from the defect that there are different standards of notification in different areas, as a result of which the notification rate is influenced by many factors other than the true incidence of disease.

Prevalence surveys undertaken to identify all cases of tuberculosis in defined communities reveal many more with active disease than does routine case notification. Prevalence surveys in the Transkei suggested that in that community less than one-third of all cases of open tuberculosis were diagnosed and notified. As prevalence surveys are difficult and expensive to conduct and need to be repeated to assess trends within communities, alternative means of assessing trends in tuberculosis have been sought.

The annual risk of infection, an index calculated from the rate of tuberculin conversion in a defined representative group of children, is recognized as being a more sensitive method of expressing the status of tuberculosis in any community as it reflects the rate of spread of tuberculosis infection. It has the advantage that it is a generation ahead of notification data in its ability to monitor tuberculosis trends. Studies in South Africa have shown great variation in trends of the annual rate of infection in different population groups and also in the same groups within different parts of the country (see Chapter 4).[1, 10, 32]

In many parts of the world today, and in the United States less than 50 years ago, most people become infected with *Mycobacterium tuberculosis* in childhood. In an autopsy study of more than 1 000 New Yorkers who died suddenly and unexpectedly between 1944 and 1947, 88 per cent of those aged 60 years or older, and 80 per cent of those between 40 and 59 years of age had evidence of previous tuberculous infection.[13] The incidence of disease remains very variable within and between countries. For example, in the United States the notification rate ranges from 8,8 per 100 000 per year in Wichita to 54,5 per 100 000 per year in San Francisco. Death rates from tuberculosis in 1973 ranged from one per 100 000 population in Australia, 1,8 in the United States, 6,3 in France, to 11 in Japan and 27,7 per 100 000 in Hong Kong.[13] The wide variations in South Africa are well known and are described in Chapter 4.

CLINICAL FEATURES

Primary tuberculosis is seldom associated with significant clinical symptoms, although a small percentage of patients may have peripheral manifestations such as erythema nodosum or phlyctenular conjunctivitis. The diagnosis in asymptomatic contacts is usually made from a chest radiograph or by observing Mantoux skin test conversion. Progressive primary tuberculosis in Africa is often associated with massive enlargement of mediastinal and cervical lymphadenopathy, which can result in compressive effects and sinus formation.

Post-primary tuberculosis may be due to either reactivation or exogenous re-infection, but these two mechanisms are not easily distinguished clinically. Although apical and sub-apical regions of the lung are classically considered to be the common sites, any portion of the lung can be involved and it is well recognized that lower lobe, endobronchial and pleural tuberculosis are quite common in the elderly.[19] Most cases of tuberculous disease seen in adults represent reactivation of previous dormant foci, although in institutions such as shelters for the homeless (where overcrowding and malnutrition are common) exogenous re-infection is more common than had previously been thought to be the case.[20] The incidence of tuberculosis is also extremely high in such shelters — up to 150–300 times the national average. This is further complicated by the high incidence of infection with primary drug resistant organisms.

Reactivation and organ tuberculosis

The proportions of reactivation tuberculosis affecting different organs in South Africa (obtained from notification data) and in the United States are difficult to compare as they are recorded using different sub-categories. Pulmonary tuberculosis accounts for the vast majority of all cases in all countries, but especially in developing countries. In developed countries the rate of decline of notified organ tuberculosis has been lower than that of pulmonary tuberculosis, and this pattern may also be influenced by the frequency of extra-pulmonary tuberculosis in patients with AIDS. The frequency with which some investigations are helpful in the diagnosis of organ tuberculosis is summarized in Table 6.1.

Pulmonary tuberculosis

The clinical manifestations of reactivation pulmonary tuberculosis are very variable. They range from a low grade inflammatory process, with minimal acute local or systemic manifestations, which may, over a long period of time, lead to unilateral or bilateral upper lobe fibrosis with considerable impairment of lung function, to a very rapidly progressive form of cavitating lung disease associated with pronounced local symptoms and systemic manifestations. This spectrum reflects the variable relationship between the virulence of the organism and the host response.

Symptoms due to the local effects of the disease process include cough, haemoptysis (which can range from recurrent minor to major life-threatening haemoptysis), chest pain and dyspnoea. General symptoms include malaise, lethargy, fever, weight loss, night sweats, and anorexia. Physical signs may be minimal or pronounced according

Table 6.1
Range of results of investigations in patients with organ tuberculosis

	PLEURAL TUBERCULOSIS	PERITONEAL TB (WITH ASCITES)	MENINGEAL TB	PULMONARY TB	GENITO-URINARY TUBERCULOSIS
Positive Mantoux	70%	<65%	<65%	±80%	±80%
Fever	>85%	100%	100%	40%	<10%
AFB's					
— direct stain	—	>5%	<20%	±50%	±80%
— culture	<50%	±80%	>85%	±95%	±80%
— biopsy plus culture	>85%	>85%	—		

to the degree and the nature of local damage produced, such as pleural effusion, lobar consolidation, cavitation or fibrosis.

The range of usual and unusual radiographic features[22] is described in many publications and in detail in Chapter 13. The differential diagnosis of radiographic abnormalities will depend on the pattern of the abnormality but common considerations include carcinoma, sarcoidosis, allergic broncho-pulmonary aspergillosis, pneumoconiosis, pneumonia due to a variety of agents (including fungi), pulmonary vasculitis, lymphoma, and extrinsic allergic alveolitis. As the definitive diagnosis of pulmonary tuberculosis rests on finding *Mycobacterium tuberculosis* in the sputum, every attempt should be made to identify the organism on direct stains or culture. Cowie and Escreet, in their study of 300 patients with newly diagnosed pulmonary tuberculosis in the gold mines of the Orange Free State, showed that in the presence of a suspicious radiograph, a normal erythrocyte sedimentation rate, a negative Heaf test and the absence of symptoms are not reliable factors for excluding the diagnosis.[6]

When tuberculosis is suspected and the direct sputum smear is negative, an alternative to waiting six weeks for the results of sputum culture or to treating the patient until these results are available, is to perform fibre-optic bronchoscopy and obtain brushings and biopsies from the involved area of the lung. Several workers have shown the value of this approach in making an early definitive diagnosis, but it should be noted that, even with this technique, the diagnosis is not made in all patients in whom tuberculosis is subsequently proven.[29, 31]

As indicated above, the evolution of tuberculosis lesions in the lung is very variable. Hence in some patients, in whom the host response is adequate, the disease remains localized and may even resolve without treatment, leaving some destruction of lung tissue and a few persisting viable organisms which may again reactivate at a later date. If disease is progressive, the lesion spreads through the lung by destruction of tissue (caseation and cavitation), may rupture into a bronchus and spread to other parts of the lung, or disseminate widely via the lympho-haematogenous route to involve many organs. Endobronchial involvement can result in bronchial obstruction and bronchiectasis. Rupture of a cavity or large caseous lesion into the pleural space results in a pyopneumothorax with bronchopleural fistula. Acid-fast bacilli are usually evident on direct examination of aspirated material and surgical drainage is often required.

Slight and recurrent haemoptysis is usually the result of mucosal involvement, but massive and life-threatening haemoptysis can occur when a pulmonary artery traversing a tuberculous cavity is eroded.

Residual, open healed cavities have a tendency to become colonized with fungus of the Aspergillus species, the growth of which can lead to the formation of an aspergilloma (fungal ball). This local growth is accompanied by the development of circulating IgG antibodies to the aspergillus fungus. A British Thoracic Association survey in the United Kingdom showed that 30 per cent of patients with open healed tuberculous cavities had positive serology but no clinical evidence of aspergillomas.[2] Another 15 per cent had chest radiograph appearances of fungus balls, and in 10 per cent of these patients the course was complicated by recurrent, severe or life-threatening haemoptysis. The role of surgery in such cases is often debated, in particular where lung function is severely impaired. In those patients with adequate lung function surgery is associated with a better long term prognosis than is conservative treatment.[9]

Lymph node tuberculosis

In Britain 75 per cent of patients with lymph node tuberculosis are African or Asian immigrants. Cervical lymphadenitis makes up 50 per cent of non-pulmonary tuberculosis in this group but is often associated with tuberculosis of the lungs or other organs. Clinically the onset is usually insidious, but progression to chronic discharging sinuses and ultimately to unsightly scars (scrofula) is a common outcome in the absence of treatment. The bacilliary load is usually low and positive cultures are obtained in about 60 per cent of patients. Lymph nodes may enlarge in size, new glands may enlarge on therapy in up to 25 per cent of patients, and breakdown may even occur in some while on treatment. Excision or aspiration after the start of chemotherapy may be required in up to 20 per cent of patients. Long term results are good although up to 13 per cent of patients still have enlarged (asymptomatic) nodes at the end of successful treatment.[3]

Mediastinal lymphadenopathy is less common than cervical or axillary lymphadenopathy and is transient in some patients. In others it is more persistent and conditions such as sarcoidosis, lymphoma and metastatic carcinoma enter the differential diagnosis.

Pleural tuberculosis

Once considered to be almost always a manifestation of primary tuberculosis affecting predominantly children and young adults, pleural tuberculosis is now a recognized manifestation in older patients with concomitant pulmonary tuberculosis. A distinction needs to be made between tuberculosis effusions and effusions due to other diseases (cirrhosis with ascites, cardiac failure, rheumatoid arthritis, and lymphoma) in these patients. Pleural biopsy (with culture of fluid and biopsy material) is needed to make a definitive diagnosis.[8]

Pleural tuberculosis and its complications comprised 4,3 per cent of general thoracic surgical patients seen at the Natal University Cardiothoracic Unit during the 20 years between 1966 and 1985. Odell has reported and reviewed the role of the thoracic surgeon in the investigation and surgical management of such patients.[21] On those few occasions when pleural effusions do not resolve on medical therapy, decortication is only recommended if the pleural fibrosis is significantly impairing lung function. It is not recommended until patients have received chemotherapy for at least four months or sputum results, previously positive, have been negative for four months.[21] The surgical management of pleural complications of tuberculosis, only rarely seen in developed countries, is demanding and requires considerable experience and skill. It is well described by Odell.[21]

Genito-urinary tuberculosis

Reactivation of dormant organisms in the cortex of the kidney leads to the spread of infection into the renal pelvis and from there into the ureter and bladder. Twenty per cent of patients are asymptomatic. Ulceration and fibrosis in the urethra result in hydronephrosis and impairment of renal function, and in the bladder causes shrinkage in size with consequent urinary symptoms.

Clinical manifestations include frequency, dysuria, microscopic haematuria, ureteric colic, loin pain, backache, chronic renal insufficiency and extension of cold abscesses to the loin. Two-thirds of patients have abnormal chest radiographs.

The diagnosis should be suspected in the context of sterile pyuria or microscopic haematuria. Bacteriological studies are required for confirmation. Intravenous pyelography reveals the site and extent of involvement and may show both non-specific abnormalities such as cortical scarring, dilatation of calyces, papillary cavities and other more specific features, including renal calcification, cavitation and urethral strictures with a classical beaded appearance.

In the male, painless or symptomatic scrotal swelling occurs with nodular swelling of the epididymis, vas deferens or seminal vesicles. Prostatic involvement may also occur, and the development of skin sinuses is common.

In the female, infertility arising from the involvement of the Fallopian tubes and endometrium is the most common result. Dyspareunia, pelvic pain, menstrual disturbances and vaginal discharge are other manifestations.

Abdominal tuberculosis[11, 17, 25, 28]

Although any part of the gastrointestinal tract may be involved, the most common sites of tuberculous involvement are the distal ileum and ileocaecal regions. Small bowel, ileocaecal and colonic tuberculosis account for about 40 per cent of all cases of abdominal tuberculosis; tuberculous ascites and plastic peritonitis for about 50 per cent; and mesenteric tuberculous lymphadenitis for the remaining 10 per cent. Prior to the chemotherapy era autopsy data showed that there was involvement of the bowel in up to 80 per cent of patients who died of TB, and radiological studies showed that the incidence of bowel tuberculosis was directly proportional to the extent of pulmonary tuberculosis. In more recent studies less than 50 per cent of patients presenting with intestinal tuberculosis have had radiographic evidence of active pulmonary disease. Reactivation of organisms previously spread by the haematogenous route to the bowel, rather than by infection of the bowel from swallowed organisms, now seems the more likely pathogenic sequence under these circumstances.

Marks and colleagues have described the clinical features of abdominal tuberculosis as being 'varied, deceptive and generally non-specific', the wide spectrum of presentation ranging from relatively mild abdominal symptoms to an acute life-threatening emergency. In a twenty-year experience of 242 patients at Cape Town's Groote Schuur Hospital weight loss, abdominal pain and fever were the most frequent findings, occurring in 60–80 per cent of patients, with diarrhoea as a symptom in about 30 per cent, and vomiting and constipation in 20 per cent. An abdominal mass was palpable in 25 per cent and ascites was a feature in almost 50 per cent of patients. Routine investigations were usually non-specific, with the ESR being normal in 22 per cent of patients and the Mantoux test positive in only 57 per cent of patients tested. Active pulmonary disease and/or pleural effusion were present in less than 40 per cent of patients on whom a chest x-ray had been performed.[17]

Dysphagia is usually the presenting symptom of oesophageal tuberculosis, although this is the least common site in the gastrointestinal tract. Tuberculosis of the stomach is also rare but the clinical, radiological and even gastroscopic features may simulate peptic ulceration or malignant disease. Pyloroduodenal obstruction due to extrinsic compression by massive caseating glands is unusual but is the commonest cause of pyloroduodenal obstruction in the South African black and may be confused with carcinoma of the pancreas.

Small bowel tuberculosis, which accounts for 36 per cent of patients with abdominal tuberculosis, may present either with malabsorption syndrome or with features of small bowel obstruction. Ileocaecal tuberculosis presenting as a tender abdominal mass needs to be differentiated from Crohn's disease, caecal carcinoma, amoeboma and appendix abscess.

Patients with colonic tuberculosis may present with features of a dysenteric illness, a colonic mass, an anorectal lesion, or any combination of these.

Tuberculous mesenteric adenitis in the absence of obvious bowel involvement may simulate a variety of disorders, including pancreatic carcinoma and abdominal lymphoma. Presentation may be with weight loss, abdominal pain, and variable constitutional symptoms, while in approximately 80 per cent of cases there will be a palpable mass in the epigastrium, central abdomen or right iliac fossa.

Tuberculous peritonitis may present either with clinical ascites or with the chronic, plastic variety of the disease. Weight loss, abdominal distension, abdominal pain and tenderness are common clinical features. Most complications of abdominal tuberculosis are related either to malabsorption or to the effects of obstruction and/or perforation of the bowel.

Diagnosis is dependent on knowledge of the protean manifestations of abdominal involvement in tuberculosis, the consideration and possibility of tuberculosis in the differential diagnosis of a wide variety of disorders, and the use of appropriate investigations. Radiology, although non-specific, plays an important role and the chest x-ray may provide a clue in up to 40 per cent of patients. As in other forms of organ tuberculosis, routine haematological and biochemical tests are of little diagnostic value. The diagnosis rests on finding acid-fast bacilli on direct staining or culture, or on the typical histopathological picture in an appropriate tissue biopsy.

The distinction between tuberculosis and Crohn's disease and the diagnostic criteria for abdominal tuberculosis are discussed in detail by Marks and colleagues.[17]

The diagnostic value of measuring adenosine deaminase levels (ADA) in ascitic fluid has been reported by Voigt and colleagues.[28] In a retrospective case control study the sensitivity and specificity of ADA above 32,3 u/l were 98 per cent and 95 per cent respectively. In a follow up prospective study of 64 patients with ascites (11 found to have tuberculosis), ADA had a sensitivity of 100 per cent and specificity of 96 per cent in discriminating tuberculosis from other causes of ascites.[28] False negative results were noted in only two patients, both alcoholics with tuberculosis. False positives occurred in two patients with malignant ascites and one with pancreatitis.

Modalities of therapy which may need to be considered over and above conventional antituberculous drugs include parenteral chemotherapy and intravenous hyperalimentation in patients with diffuse bowel involvement, surgery for bowel perforation, acute intestinal obstruction, or (in some patients) to establish the diagnosis. There is probably little place for extensive resection of bowel, although limited resections may be justified in some patients.

The appreciable mortality in patients with abdominal tuberculosis, despite the advent of safe and effective antituberculous drugs, is largely due to serious complications, such as perforated bowel, and the late presentation of many desperately ill patients, many of whom suffer from predisposing conditions such as cirrhosis or alcoholism. Patients with uncomplicated abdominal tuberculosis usually respond dramatically to appropriate drug therapy.

Disseminated tuberculosis[16, 23]

Disseminated tuberculosis may result from the haematogenous spread of tubercle bacilli that directly follows a primary infection (usually in children), from the rupture of a reactivated old focus into the lymphatic or blood-streams, or as a terminal event in a patient with extensive organ tuberculosis. The outcome of such dissemination, clinically and pathologically, varies with the size of the bacillary load and the state of the host defences, and ranges from the very rare acute fulminating form of non-reactive tuberculous septicaemia to the more common classic miliary tuberculous picture. The acute non-reactive form is characterized by extensive tissue necrosis containing numerous mycobacteria and little cellular response, whereas the more chronic reactive type shows a marked cellular response with numerous well-formed tubercles and fewer organisms. Between these extremes lies a spectrum of pathological features. Clinically, the cases closest to the non-reactive end of the spectrum are the ones most likely to be missed in life because of the absence of the miliary chest radiograph.

There have been many reports of disseminated tuberculosis that have only been diagnosed at necropsy, and this form of the disease has been labelled 'cryptic disseminated tuberculosis'. It is also well documented that miliary lesions in the lung are not always accompanied by a miliary pattern on the chest radiograph, although careful inspection of an under-penetrated film may reveal miliary shadows in such patients. Patients with miliary lung lesions may also have an atypical radiographic pattern with unevenly distributed, irregularly shaped nodules, unlike the classic miliary pattern of evenly distributed lesions of less than 2 mm in diameter. Therefore, neither the apparently normal chest radiograph nor the atypical miliary-like picture should be considered to exclude the diagnosis of disseminated tuberculosis in an appropriate clinical setting.

In a retrospective study of 62 cases of disseminated tuberculosis seen over a six-year period in a large teaching hospital, approximately a quarter of the patients had a short history of less than a month, but 17 per cent had had symptoms for longer than six months.[23] The clinical presentations were non-specific. Respiratory symptoms were common, two-thirds of the patients having had a cough (half of these productive) and one-third complained of dyspnoea. Adventitious chest sounds and tachypnoea were frequently found in association with these symptoms. Fever, usually low grade, was almost always present (95 per cent), hepatomegaly was a common finding (62 per cent), but splenomegaly was uncommon (12 per cent) as in other series. The systemic effects and chronicity of the illness were evident from the loss of appetite and weight, with physical evidence of wasting (50 per cent), hypo-albuminaemia (89 per cent), hyponatraemia (51 per cent) and haemoglobin of less than 10 g/dl (35 per cent). As in other series, headache had a high degree of specificity for meningeal involvement. Negative responses to tuberculin skin tests shortly after admission to hospital were recorded in 62 per cent. Previous series have reported negative reactions in 40 per cent of patients with cryptic tuberculosis and in over 30 per cent of patients with miliary tuberculosis. The diagnosis of disseminated tuberculosis was suspected in life in 94,7 per cent of patients with a miliary or miliary-like chest radiograph, and a definitive diagnosis was made during life in 74 per cent. Of the patients without radiographically visible miliary lesions, 15 had other lesions on the chest radiograph. Tuberculosis was considered during life in only 67 per cent of patients without a miliary pattern, while a definite diagnosis of tuberculosis was made during life in only 25 per cent.

None of the patients in this series had gross haematological abnormalities, such as pancytopenia, aplastic anaemia, lymphocytosis or leukemoid reaction. Haemoglobin levels less than 10 g/dl were found in 34,5 per cent, white cell count of less than $4x10^6/l$ in 12,3 per cent and a similar percentage had white cell counts above $12x10^6/l$. A third of the patients had abnormal differential white counts and all had neutrophilia. Only four patients showed an absolute lymphopenia and only three had a platelet count of less than $100x10^6/l$. The ESR ranged from 4 to 150 mm in the first hour, and almost a third of the patients had an ESR of more than 100 mm. Although there were no patients with pancytopenia, three had a combination of relatively low haemoglobin levels, white cell and platelet counts. Bacteriological confirmation of the diagnosis was obtained most frequently from sputum (31 per cent of 39 patients), bronchial brushings (100 per cent of three patients), pleural biopsy (50 per cent of four patients) and lung biopsy (100 per cent of two patients).

Twenty five of the 62 patients (40 per cent) had associated conditions which could have predisposed them to the development of severe tuberculosis. These included alcoholism, malnutrition, diabetes, and cytotoxic or deep x-ray therapy for malignant disease. Of the 38 patients with a miliary-like pattern on the chest radiograph, 53 per cent died, as compared with 83 per cent of patients without miliary shadowing.

In a more recent study of 109 patients with miliary tuberculosis treated in the rifampicin era (1978–87), predisposing conditions were present in 42 per cent of patients.[16] Clinical features were similar to previously reported series. Fibre-optic bronchoscopy was diagnostic in 44 of 51 patients (86 per cent), bone marrow examination in 19 of 22 patients (86 per cent), and liver biopsy in all 10 patients in whom this investigation was done. Twenty four per cent of patients died of miliary tuberculosis, a median of six days after starting treatment. Stepwise logistic regression identified age (over 60 years), lymphopenia, thrombocytopenia, hypo-albuminaemia, elevated transaminases and treatment delay as

Table 6.2
Frequency of positive diagnosis of tuberculosis in patients with disseminated disease[16]

	SPUTUM	BRONCHIAL BRUSHINGS	TRANS-BRONCHIAL BIOPSY	BONE MARROW BIOPSY	LYMPH NODE	LIVER BIOPSY
	(n64)	(n51)	(n48)	(n22)	(n9)	(n11)
AFB stain (Ziehl-Neelsen)	33%	27%	27%	0	56%	27%
AFB culture*	62%	55%	52%	21%	100%	50%
Histology-Granulomata	—	—	63%	82%	100%	100%
Caseation	—	—	42%	41%	100%	45%

* Culture not obtained in all patients in each group

independent predictors of mortality. Tuberculin skin tests were positive in 20 of 47 recorded cases (43 per cent). Twelve patients, all of whom were shown to have haematogenous dissemination, did not have miliary nodules on the chest radiograph. Other common radiological features included pleural reactions, hilar or mediastinal lymphadenopathy, evidence of previous tuberculosis, confluent shadowing, cavities, and spontaneous pneumothorax. In 20 patients in whom follow-up chest radiographs to resolution were available, the mean time for resolution was 18,7 weeks (range 1–44 weeks). Bacteriological analysis of body fluids and biopsy results are shown in Table 6.2.

The temperature response to therapy could be adequately assessed in 55 patients and the median duration for complete resolution of pyrexia was seven days (range 1–55 days), while 76 per cent were afebrile within 14 days. Twenty eight patients died whilst receiving treatment, and this was due to miliary tuberculosis in 26. Median time from commencing treatment to death was six days and 22 patients died within two weeks of commencing treatment.

Complications in this group of patients included central nervous system complications (seizures and hydrocephalus requiring shunting), the adult respiratory distress syndrome, deep vein thrombosis or pulmonary embolism, pericardial tamponade, and Addison's disease.

It is clear from both these series of patients at Groote Schuur Hospital that delayed treatment in miliary TB is associated with increased mortality. There is thus a need for rapid diagnosis, but treatment in severely ill patients should be commenced as soon as the diagnosis is considered.

HIV INFECTION AND TUBERCULOSIS

In the 31 year period from 1953 to 1984 the number of reported cases of tuberculosis in the United States decreased by 73,6 per cent, but this reduction was much greater among whites than among other races.[24] The ratio of the annual risk of tuberculosis among other-than-whites to the risk among whites rose continuously from 2,9 in 1953 to approximately five in 1984.

Beginning in 1985, the decline in the number of reported cases has been reversed and an increase in the number of cases of tuberculosis is being reported. Although such recent increases have been reported from many localities in the United States, the increase in New York city has been most marked. In 1978 tuberculosis in New York city accounted for 4,6 per cent of all cases of TB in the United States, but by 1987 the proportion had more than doubled to 9,8 per cent. The observation that this increase is almost exclusively limited to non-Hispanic blacks and Hispanics in the 20 to 54 year-old age group has been interpreted as evidence that endogenous reactivation of a latent tuberculous infection is caused by a factor that is particularly prevalent in this group of young adults. Infection with the human immunodeficiency virus is a strong contender, and matching of tuberculosis and AIDS registries has shown that in New York city four per cent of patients and in Florida 10 per cent of patients with AIDS had histories of tuberculosis. Tuberculosis preceded the diagnosis of AIDS in a large proportion of cases (up to 50 per cent) suggesting that this infection arises at the point where there is a milder degree of HIV-induced immune deficiency than later in the natural history when this is more profound, and less virulent organisms commonly produce clinical disease.[24]

The hypothesis that tuberculosis in HIV-infected persons results from reactivation of a primary infection is supported by data from a follow-up study of a cohort of drug abusers whose HIV and tuberculin skin test status were known. Of those who were both HIV and tuberculin positive, approximately 14 per cent developed tuberculosis as compared with 0,3 per cent of those who were only HIV positive.[26]

Immigration of people to the United States from countries with high tuberculosis prevalence, as well as poverty and homelessness, are other contributing factors to the reversal in the trend of tuberculosis in the United States.[24]

The implications of these observations are potentially very serious for the African continent where tuberculosis remains a major and growing problem and HIV infection is on the increase. It has been estimated that two per cent of Zairians develop active tuberculosis during their adult lives. HIV sero-prevalence surveys in adults in Kinshasha showed a positive rate of four to six per cent in the general population, 17 per cent in a 1987 sero-survey of 509 consecutive patients with an initial diagnosis of pulmonary tuberculosis seen at an outpatient TB diagnostic centre, and up to 40 per cent in hospitalized sanatorium patients. The death rate was 21 per cent in 84 HIV sero-positive sanatorium patients in 1987 who were followed for two months after admission, as compared with nine per cent

in 128 HIV negative patients.[5] In Uganda, one of the first countries in Africa to collaborate with the WHO in setting up a national AIDS control programme, 8 000 cases of AIDS had been reported by 1989.[12] The gravity of the AIDS problem in Africa is reflected in the very high rate of seropositivity in some groups (e.g. 67 per cent in barmaids and 32 per cent in truck drivers in Uganda).[12] It has been estimated that there could be 40 000 to 50 000 new cases of HIV-induced tuberculosis each year in addition to the usual 16 000 new cases that had been reported annually in Uganda before the HIV epidemic.[12]

Studies of mycobacterial disease among adult patients with AIDS have shown that many have severe and unusual manifestations of infection with *Mycobacterium tuberculosis* which often includes extrapulmonary and disseminated disease.[4, 14, 27] This picture is complicated by the fact that many patients with AIDS were also drug abusers. Although the diagnosis of tuberculosis most commonly precedes the diagnosis of AIDS, in some patients both diagnoses may be made concurrently while in others the diagnosis of AIDS may precede the development of tuberculosis. In 29 patients with AIDS who also had tuberculosis, 72 per cent had predominantly extrapulmonary tuberculosis, 55 per cent had disseminated disease, 35 per cent had peripheral lymph node and 27 per cent bone marrow involvement.[27] In another study more than 50 per cent of intravenous drug abusers with AIDS and clinically significant lymphadenopathy, had tuberculous adenitis on biopsy.[14] Hilar, mediastinal and paratracheal lymphadenopathy are more common in association with tuberculosis in AIDS patients than in those without. Histologic non-reactive tuberculosis with poor or absent granuloma formation is relatively common.

Radiographically most patients with AIDS and tuberculosis have a disease suggestive of progressive primary tuberculosis and only a minority have the classical apical infiltrates of reactivation disease. Lower lobe infiltrates, considerable lymphadenopathy and air-fluid levels in cavities are common features. The presence of extrapulmonary tuberculosis in 72 per cent of patients is at least three times higher than in patients without AIDS. Despite the state of the immune system, most patients with AIDS respond well to conventional antituberculous treatment: a small proportion do not respond adequately and the death rate, as mentioned above, is higher in patients with AIDS.

Recent descriptions of endobronchial tuberculosis in patients with AIDS adds another dimension to the presentation and natural history of tuberculosis in these patients.[30] Despite involvement of the bronchial mucosa, sputum is often negative for acid-fast bacilli and biopsies often fail to reveal granulomas. Cultures are important as bronchoscopic appearances closely resemble those of bronchogenic carcinoma.[15] Despite rapid progression of disease prior to diagnosis, patients usually respond well to anti-tuberculous chemotherapy and this again emphasizes the need for prompt and accurate diagnosis.

TUBERCULOSIS AND MALIGNANCY[7]

Carcinoma may complicate tuberculosis by developing in a scar of previous disease. Similarly, tuberculosis may complicate carcinoma by reactivation due to immune suppression. Patients with tuberculosis have up to a twenty-fold increased risk of carcinoma and this applies in particular to patients with carcinoma of the lung, in whom the diagnosis of tuberculosis often ante-dates the diagnosis of carcinoma. Tuberculosis may also occur with Hodgkin's and non-Hodgkin's lymphomas and in particular after immunosuppressive treatment.

CONCLUSION

Tuberculosis remains a major scourge throughout the world, but most especially in developing countries. The range of clinical manifestations it produces are protean, but knowledge of these combined with early diagnosis and appropriate modern management have greatly transformed the prognosis for the individual patient over the last 50 years.

REFERENCES

1 Benatar S R, 1982. Tuberculosis in the 1980s, with particular reference to South Africa. *South African Medical Journal*. 62, 359–64.
2 British Thoracic and Tuberculosis Association, 1970. Aspergilloma and residual tuberculous cavities. The results of a survey. *Tubercle*. 51, 227–45.
3 Campbell I A & Dyson A J, 1977. Lymph node tuberculosis, a comparison of various methods of treatment. *Tubercle*. 58, 171–9.
4 Chaisson R E, Schecter G F, Theuer C P *et al.*, 1987. Tuberculosis in patients with the acquired immunodeficiency syndrome. Clinical features, responses to therapy and survival. *American Review of Respiratory Diseases*. 136, 570–4.
5 Colebunders R L, Ryder R W, Nzilambi N *et al.*, 1989. HIV infection in patients with tuberculosis in Kinshasha, Zaire. *American Review of Respiratory Diseases*. 139, 1082–5.
6 Cowie R L & Escreet B C, 1980. The diagnosis of pulmonary tuberculosis. *South African Medical Journal*. 57, 75–7.
7 Ellner J J, 1989. Tuberculosis. In: Kelley W N (ed.). *Textbook of Internal Medicine*. Philadelphia: J B Lippincott Co.
8 Epstein D M, Kline S M, Albelda S M & Miller W T, 1987. Tuberculous pleural effusions. *Chest*. 91, 106–9.
9 Faulken S L, Vernon R, Brown P B *et al.*, 1978. Haemoptysis and pulmonary aspergilloma, operative versus non-operative treatment. *Annals of Thoracic Surgery*. 25, 389–92.
10 Fourie P B, 1983. Prevalence and annual rate of tuberculosis infection in South Africa. *Tubercle*. 64, 181–2.
11 Gilinsky N H, Marks I N, Kottler R E & Price S K, 1983. Abdominal tuberculosis, a 10 year review. *South African Medical Journal*. 64, 849–57.

12 Goodgame R W, 1990. AIDS in Uganda — clinical and social features. *New England Journal of Medicine.* 323, 383–9.

13 Harris H W & McClement J H, 1983. Pulmonary tuberculosis. In: Hoeprich P D (ed.). *Infectious Diseases.* 3rd ed. Philadelphia: Harper and Row.

14 Hewlett D Jr, Duncanson F P, Jagadha V, Lieberman J, Lenox T H & Wormser G P, 1988. Lymphadenopathy in an inner-city population consisting principally of intravenous drug abusers with suspected acquired immunodeficiency syndrome. *American Review of Respiratory Disease.* 137, 1275–9.

15 Ip M S M, So S Y, Lam W K & Mok C K, 1986. Endobronchial tuberculosis revisited. *Chest.* 89, 727–30.

16 Maartens G, Willcox P A & Benatar S R, 1990. Miliary tuberculosis: Rapid diagnosis, haematological abnormalities and outcome in 109 treated adults. *American Journal of Medicine.* 89, 291–6.

17 Marks I N, Kottler R E & Gilinsky N H, 1983. Abdominal tuberculosis. In: Jewell D P & Shepherd H A (eds). *Topics in Gastroenterology II.* Oxford: Blackwell Scientific Publications.

18 McKeown T, 1979. *The Role of Medicine.* Oxford: Blackwell Scientific Publications.

19 Morris C D W, 1989. The radiography, haematology and biochemistry of pulmonary tuberculosis in the aged. *Quarterly Journal of Medicine.* 266, 529–35.

20 Nardell E, McInnes B, Thomas B & Weidhaas S, 1986. Exogenous re-infection with tuberculosis in a shelter for the homeless. *New England Journal of Medicine.* 315, 1570–5.

21 Odell J, 1990. Pleural tuberculosis. In: Deslaurieux J & Lacquet L K (eds). *Thoracic Surgery: Surgical Management of Pleural Diseases.* Vol. 6. St Louis, C V Mosby Co..

22 Palmer P E S, 1979. Pulmonary tuberculosis — usual and unusual radiographic presentations. *Seminars in Roentgenology.* 14(3), 204–43.

23 Prout S & Benatar S R, 1980. Disseminated tuberculosis, a study of 62 cases. *South African Medical Journal.* 58, 835–42.

24 Rieder H L, Cauthen G M, Kelly G D, Bloch A B & Snider P E, 1989. Tuberculosis in the United States. *Journal of the American Medical Association.* 263, 385–9.

25 Segal I, 1984. Intestinal tuberculosis, Crohn's disease and ulcerative colitis in an urban black population. *South African Medical Journal.* 65, 37–44.

26 Selwyn P A, Hartel D, Lewis V A *et al.,* 1989. A prospective study of the risk of tuberculosis among intravenous drug users with human immunodeficiency virus infection. *New England Journal of Medicine.* 320, 545–50.

27 Sunderam G, McDonald R J, Maniatis T, Oleske J, Kapila R, Reichman L B, 1986. Tuberculosis as a manifestation of the acquired immunodeficiency syndrome (AIDS). *Journal of the American Medical Association.* 256, 362–6.

28 Voigt M, Trey C, Lombard C *et al,* 1989. Diagnostic value of ascites adenosine deaminase in tuberculous peritonitis. *Lancet.* 1, 751–4.

29 Wallace J M, Deutsch A L, Harrell J H & Moser K M, 1981. Bronchoscopy and transbronchial biopsy in evaluation of patients with suspected active tuberculosis. *American Journal of Medicine.* 70, 1189–94.

30 Wasser L S, Shaw G W & Talavera W, 1988. Endobronchial tuberculosis in the acquired immunodeficiency syndrome. *Chest.* 94, 1240–4.

31 Willcox P A, Benatar S R & Potgieter P D, 1982. Use of the flexible fibreoptic bronchoscope in diagnosis of sputum-negative pulmonary tuberculosis. *Thorax.* 37, 598–601.

32 Yach D, 1988. Tuberculosis in the western Cape health region of South Africa. *Social Science and Medicine.* 1988, 27, 683–9.

CHAPTER 7

Tuberculous pericarditis

P J Commerford and J I G Strang

INTRODUCTION

Tuberculous pericarditis, arguably one of the most important and common bacteriological infections of the heart, receives scant attention in the world literature and even in many major cardiology texts. It is uncommon in the United States and Europe, but remains an important cause of morbidity and mortality in countries where tuberculosis is endemic. In one series, tuberculosis was considered to be the cause of the effusion in 56 per cent of 52 consecutive unselected patients with pericardial effusion referred for diagnostic pericardiocentesis at Cape Town's Groote Schuur Hospital.

Unfortunately, the clinical diagnosis is often missed and patients with a treatable and curable form of heart disease are misdiagnosed as 'cardiomyopathy' or 'heart failure — cause undetermined'. For this reason, no apology is made for re-emphasizing the importance of careful clinical examination and the value of simple, readily available special investigations when evaluating patients with the symptoms and signs of heart failure in the South African context. Regrettably tuberculous pericarditis is still common in this country and the diagnosis must be considered and excluded in all patients presenting with dyspnoea, raised venous pressure, hepatomegaly, ascites and peripheral oedema. This is particularly important when cursory examination has revealed 'no abnormality of the heart' or ventricular function has been reported to be 'normal'.

Unresolved problems include the role of diagnostic pericardiocentesis as opposed to open pericardial drainage and biopsy, the difficulty of establishing a bacteriological or histological diagnosis, and the timing of pericardiectomy. The clinical diagnosis of constrictive pericarditis may be difficult and its differentiation from restrictive cardiomyopathy almost impossible, despite the use of sophisticated special investigations.

PATHOLOGY AND PATHOGENESIS

Pericardial involvement usually develops by retrograde spread from peritracheal, peribronchial or mediastinal lymph nodes or by haematogenous spread from the primary tuberculous infection.[3, 4, 18] The pericardium is involved infrequently by breakdown and contiguous spread from a tuberculous lesion in the lung or by haematogenous spread from distant secondary skeletal or genito-urinary infections.[1]

Viable acid-fast bacilli, fibrin deposits and granuloma formation are followed by the development of a pericardial effusion,[18] which is usually haemorrhagic but may be serous. Polymorphonuclear leucocytes are said to be present early in the development of the effusion, but later at the time of clinical presentation they are replaced by monocytes, lymphocytes and plasma cells. The rate of accumulation of fluid is variable. If the effusion develops slowly, even large effusions may be well tolerated, but rapid accumulation of even relatively small effusions may cause haemodynamic compromise and tamponade. The demonstration of complement-fixing antimyolemmal and antimyosin type antibodies in 75 per cent of patients with acute tuberculous pericarditis has been cited as being possible evidence that cytolysis mediated by antimyolemmal antibodies may contribute to the development of exudative tuberculous pericarditis.[15]

As the effusion is absorbed the pericardium thickens and a thick fibrinous exudate is deposited on the visceral and parietal pericardium. The pathology is very

Table 7.1
Physical signs documented by a single observer in 88 patients with tuberculous pericardial effusion and 67 patients with constrictive pericarditis[20]

	PERICARDIAL EFFUSION (N=88)	CONSTRICTIVE PERICARDITIS (N=67)
1. Sinus tachycardia	68 (77%) (transient AF in 3)	47 (70%) (persistent AF in 2)
2. Significant pulsus paradoxus	32 (36%)	32 (48%)
3. Raised jugular venous pulse	74 (84%)	67 (100%)
4. Apex palpable	53 (60%)	39 (58%)
5. Soft heart sounds	69 (78%)	51 (76%)
6. Hepatomegaly	84 (95%)	67 (100%)
7. Ascites	64 (73%)	60 (89%)
8. Oedema	22 (25%)	63 (94%)
9. Increased cardiac dullness	83 (94%)	17 (25%)
10. Pericardial friction rub	16 (18%)	—
11. Tamponade	3 (3%)	—
12. Pericardial knock	—	14 (21%)
13. Third heart sound	—	30 (45%)
14. Sudden inspiratory splitting of S^2	—	24 (36%)

AF = Atrial fibrillation

variable and may range from a serous effusion, with a few strands of fibrin, to the more common haemorrhagic effusion. Two dimensional echocardiographic appearances of porridge-like material filling the pericardial cavity presumably reflect a fibrinous exudate with a very high protein content. With further resolution, a granulomatous reaction with caseation develops and the effusion may become loculated. Fibrous tissue and collagen finally replace the granulomatous reaction and may become calcified, encasing the heart in a fibro-calcific skin which impedes diastolic filling and causes the classical clinical syndrome of constrictive pericarditis.

However, all this is to some extent hypothetical, based on individual 'windows of observation' in the course of a chronic illness, and on clinical observation in countries where tuberculosis is endemic. A characteristic course can be recognized where patients are identified with a large effusion but little evidence of constriction. The heart shadow then decreases in size and signs of constriction become apparent even when it

is moderately enlarged, in an effusive-constrictive phase.[7] In some patients signs of chronic constriction develop insidiously over the course of months and years without a preceding identifiable illness, and in countries where tuberculosis is uncommon this illness is usually considered to be idiopathic. In areas and populations where the disease is common, 'idiopathic' constrictive pericarditis is often attributed to pericardial tuberculosis.

Several important questions remain. Does a pericardial effusion always precede the development of the fibro-caseous effusive-constrictive syndrome? Do some pericardial effusions resolve spontaneously? Is it correct to incriminate a tuberculous aetiology in the majority of patients presenting with dense fibrous or calcific constriction in countries where tuberculosis is endemic?

CLINICAL FEATURES

Clinical manifestations are extremely variable and depend on how far advanced the disease is when the patient presents, and on the systemic reaction to infection.

They will obviously be different in the effusive, effusive-constrictive and constrictive phases. The physical signs elicited by a single observer in a large series of patients with effusion and constriction are recorded in Table 7.1.[20]

Effusion

The condition is said to develop slowly with non-specific symptoms of systemic infection, such as low-grade fever, night sweats, malaise, anorexia and loss of weight. Not all patients have these features, and some may appear remarkably healthy, well-nourished and have no features of systemic disease. Occasionally the disease takes a fulminant course with marked systemic symptoms, a high fever and rapid progression to tamponade or constriction. If the effusion is large, patients may complain of dyspnoea or a dull heavy retrosternal discomfort. Typical pericardial pain is uncommon.[10]

Physical examination may reveal tachypnoea and fever with evidence of recent weight loss.

The effusion itself may be silent clinically, but if the fluid accumulation causes a rise in intrapericardial pressure and cardiac compression, then the symptoms and signs of cardiac tamponade develop. Several factors influence the development of increased intrapericardial pressure secondary to a pericardial effusion,[5] including the volume of fluid, its rate of accumulation and the physical characteristics of the pericardium. The pericardial space normally contains between 15 and 50 ml of fluid, but if additional fluid accumulates slowly, allowing the pericardium to stretch, one to two litres of fluid may be accommodated without a rise in pressure. Rapid accumulation of relatively small volumes of fluid in the unstretched pericardial space may precipitate serious haemodynamic compromise and tamponade. It is important to appreciate this in order to understand clinical presentations.

Pericardial effusion without cardiac compression

Patients with pericardial effusions that do not cause cardiac compression may have no symptoms apart from a vague sensation of a dull ache or oppression in the chest. Large effusions may compress adjacent structures, causing cough due to bronchial or tracheal compression, or dyspnoea due to compression of lung parenchyma.

A small effusion without cardiac compression may produce no abnormal physical signs apart from a pericardial friction rub. When a large pericardial effusion is present, cardiac dullness may be increased and may be detected to the right of the sternum, the apex beat may be impalpable and the heart sounds soft and muffled. A large effusion compressing the left lower lobe bronchus may cause signs of consolidation at the left base (Ewart's sign). Coexistent pleural effusions may also be detected. A pericardial friction rub may be heard even in the presence of a large effusion. Abnormalities of pulse, blood pressure and jugular venous pressure do not occur when the intrapericardial pressure is not raised.

While tuberculous pericarditis may cause effusions which do not produce cardiac compression, it is more common for there to be at least some degree of cardiac compression, which may be severe causing tamponade.

Pericardial effusion with cardiac compression: cardiac tamponade

Intrapericardial pressure is normally similar to intrapleural pressure and lower than ventricular diastolic pressures. When fluid accumulation in the pericardial space causes the pressure to rise to the same level as the right atrial and right ventricular diastolic pressure the transmural pressure distending these cardiac chambers is reduced to almost zero, and cardiac tamponade results.[9] Further elevations of intrapericardial pressure will cause right ventricular pressure to rise to left ventricular diastolic pressure. Thereafter all three pressures rise together and systemic arterial pressure falls. The clinical syndrome of cardiac tamponade then develops. The findings on physical examination will depend on the degree of elevation of pericardial pressure and the length of time the abnormality has been present. With severe compression, patients are extremely ill and complain of dyspnoea. Peripheral oedema, hepatomegaly and ascites will be present.

In addition to the signs of a pericardial effusion outlined above, abnormalities of the pulse and venous pressure will be detected. The jugular venous pressure will be raised with a characteristic waveform, consisting of a prominent systolic 'x' descent and absent diastolic 'y' descent. However, this may be difficult to appreciate at the bedside in an ill patient with a tachycardia who is breathing rapidly and using accessory muscles of respiration. The peripheral arterial pulse is rapid and of small volume.

Pulsus paradoxus is characteristic and is critical in making a diagnosis. This is detected on physical examination as an inspiratory decrease in amplitude of the palpated pulse, and is best sought in a large pulse such as the femoral. Complete disappearance of the palpated pulse during inspiration (total paradox) occurs during severe compression. The sign may be difficult to detect in a patient with a marked tachycardia and tachypnoea. The magnitude of the paradoxus can be estimated by using a sphygmomanometer.

Pulsus paradoxus must be measured carefully. The sphygmomanometer cuff should be inflated above the systolic pressure and slowly deflated until the Korotkoff sounds are heard during expiration only. The cuff should then be deflated further to the point at which Korotkoff sounds are heard equally well in inspiration and expiration. The measured pulsus paradoxus is then the difference between these two pressures. Ten mmHg of paradoxus is usually considered abnormal. However, the absolute value may not be an accurate indication of the severity of compression (particularly in patients with a very small pulse volume) and some suggest that the ratio of the magnitude of the paradoxus to the pulse volume should be considered. It is significant if it equals or exceeds half the pulse pressure.[12]

Constrictive pericarditis

The clinical features of constrictive pericarditis depend on how long the process has been present, how severe it is and whether or not there is an active inflammatory process. Patients with only modest elevations of systemic venous and right atrial pressures will also have only modest elevation of the left ventricular end diastolic pressure. Under these circumstances the predominant symptoms will be those secondary to systemic venous congestion and include oedema, abdominal swelling and abdominal discomfort secondary to hepatomegaly and ascites. If both left and right heart filling pressures are raised significantly then symptoms of pulmonary venous congestion, including dyspnoea on exertion and orthopnoea, will be present.

Examination will confirm evidence of systemic venous congestion with elevation of the jugular venous pressure, hepatomegaly, ascites and peripheral oedema. Frequently the severity of hepatomegaly and ascites is out of proportion to the degree of peripheral oedema and such patients are sometimes misdiagnosed as suffering from hepatic cirrhosis.

However, in constrictive pericarditis the jugular venous pressure is always raised, although a casual examination of the neck may miss this important feature. The waveform is characteristic with rapid 'x' and 'y' descents. In very severe cases of pericardial constriction the neck veins may appear to be non-pulsatile and the abnormality may only be detected when the patient is in the upright position.

In patients with severe constrictive pericarditis, palpation of the praecordium usually reveals a palpable third heart sound, diastolic lift or pericardial knock, occurring about 120 mS after the aortic component of the second heart sound, and corresponding in timing to the sudden cessation of ventricular filling and the early diastolic plateau of the diastolic ventricular volume curve. It becomes more prominent during inspiration. It will only be detected if palpation is performed carefully and will be missed if praecordial events are not related to a reliable marker of ventricular systole such as the upstroke of the carotid pulse.

Once significant constriction occurs the arterial pulse is of small volume and the pulse pressure is reduced. Pulsus paradoxus can usually be detected, and if not detectable on palpation, then it should always be sought with a sphygmomanometer as described above.

The auscultatory signs are subtle, and will often be missed by the inexperienced observer unless sought specifically. A high pitched early diastolic sound, commonly described as an early third heart sound, will often be heard along the left sternal border in rigid constrictive pericarditis. This coincides with the diastolic lift, is accentuated by inspiration, and the stethoscope will be seen to move coincident with this sound. Sudden (instantaneous) splitting of the second heart sound in constrictive pericarditis was described many years ago,[2] and it remains a valuable clue to those experienced in its recognition. Sophisticated echocardiographic and Doppler studies have clarified the mechanism of this physical sign with the demonstration that there is a marked decrease in early mitral flow velocity on the first beat after the onset of inspiration. The tricuspid flow velocity shows reciprocal changes with an increase on the first beat of the inspiration. These abnormalities can be reversed by pericardiectomy.[13]

Effusive constrictive pericarditis

While the clinical syndromes of pericardial effusion, with or without cardiac tamponade, and classical constrictive pericarditis are seen in patients with tuberculous pericarditis, a mixed form (the so-called effusive-constrictive variety) is well-recognized[25] and may, in fact, be the most common clinical presentation in South Africa. In this condition there is increased pericardial pressure due to a pericardial effusion in the presence of visceral pericardial constriction.[11] The characteristic of this condition is persistent elevation of the right atrial and jugular venous pressure after aspiration of pericardial fluid and restoration of pericardial pressure to zero. Effusive constrictive pericarditis may be a stage in the development of classic constrictive pericarditis.

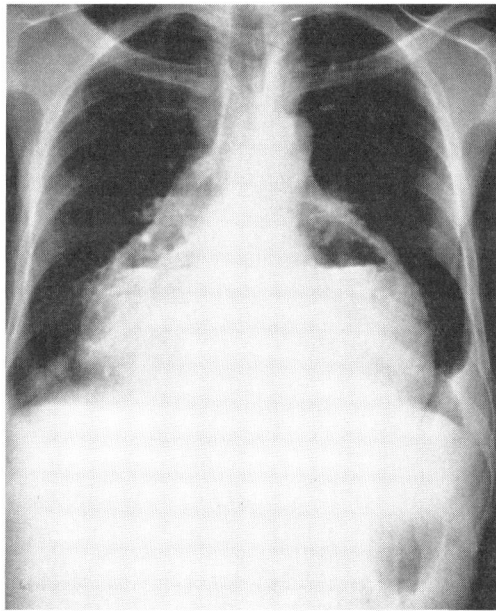

Figure 7.1. (a) Pre-treatment chest radiograph of a patient with a proven tuberculous pericardial effusion, following pericardiocentesis and introduction of air. The thickened pericardium is common, but is not specific to tuberculous pericarditis. Note the clear lung fields.

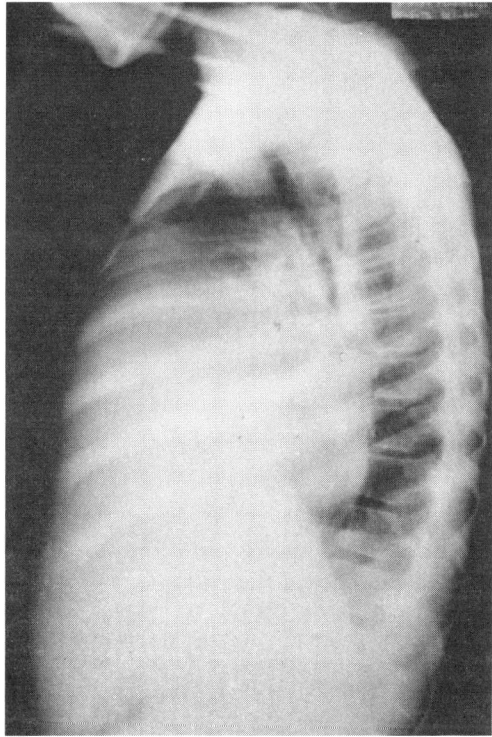

Figure 7.1. (b) Lateral chest radiograph of a child with a large pericardial effusion, showing reduction in the retrosternal space.

Physical findings are similar to those found in pericardial effusion with pulsus paradoxus and raised venous pressure, and the venous pressure waveform is intermediate between that seen in effusion and that seen in constriction.[11] However, unlike effusion a diastolic knock may be detected on palpation and an early third heart sound on auscultation. It is in patients with the effusive-constrictive syndrome that echocardiography may show a pericardial effusion between thickened pericardial membranes, with fibrinous pericardial bands apparently causing loculation of the effusion.

INVESTIGATION AND DIAGNOSIS

Three investigations are commonly used to diagnose pericarditis: chest radiography, electrocardiography and echocardiography. Echocardiography is the most useful, but may be unavailable where the disease is most common.

Pericardial effusion

Chest radiography

An enlarged globular cardiac shadow with a clear margin, due to impaired movement of the distended pericardium, is characteristic (Figure 7.1a). Pleural effusion is common, while pulmonary venous congestion is unusual. There is evidence of associated pulmonary tuberculosis in the minority. In the Transkei pericarditis study, pleural effusion was present in 39 per cent of 198 patients, but changes suggestive of active pulmonary tuberculosis were present in only 30 per cent, and only 11 per cent had sputum-positive tuberculosis.[23] With large pericardial effusions, a lateral chest radiograph shows diminution of the retrosternal space (Figure 7.1b).

Electrocardiography

Electrocardiography is useful only in that it may suggest a cardiac abnormality. Traditionally, the QRS complexes are described as small, with generalized T-wave inversion. However, in the Transkei study, QRS complex voltages on ECG were reduced in 19 per cent, and there were generalized T-wave abnormalities in 90 per cent of 187 patients. Eight patients had atrial fibrillation which was transient, the remainder were in sinus rhythm.[23] Electrical alternans was seen in two patients on admission.

Echocardiography

Two dimensional and M-mode features of pericardial effusion are well described.[8] The two dimensional (sector scanning) technique is the easier of the two and even an inexperienced operator can learn to diagnose a pericardial effusion. Typically, the pericardial effusion is moderate or large in size, and fibrinous strands extend into it from the visceral and parietal surfaces of the pericardium (Figure 7.2). Confirmation of a pericardial effusion by echocardiography gives no clue as to its aetiology and, since amoebiasis occurs in populations affected by tuberculous pericarditis, it is essential to scan the liver in the subcostal view during echocardiography, to exclude amoebic liver abscess as the cause. Although uncommon, amoebic pericarditis is a condition which is likely to be fatal if not treated specifically.[21] In the diagnosis of pericardial effusion, echocardiography is so simple, fast and certain that all other sophisticated investigations, such as cardiac catheterization with the injection of radio-opaque contrast medium or carbon dioxide into the right ventricle, to assess the distance between the parietal pericardium and the endocardium, are of historical interest. The value of echocardiography in the diagnosis of pericardial effusion is such that it should be available in all hospitals in which the condition is seen regularly.

Pericardiocentesis

This is safe in the presence of all but the smallest effusions but ideally it should not be done without confirmation by echocardiography. This is especially important in the presence of a pericardial rub, because usually the anterior surface of the heart is rubbing against the anterior surface of the visceral pericardium making the procedure more hazardous. In an emergency, life-saving pericardiocentesis may be required on clinical grounds alone. The subcostal route is best, since the needle enters the most dependent part of the pericardium, does not cross the pleural space, is away from the advancing surface of the heart, and is aimed at the inferior surface of the heart,

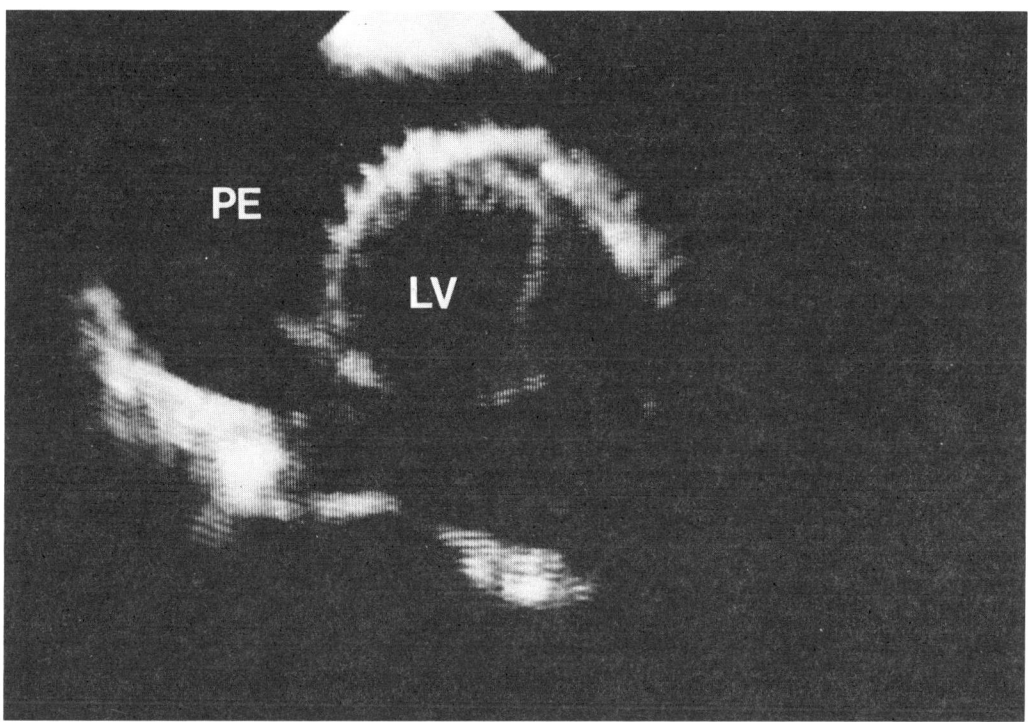

Figure 7.2. Two dimensional echocardiograph, apical four chamber view. A large pericardial effusion surrounds the heart and numerous fibrinous strands are present on the visceral pericardium. LV = left ventricle, PE = pericardial effusion.

where it is least likely to damage a coronary artery. The risk of causing a pneumothorax if the pleura is crossed when using another route is small, but contamination of the pleura if the effusion is purulent or due to amoebiasis is serious. Ideally, the patient should be connected to a cardiac monitor and have an intravenous infusion during the procedure, and atropine 0,5 mg intravenously should be given to try to prevent a vaso-vagal attack.

Pericardiocentesis is indicated to establish the cause of a pericardial effusion and to relieve tamponade. Tamponade was present in 10 per cent of 198 patients on admission in the Transkei study.[23] Eighty per cent of tuberculous pericardial effusions are blood stained, often heavily, but the fluid does not clot on standing and spreads rapidly on gauze or a paper towel, with a wide halo, unlike blood which spreads more slowly with a narrow halo. If there is any doubt, a haemoglobin estimation of the fluid, with a simultaneous estimation from the patient's venous blood will settle the matter. The remainder are straw coloured, clear or turbid.

Culture of tubercle bacilli from pericardial effusions can be improved considerably by inoculation into double strength Kirchner culture medium at the bedside. In the Transkei study this resulted in the culture of tubercle bacilli from 59 per cent of 189 pericardial effusions, a far higher figure than had been previously obtained.[23] Pericardial fluid can be examined for the presence of malignant cells. If purulent, immediate Gram-stain and early surgical drainage are required.

Elevated levels of adenosine deaminase have been reported in the pericardial fluid of a small number of patients with tuberculous pericarditis.[16] The experience at Groote Schuur Hospital with a larger group of patients tends to confirm this and assay of adenosine deaminase may be of value in establishing the tuberculous aetiology of a pericardial effusion.

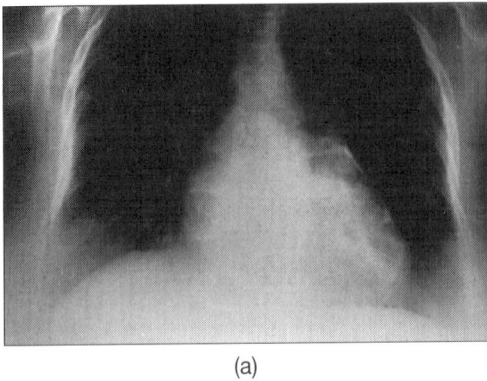

(a)

(b)

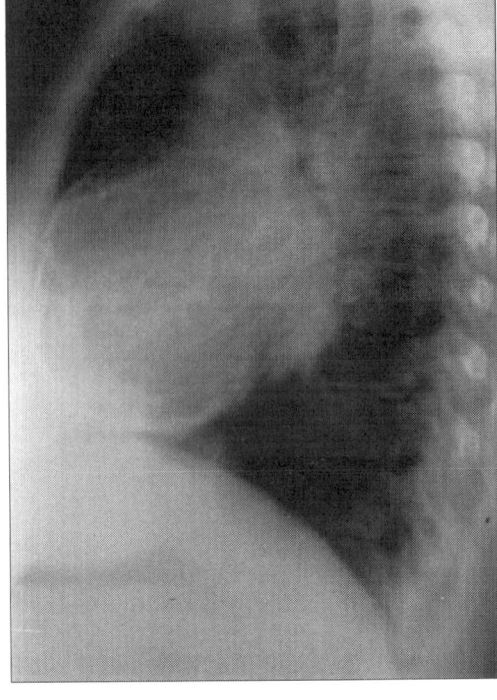

Figure 7.3. Chest radiographs of a patient with constrictive pericarditis showing calcification of the pericardium which is more obvious in the lateral view (b).

Pericardial biopsy and drainage

Pericardial biopsy and drainage by inferior pericardiotomy is a minor operation for a surgeon and can be done under local anaesthesia if general anaesthesia is not available.[6, 14] It has the advantage of draining the pericardium completely and may give histological confirmation of the cause of pericarditis. In the Transkei study, further pericardiocentesis for haemodynamic reasons was necessary in 23 per cent of patients who did not have an open drainage on admission. Culture of the fluid confirmed tuberculosis more often than did histology of the pericardium.[23] The decision to undertake pericardial biopsy and drainage or pericardiocentesis depends on local facilities, but in practices in which tuberculosis is not common, biopsy and drainage is preferable because of the greater likelihood of malignancy. Tamponade is a life-threatening condition and if staff are unable to perform pericardiocentesis, open drainage is safer and prevents recurrence of pericardial effusion.

The examination of sputum for tubercle bacilli and biopsy of lymph nodes may produce additional supportive evidence of tuberculosis as the cause of pericarditis, but it is worth re-emphasizing that sputum positive tuberculosis and chest radiograph appearances compatible with tuberculosis are seen in the minority of patients. Their absence does not reduce the likelihood of a tuberculous aetiology in a susceptible population.

Constrictive pericarditis

Most patients with constrictive pericarditis in southern Africa have the sub-acute variety, in which a thick fibrinous exudate (which may contain small locules of fluid) fills the pericardial sac, compressing the heart and causing a circulatory disturbance. Again, chest radiography and electrocardiography give clues to the diagnosis, but echocardiography is definitive.

Chest radiography

The sub-acute nature of the disease means that calcification of the pericardium will be absent in the majority and was found in less than five per cent in Transkei[20] (Figure 7.3).

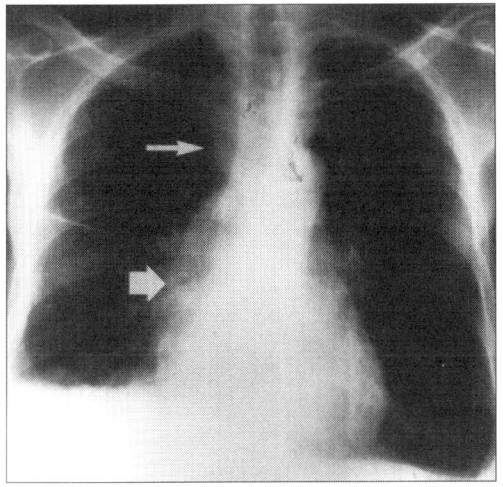

Figure 7.4. Chest radiograph of a patient with sub-acute constrictive pericarditis (same patient as in Figure 7.1(a), who developed constriction). The lower arrow indicates the convex right heart border rising from the diaphragm and the upper arrow indicates the distended superior vena cava.

The chest radiograph findings, while non-specific if taken individually, are characteristic when taken in conjunction. In the Transkei study, 70 per cent of 143 patients had a cardiothoracic ratio greater than 55 per cent but in only six per cent was it greater than 75 per cent.[24] The right heart border shows a characteristic appearance, with a convex curve rising from the diaphragm upwards to where the shadow of the distended superior vena cava appears as a soft vertical line adjacent to the mediastinum. The normal notch at the root of the right lung is absent.

This appearance was described 40 years ago in Britain,[19] while in the Transkei study it was noted in 71 per cent of 112 patients presenting with constrictive pericarditis. The left heart border may be straight, and pleural effusion is common. Bilateral pleural effusions were seen in 80 per cent of 112 patients with constriction, on admission, in the Transkei study, the majority being either moderate sized or small. Lung changes suggestive of active tuberculosis were noted in only 14 patients, while

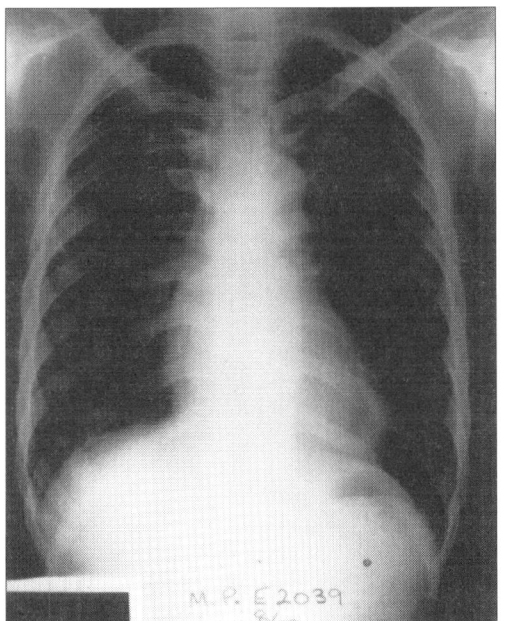

Figure 7.5. Chest radiographs of a patient with sub-acute constrictive pericarditis, relieved by pericardiectomy. **(a)** A pre-operative film which looks remarkably normal, but was taken seven weeks after

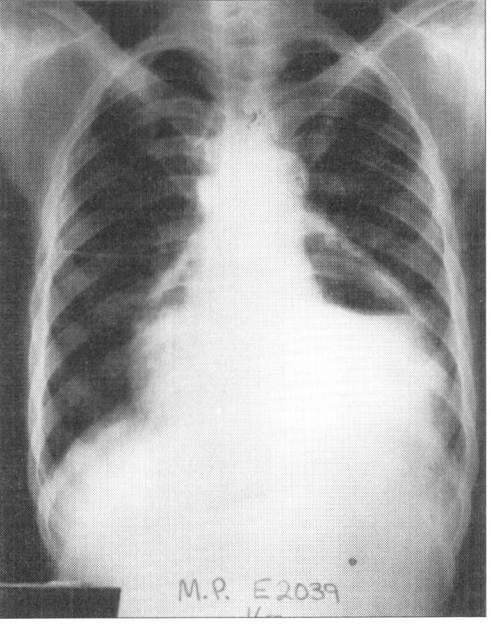

Figure 7.5. (b) when the patient had a pericardial effusion. Note the clear lung fields.

sputum examination for tubercle bacilli was positive in 14. Figure 7.4 shows the characteristic appearance of sub-acute constrictive pericarditis in a patient whose pericardium was surgically removed for severe constriction. The chest radiograph may look remarkably normal, as in Figure 7.5a. The radiograph is that of a patient with constrictive pericarditis, confirmed by pericardiectomy, whose initial chest radiograph, showing a pericardial effusion appears in Figure 7.5b.

Electrocardiography

Non-specific but generalized T-wave changes were seen in 107 of 108 patients in the Transkei study, but low-voltage complexes occurred in only a third of them.[24] Atrial fibrillation occurred in less than five per cent of patients, was persistent, and usually occurred with a calcified pericardium. As with pericardial effusion, the ECG is useful only in drawing attention to the presence of a cardiac abnormality.

Echocardiography

This is particularly valuable in confirming the diagnosis of subacute constrictive pericarditis. Typically, a thick fibrinous exudate is seen in the pericardial sac and is associated with diminished movements of the surface of the heart, normal sized chambers, absence of valvular heart disease and absence of myocardial hypertrophy.[22] The inferior vena cava is greatly dilated as are the intrahepatic veins. In time the pericardial exudate condenses into a thick skin surrounding the heart, which usually, but not always, can be distinguished from myocardium.

Movement of the interventricular septum to the left on inspiration is commonly seen in constrictive pericarditis and may be responsible in part for pulsus paradoxus.[22]

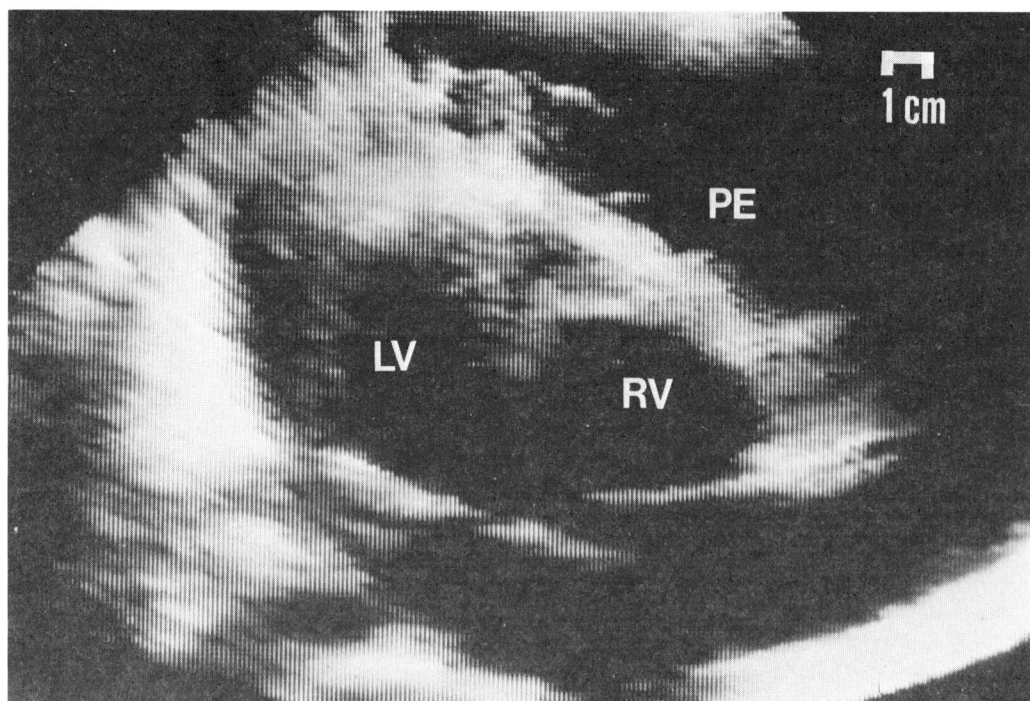

Figure 7.6. Patient with effusive-constrictive pericarditis, who subsequently had pericardiectomy for severe constriction. Two dimensional echocardiograph, apical four chamber view. Note the very thickened visceral pericardium with fibrinous strands extending into the effusion. The posterior surface of the heart is immobilized by attachment to the posterior parietal pericardium. Surface movements of the heart were diminished. LV = left ventricle. RV = right ventricle. PE = pericardial effusion.

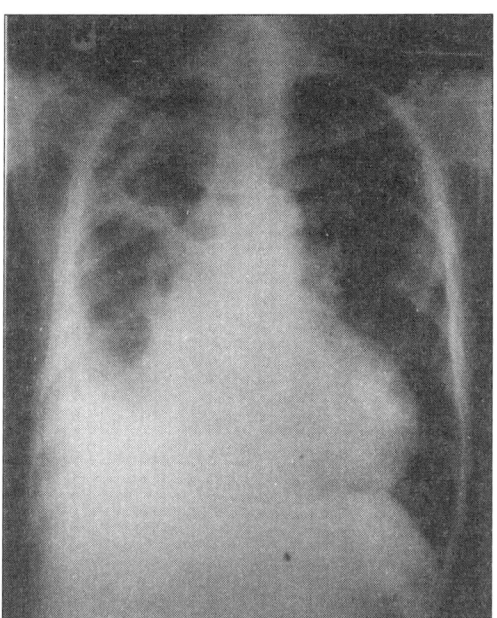

Figure 7.7. Chest radiograph of a patient with effusive-constrictive pericarditis, who had a pericardial knock and whose condition was confirmed by echocardiography. The heart shadow is more suggestive of myocardial disease than pericarditis.

In the context of 'congestive cardiac failure of unknown cause' the findings described, if not associated with a pericardial exudate or obvious pericardial thickening, can be due only to a restrictive cardiomyopathy, a rare disease compared with constrictive pericarditis. The only other explanation is that the echocardiogram has not detected an abnormal pericardium. It is unclear how frequently this occurs. However, recent reports claim that Doppler and M-mode echocardiography can distinguish the two accurately.[13, 17] Despite these advances, the ability of any test to differentiate constrictive pericarditis from restrictive cardiomyopathy remains to be proven in a large number of patients, and occasionally it may be necessary to proceed to diagnostic thoracotomy before constrictive pericarditis can be excluded. Acyanotic cor pulmonale is another condition which may mimic constrictive pericarditis clinically, but echocardiographic demonstration of enlargement of the pulmonary artery and right sided chambers will distinguish it from constriction.

Effusive-constrictive pericarditis

Echocardiography is the most useful investigation for confirming the coexistence of pericardial effusion and constriction because, although the cardiac shadow is enlarged radiographically (due to the effusion), the haemodynamic disturbance is a result of constriction by the visceral pericardium (Figure 7.6). Therefore, in addition to a pericardial effusion, thickening of the visceral pericardium is seen and the surface movements of the heart are diminished. A rapid outward movement of the cardiac apex (the pericardial knock) is sometimes seen and the inferior vena cava is very distended. Figure 7.7 illustrates how conventional chest radiography can be misleading in pericardial disease.

MANAGEMENT
Pericardial effusion

Pericardial effusion which is bloody or straw coloured should be managed as a tuberculous effusion when it occurs in a population in which tuberculosis is common, unless there is evidence suggesting a non-tuberculous cause. Standard anti-tuberculosis drugs should be given in doses according to the patient's body weight and age. Pericardiocentesis should be done on haemodynamic grounds after the initial diagnostic aspiration. If it is required more than twice for this reason, inferior pericardiotomy and drainage should be undertaken. Good results were obtained using streptomycin, isoniazid, pyrazinamide and rifampicin in the Transkei study. All four drugs should be given for two months, continuing rifampicin and isoniazid for up to six months. This study was the first to investigate the possible benefit of additional prednisolone in the management of tuberculous pericarditis in a prospective, randomized double-blind controlled trial. The study also investigated the value of complete open surgical drainage on admission. Prednisolone reduced the risk of death from pericarditis and reduced the need for repeat pericardiocentesis but did not significantly reduce the need for pericardiectomy for constriction. Complete open drainage on admission made further pericardial drainage unnecessary, but did not influence the need for pericardiectomy for constriction, or the risk of death.[23] During two years of follow-up, 17 of 198 patients developed constriction requiring pericardiectomy. An important consideration when using prednisolone is that rifampicin induces the metabolism of corticosteroids, and so greater benefit may be gained by using larger doses than have been used in the past, i.e. 120 mg daily, rather than 60 mg for adults. Apart from 16 patients who died from pericarditis, all but three were well at 24 months. A period of constriction which resolves within six months occurs in about 10 per cent of patients presenting with pericardial effusion, when they are treated with anti-tuberculosis drugs.

Constrictive pericarditis

Management of tuberculous pericardial constriction involves the use of anti-tuberculosis drugs and pericardiectomy for persistent constriction. Drugs are used in the same way as for pericardial effusion and by 24 months, 89 per cent of 114 patients in the Transkei study were well. They were randomly allocated to receive either prednisolone or placebo in addition to anti-TB drugs for the first 11 weeks, and improvement was significantly more rapid in the prednisolone group (as shown by the rate at which the level of physical activity became normal and by the rate of fall in the mean pulse rate and jugular venous pressure). Fewer of the prednisolone patients died from pericarditis and fewer required pericardiectomy. At 24 months more of the prednisolone patients had achieved favourable status than had those receiving placebo, but none of these differences were statistically significant. Twenty-nine of 114 patients required pericardiectomy for persistent or worsening constriction.[24]

Constriction will resolve on anti-TB treatment within six months in most patients and further resolution may occur after treatment has stopped.

Pericardiectomy for constrictive pericarditis is advised if there is clinical evidence of significant cardiac compression. Persistently raised venous pressure, hepatomegaly or ascites are an indication of such compression. Indications for pericardiectomy can be summarized as follows:

1. If not associated with calcification of the pericardium:
   (a) if static haemodynamically or deteriorating after four to six weeks of anti-tuberculosis treatment;
   (b) if improving after six months of anti-tuberculosis treatment; if justified on haemodynamic grounds. If not urgent and if the patient is not keen on surgery, observation should continue for up to one year as further improvement may occur. The results of surgery are good, but the signs of constriction may persist for three to four months post-operatively.
2. If associated with calcification of the pericardium, surgery should be undertaken with anti-tuberculosis cover, assuming that there is no evidence of activity elsewhere. In some patients with calcification of the pericardium and atrial fibrillation, both of which suggest chronic disease, a bad post-operative course may be explained by myocardial atrophy.

Effusive-constrictive pericarditis

Management of effusive-constrictive pericarditis is a problem because pericardiocentesis does not relieve the impaired filling of the heart and surgical removal of the fibrinous exudate coating the visceral pericardium is not possible. Anti-tuberculosis drugs should be given and serial echocardiography performed to detect the development of a pericardial skin which is amenable to surgical stripping. The place of corticosteroids in such patients is unknown.

Echocardiography can play an important part in the prospective study of the history of such disease as it allows monitoring of the abnormal structure and function of the pericardium.

PERICARDITIS AND CARDIOMYOPATHY: A DIAGNOSTIC PROBLEM

Sometimes it is difficult to differentiate pericardial effusion from dilated cardiomyopathy, and constrictive pericarditis from restrictive cardiomyopathy. With regard to dilated cardiomyopathy, confusion is likely only if the chest radiograph is seen before the patient. The quality of the pulse, palpation of the apex and praecordium and auscultation are particularly helpful distinguishing features. Pulsus alternans does not occur in pericarditis and the diffuse, dyskinetic impulse of the left ventricle (or of both ventricles in dilated cardiomyopathy) is characteristic. A summation gallop and murmurs of atrioventricular valvular regurgitation are also common in this condition. The ECG in dilated cardiomyopathy shows evidence of ventricular hypertrophy and strain and may show bundle-bunch block. Echocardiography differentiates the two conditions.

Distinguishing restrictive cardiomyopathy from constrictive pericarditis can be very difficult and occasionally the matter can be settled only at thoracotomy when full investigation has been inconclusive. This is justified since surgically correctable constriction should not be missed and, if restrictive cardiomyopathy is found, an adequate myocardial biopsy can be obtained. Recent reports[13, 17] of echocardiographic features differentiating the conditions are encouraging, but require validation.

REFERENCES

1 Auerbach O, 1950. Pleural, peritoneal and pericardial tuberculosis. *American Review of Tuberculosis*. 61, 845.
2 Beck W, Schrire V & Vogelpoel L, 1962. Splitting of the second heart sound in constrictive pericarditis, with observations on the mechanism of pulsus parodoxus. *American Heart Journal*. 64, 765–78.
3 Bellet S, McMillan T M & Gouley G A, 1934. Tuberculous pericarditis. Clinical and pathological study based upon a series of 17 cases. *The Medical Clinics of North America*. 18, 201
4 Bialock A & Levy S, 1937. Tuberculous pericarditis. *Journal of Thoracic Surgery*. 7, 132
5 Braunwald E, 1980. In: *Heart Disease. A Textbook of Cardiovascular Medicine*. Philadelphia: W.B. Saunders and Co.
6 Cassel P & Cullum P, 1967. Technique of pericardial biopsy. *British Journal of Surgery*. 54, 620–6.
7 Chesler E, 1981. *Schrire's Clinical Cardiology*. 4th ed. Bristol: John Wright and Sons.
8 Feigenbaum H. *Echocardiography*. 4th ed. Philadelphia: Lea and Febiger.
9 Fowler N O, 1978. Physiology of cardiac tamponade and pulsus paradoxus. Physiologic, circulatory and pharmacologic responses in cardiac tamponade. *Modern Concepts in Cardiovascular Disease*. 47, 115.
10 Hageman J H, D'Esopo N D & Glenn W W L, 1964. Tuberculosis of the pericardium, a long-term analysis of forty-four cases. *New England Journal of Medicine*. 270, 327.
11 Hancock E W, 1971. Subacute effusive-constrictive pericarditis. *Circulation*. 43, 183–92.
12 Hancock E W, 1979. Cardiac Tamponade. *The Medical Clinics of North America*. 63(1), 223–37.
13 Hatle L K, Appleton C P & Popp R L, 1989. Differentiation of constrictive pericarditis and restrictive cardiomyopathy by Doppler echocardiography. *Circulation*. 79, 357–70.
14 Hofmeyr G H & Purry N A, 1979. Inferior pericardiotomy in the treatment of pericardial effusion. *South African Medical Journal*. 55, 280–4.
15 Maisch B, Maisch S & Kochsiek K, 1982. Immune reactions in tuberculous and chronic constrictive pericarditis. Clinical data and diagnostic significance of antimyocardial antibodies. *American Journal of Cardiology*. 50, 1007–13.
16 Martinez-Vazquez J M, Ribera E, Ocana I, Segura R M, Serrat R & Sagrista J, 1986. Adenosine deaminase activity in tuberculous pericarditis. *Thorax*. 41, 888–9.
17 Morgan J M, Raposo L, Clague J C, Chow W H & Oldershaw P, 1989. Restrictive cardiomyopathy and constrictive pericarditis, non-invasive distinction by digitised M-mode echocardiography. *British Heart Journal*. 61, 29–37.
18 Peel A A F, 1948. Tuberculous pericarditis. *British Heart Journal*. 10, 195.
19 Shanks S & Kerley P. *A Text-book of X-ray Diagnosis by British Authors*. Vol. 2. 2nd ed. London: H K Lewis.
20 Strang J I G, 1984. Tuberculous pericarditis in Transkei. *Clinical Cardiology*. 7, 667–70.
21 Strang J I G, 1987. Two-dimensional echocardiography in the diagnosis of amoebic pericarditis. *South African Medical Journal*. 71, 328–9.
22 Strang J I G, 1990. Echoes from the third world; two-dimensional echocardiography in a developing country. *South African Medical Journal*. 77, 85–91.

23 Strang J I G, Kakaza H H S, Gibson D G, Allen B W, Mitchison D A, Evans D J, Girling D J, Nunn A J & Fox W, 1988. Controlled clinical trial of complete open surgical drainage and of prednisolone in treatment of tuberculous pericardial effusion in Transkei. *Lancet*. (ii), 759–64.
24 Strang J I G, Kakaza H H S, Gibson D G, Girling D J, Nunn A J & Fox W, 1987. Controlled trial of prednisolone as adjuvant in treatment of tuberculous constrictive pericarditis in Transkei. *Lancet*. (ii), 1418–22.
25 Wood P, 1961. Chronic constrictive pericarditis. *American Journal of Cardiology*. 7, 48–61.

CHAPTER 8

Tuberculosis of the skin

N Saxe

INTRODUCTION

In developed countries over the past few decades the decline in frequency of tuberculous skin lesions has mirrored that of tuberculosis of other organs. However, skin tuberculosis is still seen frequently in the less developed countries where poverty, poor housing, and malnutrition contribute to the high incidence of this disease.[28, 34]

The skin lesions of tuberculosis vary both with the host response, which is modified by previous exposure and/or infection with *Mycobacterium tuberculosis,* and with the virulence and route of entry of the organism.

In the past, the classification of cutaneous tuberculosis has been complicated by the incorporation of the immune status of the host (whether primary or re-infection tuberculosis) with the different routes of entry of the organism. The simpler approach of Beyt et al.[1] has greatly enhanced the understanding of skin lesions of tuberculosis, in that they consider the pathogenesis of skin tuberculosis in the broad context of all the mycobacterial skin diseases (other than leprosy) and have correlated the plethora of older unwieldy synonyms with modern terminology. The previous cumbersome nomenclature can thus be discarded.

The steady decline of tuberculosis (and, with it, skin tuberculosis) and the consequent lack of familiarity with the tuberculids led Beyt and many other dermatologists in the western world to doubt the existence of the tuberculids.[1, 24, 33, 34] In less developed countries the full spectrum of tuberculosis, including the tuberculids, continues to manifest and the latter may be one of the most common presentations of tuberculosis of the skin.[23]

AETIOLOGY AND PATHOGENESIS

Like all mycobacteria (other than *Mycobacterium leprae*) capable of inducing skin lesions, *Mycobacterium tuberculosis* enters the skin either from an exogenous source, usually associated with trauma to the skin, or from an endogenous focus of tuberculosis by haematogenous, lymphatic or direct spread. The latter may occur from underlying lymph nodes or bone to the skin, or from sputum coming in contact with mucosal surfaces.

The immune status of the patient, together with the virulence of the organism, determines whether there is an explosive, rapid, severe reaction or whether the course is indolent and prolonged. However, many aspects of the immunology of tuberculosis remain poorly understood.

The non-tuberculous mycobacterial skin lesions are very similar to those of *Mycobacterium tuberculosis,* with their portal of entry, as a rule, being exogenous following trauma, particularly in the immunocompromised host.

CLASSIFICATION

Beyt's lucid classification achieves its clarity by focusing on the route of entry of the organism and by not complicating comprehension of the great variety of clinical manifestations by incorporating immunological factors. The skin lesions of tuberculosis range from papules and infiltrated plaques to nodules which either become crusted or verrucous or break down, ulcerate and form draining sinuses. The morphologic diversity reflects differences in host responses, organism numbers and virulence, which are all implicit in the classification. Beyt's classification has been expanded to

Table 8.1
Mycobacterial Skin Lesions other than Leprosy

CLASSIFICATION OF CUTANEOUS MYCOBACTERIOSIS ACCORDING TO PATHOGENESIS	CLINICAL TYPES OF SKIN TUBERCULOSIS	SYNONYMOUS TERMS PREVIOUSLY USED IN LITERATURE
With detectable Mycobacteria		
INOCULATION CUTANEOUS MYCOBACTERIOSIS FROM AN EXOGENOUS SOURCE		
	Tuberculous chancre	Primary Inoculation
	Warty tuberculosis	Tuberculosis primary complex
		Tuberculosis verrucosa cutis
		Verruca necrogenica
		Prosector's wart
		Tuberculosis cutis verrucosa
CUTANEOUS MYCOBACTERIOSIS FROM AN ENDOGENOUS SOURCE		
Contiguous spread	Scrofuloderma	Tuberculosis colliquativa cutis
Autoinoculation	Orificial tuberculosis	Tuberculosis cutis orificialis
		Tuberculosis ulcerosa cutis et mucosae
	Warty tuberculosis	
Haematogenous spread		
	Lupus vulgaris	Tuberculosis luposa cutis
	Acute haematogenous tuberculosis	Acute miliary tuberculosis of the skin
		Tuberculosis cutis miliaris disseminata
		Tuberculosis cutis acuta generalisata
	Tuberculous nodules or abscesses	Tuberculous gumma
		Metastatic tuberculous abscess
Without detectable Mycobacteria		
TUBERCULIDS		
	Papulonecrotic Tuberculid	
	Lichenoid Tuberculid	
	Lichen scrofulosorum	
	Erythema induratum (Bazin)	

Modified from Beyt et al.[1] Assisted by Dr Paul Strauss

include the tuberculids (Table 8.1). Confusion over the tuberculids has existed since Darier separated proven tuberculous lesions from others which became known as 'tuberculides'. It later became apparent that some of the 'tuberculides' such as those occurring on the face, are not due to tuberculosis and are probably variants of either the rosaceous process or sarcoidosis.

SKIN TUBERCULOSIS WITH DETECTABLE MYCOBACTERIA
Exogenous (inoculation) skin tuberculosis

Tuberculous chancre

The tuberculous chancre may occur in medical personnel as a result of direct inoculation of the tubercle bacillus into the skin. This usually affects the finger or hand of a patient without natural or artificially

acquired immunity to this organism. The resultant tuberculous chancre with regional lymphadenopathy constitutes the primary complex of the skin. Such lesions used to be a common complication of ritual circumcision[13] and have occurred as a result of injections with inadequately sterilized syringes, accidental inoculation,[9, 29] ear-piercing,[9] and mouth-to-mouth artificial respiration.[11]

This form of primary complex is considered rare now,[1] except in Asia. However, it may be more common than is generally believed, as in 1953 Miller[21] observed 30 cases in a five-year period in north-east England. Most patients are children but the lesions can occur in adolescents or young adults.[6, 21, 26]

The tuberculous chancre initially presents as a small papule or ragged ulcer with little tendency to heal (Figure 8.1). It is shallow with a granular or haemorrhagic base

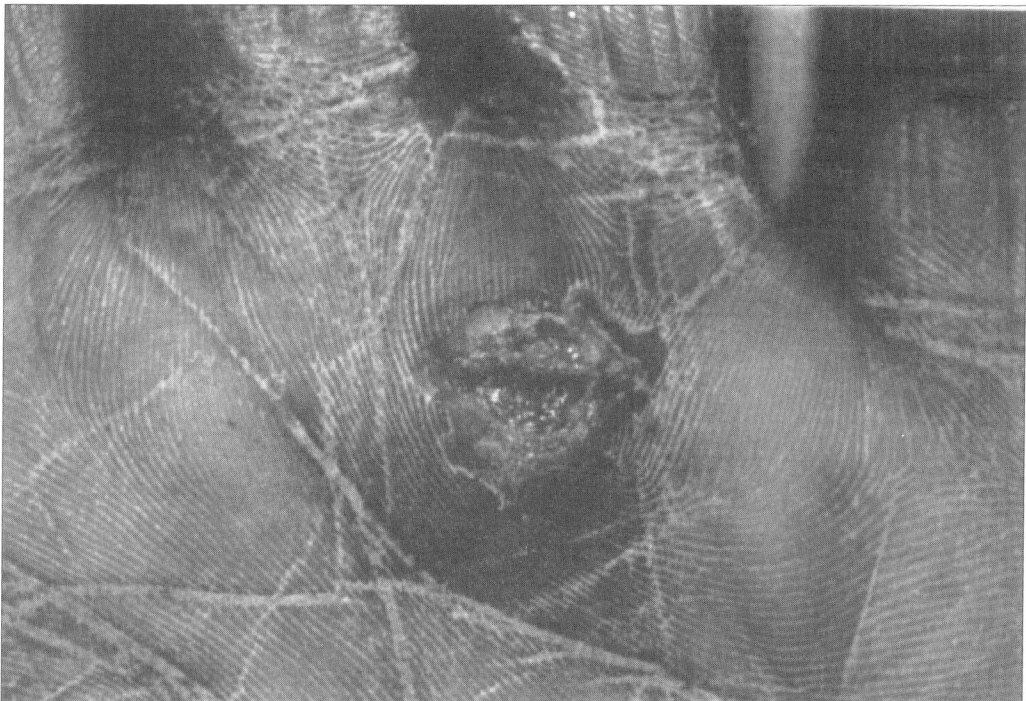

Figure 8.1. Ulcerating nodule in the palm of a nursing sister, at the site of accidental inoculation with BCG.

on which a thin adherent crust later develops. Lesions on the conjunctiva are characterized by shallow ulcers or fungating granulations.[21] In the mouth papules and ulcers occur on the gingiva or palate, and painless paronychia may occur with primary inoculation on the finger.[9] Accidental inoculation of *Mycobacterium tuberculosis* may result in a subcutaneous abscess.[12]

Within three to eight weeks painless, regional lymphadenopathy develops and may be the reason for physician consultation. A benign course is usual but the lymph nodes may break down and form cold abscesses draining onto the surface of the overlying skin with sinus formation.

The histological picture is often one of non-specific acute and chronic inflammation with necrosis and ulceration. *Mycobacterium tuberculosis* is said to be easily detected,[34] but in some cases mycobacteria are not demonstrated on histologic examination and can only be cultured from skin biopsy specimens.[1] The characteristic tuberculoid granulomas which are the most diagnostic histological feature of cutaneous

mycobacterial disease may not be found.

Any painless, unilateral localized glandular swellings in a child should raise the suspicion of tuberculosis. The presence of acid-fast bacilli or culture examination will provide the diagnosis at the stage of a small ulcer or papule before lymph node involvement becomes manifest.

There should be a high index of suspicion for tuberculosis in this clinical setting, particularly in countries where the disease is common. Catscratch fever, *Mycobacteria marinum*, sporotrichosis, actinomycosis and dental sinus (on the face) are the most important conditions to be excluded.

Warty tuberculosis

A patient with a moderate or high degree of immunity who is inoculated with tubercle bacillus will develop a more indolent warty, plaque-like form of tuberculosis. These lesions also tend to occur in medical personnel, particularly pathologists, postmortem attendants or butchers handling tuberculous cattle. Auto-inoculation with sputum may occur in a patient with active tuberculosis, and children and young adults (already infected and with some degree of immunity) may become infected exogenously from sputum by sitting or playing where the organism is present.[22, 35]

Histologic examination of warty tuberculous lesions reveals a striking pseudo-epitheliomatous hyperplasia with superficial abscess formation. The intense mixed infiltrate may show only sparse tuberculoid granulomas, and bacilli are seen only occasionally.

The usual site is the hands, but in eastern countries knees, ankles and buttocks may also be affected.[22, 35] The lesion progresses from a small indurated papule to a large, irregular hyperkeratotic verrucous plaque, purplish or red-brown in colour and with a firm consistency. At times pus may be expressed from fissures. The lesions may resemble lupus vulgaris.[20] More generalized lesions with very similar morphology can arise as a result of haematogenous spread.[3, 20]

The differential diagnosis includes warts, chromoblastomycosis, blastomycosis, actinomycosis, tertiary syphilis and lesions caused by non-tuberculous mycobacteria, particularly *Mycobacteria marinum.*

Endogenous skin tuberculosis
Contiguous spread
Scrofuloderma

Scrofuloderma results from spread to the skin surface of an underlying tuberculous focus usually from a lymph gland but sometimes from an infected bone or joint.

Clinically bluish red nodules overlying an infected gland or joint break down to ulcerate and form numerous fistulae. These communicate beneath ridges of skin, discharging pus in parts and progressing to scarring in other areas (Figure 8.2). Later, irregular densely fibrotic masses result in puckered scarring. The diagnosis is confirmed bacteriologically.

The lesions must be differentiated from actinomycosis and nocardiosis; from hidradenitis suppurativa; and, if on the face, from dental sinus.

Auto-inoculation
Orificial tuberculosis

Tuberculous lesions can occur in the mouth, pharyngeal area and tongue as a result of direct inoculation with bacteria expectorated in the sputum. Enshrined in the literature is the myth that this only occurs in very debilitated, ill patients in an advanced stage of tuberculosis, and in patients who lack immunity. However, the author has personally encountered ulcerating pharyngeal tuberculous lesions in two patients who appeared generally well and whose accompanying pulmonary tuberculosis had not been clinically suspected (Figure 8.3). Peri-anal nodules which break down and ulcerate may also be seen, resulting from the swallowing of infected sputum. This usually occurs with active pulmonary tuberculosis and is independent of tuberculosis higher in the gastrointestinal tract.

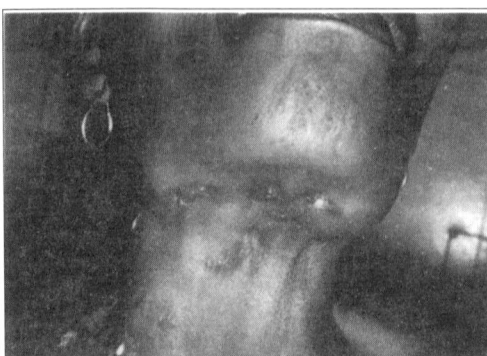

Figure 8.2. Draining sinuses of scrofuloderma under the chin and the right side of the neck.

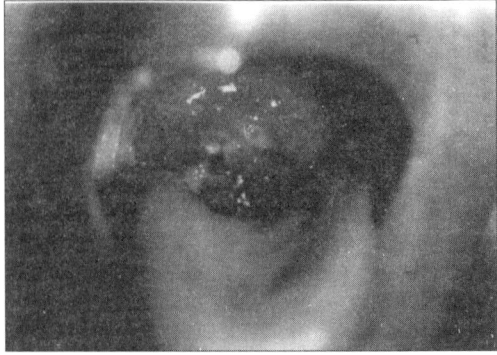

Figure 8.3. Ulcerating tuberculous nodules on the soft-palate and pharynx.

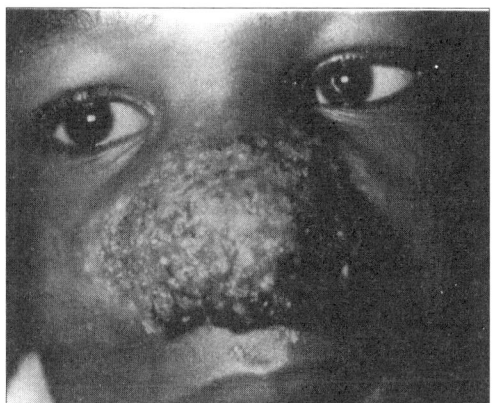

Figure 8.4. Verrucous appearance of lupus vulgaris.

Haematogenous spread

Lupus vulgaris

The word lupus, 'wolf-like', refers to the appearance that results from the destruction of the central portion of the face by tuberculosis. Biett in 1857 was the first person to report the frequent occurrence of lupus vulgaris of the nares,[32] and the term is now used in a similar way for lupus erythematosus.

Lupus vulgaris is the result of haematogenous dissemination from an endogenous focus, usually in the lungs.[15, 16] The infection runs an indolent prolonged course over many years. The lesions commence with reddish, purplish-brown infiltrated plaques which, on pressure with a glass slide (diascopy), show the characteristic yellowish 'apple-jelly nodules'. Later they extend peripherally and become more exuberant, hyperkeratotic and verrucous (Figure 8.4), at times with central atrophy, until eventually the nasal cartilage is destroyed. After many years, spontaneous healing with fibrosis may occur.

Squamous carcinoma may supervene in the chronic ulcers and thickened scars.[7] Lupus vulgaris may be associated with clinically evident tuberculosis of other organs (in one series an active focus was found in 11 per cent of patients[23]).

The histopathology is variable. Although tuberculoid granulomas are usually present in the upper dermis any feature may be absent or modified and the histology may sometimes be difficult to recognize as being tuberculosis. The histologic patterns in skin tuberculosis do not consistently correlate

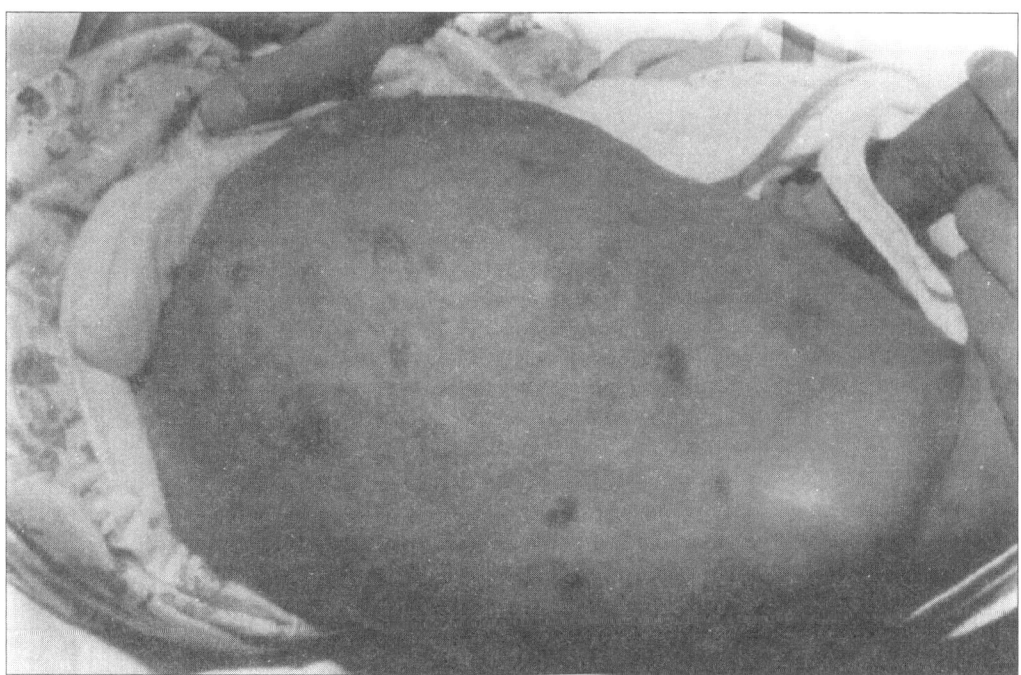

Figure 8.5. Multiple dermal and subcutaneous tuberculous nodules in a baby.

with either a particular species of mycobacteria or a specific clinical manifestation.[1] The absence of classic features of caseation necrosis and tuberculoid granulomas may lead to delays in diagnosis, particularly in developed countries where the rarity of tuberculosis causes a low index of suspicion.[32]

Leprosy, sarcoidosis and syphilis are the chief alternative causes of similar lesions, but deep fungal infection, non-tuberculous mycobacterial infections and lupoid leishmaniasis need to be considered in the differential diagnosis. In some cases lupus vulgaris may resemble psoriasis but lupus is more infiltrated and usually solitary. Bowen's disease can resemble both.

Acute haematogenous tuberculosis with nodules or abscesses

Acute haematogenous dissemination of *Mycobacterium tuberculosis* is usually a fulminant disease seen mostly in infants and children or in immuno-compromised patients. The clinical appearance is of multiple papules which may become pustular and haemorrhagic. The histological appearance is that of non-specific inflammatory cells with focal areas of necrosis and vascular thrombi containing bacilli. In the era before chemotherapy, generalized acute miliary tuberculosis was a well-recognized complication of advanced disseminated primary tuberculosis in children.[17, 18, 30]

Nodules and abscesses

In patients with a better immunity (and particularly in young children) a less acute and severe presentation is that of numerous soft nodules and subcutaneous abscesses (Figure 8.5).

Acid-fast bacilli are usually demonstrated on histologic examination.

TUBERCULOSIS WITHOUT DETECTABLE MYCOBACTERIA

Tuberculids

The tuberculids are lesions which are tuberculous but do not show evidence of the

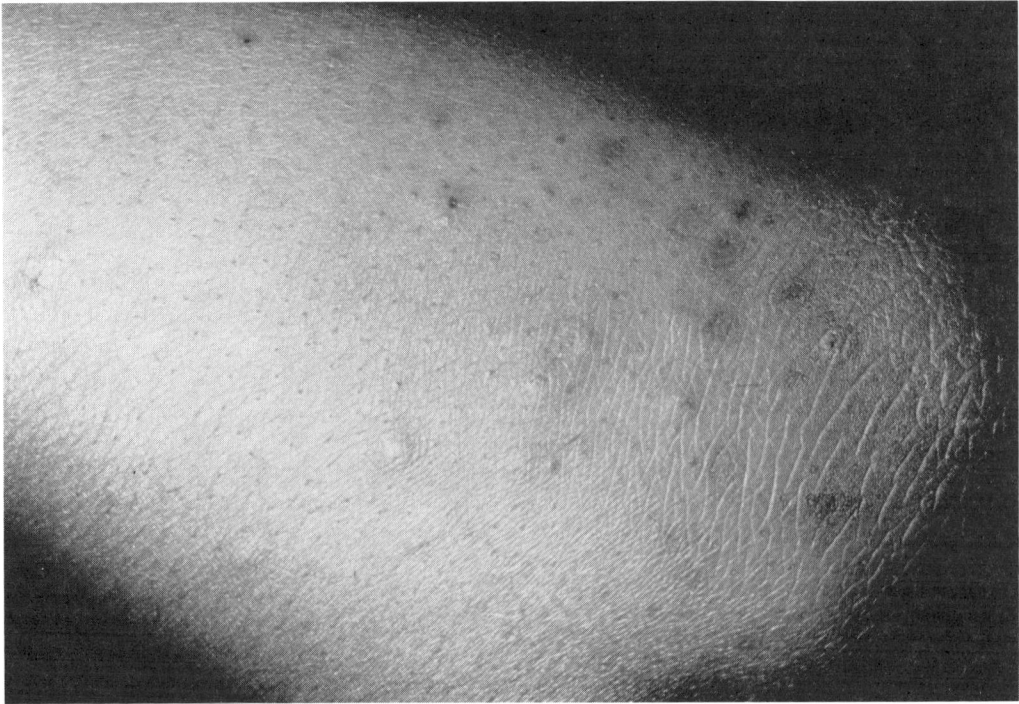

Figure 8.6. Papulonecrotic tuberculid with umbilicated papules and pitted scars over the extensor surface of the elbow and forearm.

presence of tubercle bacilli. In areas where tuberculosis is uncommon, there is doubt and scepticism about the existence of tuberculids, but in less developed countries the tuberculids not only continue to be seen,[23, 33, 35] but may be the commonest form of skin tuberculosis.[23]

Papulonecrotic tuberculid

Papulonecrotic tuberculid is an extreme form of hypersensitivity to tuberculous infection in which the tuberculin reaction is strongly positive and endarteritis and thrombosis of dermal vessels are characteristic features. The rapid response to antituberculous treatment leaves no doubt as to the aetiology.

It has been postulated that papulonecrotic tuberculid occurs in a patient who has a focus of tuberculosis from which showers of tubercle bacilli or tuberculous antigenic material are disseminated by the haematogenous route to lodge in the small vessels of the skin. The tissue-damaging (necrotizing) 'hypersensitivity' response in the patient's skin destroys the tubercle bacillus so that acid-fast bacilli are not identified on histologic examination or culture. Necrosis in lesions and skin test sites is thought to have an immunological basis, but it is not yet known which type of lymphocyte, lymphokine, macrophage or microbicidal mechanism is responsible for protection against mycobacteria.[28]

Crops of papulovesicles continue to erupt, sometimes for many years, over the extensor surfaces of the joints, the elbows, the knees, the dorsa of the hands and feet, and the ears.

The lesion starts as a papule with central vesiculation, and a haemorrhagic crust forms after a few weeks, which heals with depressed varioliform scars (Figure 8.6). The presence of pitted scars over elbows and knees is a strong clue for diagnosis in countries where tuberculosis is common.

The patient is usually clinically well, and underlying tuberculosis may be identified in only a percentage of these patients — Morrison and Fourie found a focus of

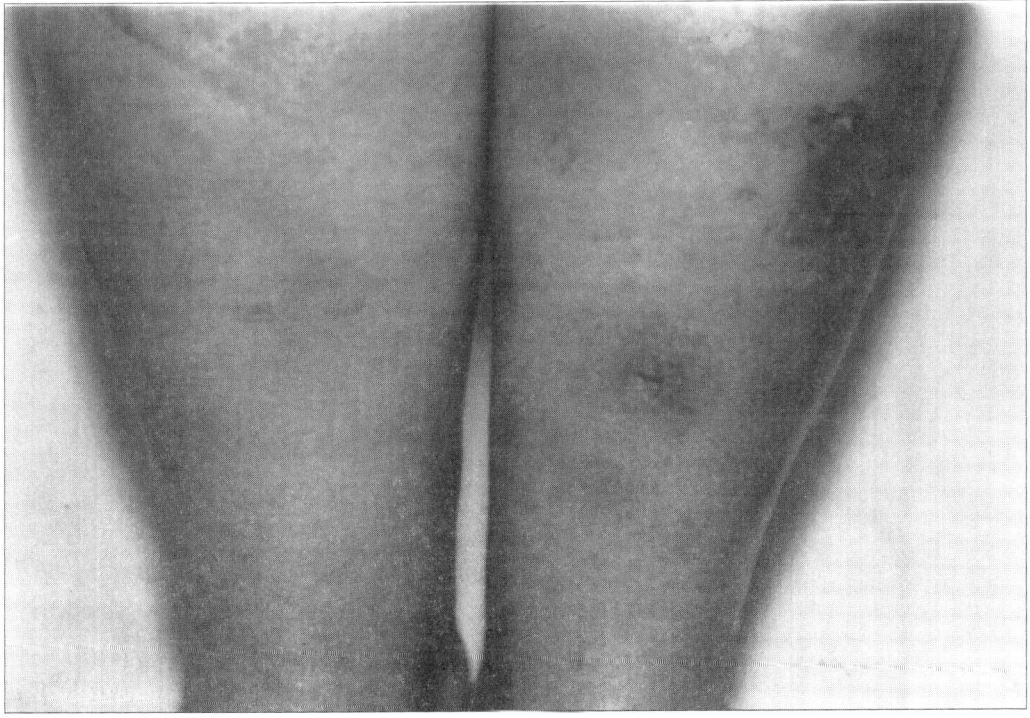

Figure 8.7. Bound-down and scarred lesions following ulceration of erythema induratum on the calves.

tuberculosis in 38 per cent of their patients with papulonecrotic tuberculid.[23] Underlying tuberculosis may be in the lung, lymph glands,[2] urogenital tract or other sites. Wilson-Jones and Winkelmann found clinical, laboratory or histologic evidence of associated tuberculosis in nine out of 12 patients.[33] The tuberculin test is positive, often with a severe — and even a necrotizing — reaction and this is a pre-requisite for the diagnosis.

The histologic appearance is characteristic and depends on the stage at which the lesion is biopsied. Wilson-Jones and Winkelmann demonstrated a lymphocytic and granulomatous vasculitis without any evidence of leucocytoclastic vasculitis in 12 patients.[33] However, in the experience of the author and her colleague, Dr H F Jordaan of the University of Stellenbosch, it is possible to demonstrate leucocytoclastic neutrophilic vasculitis in early lesions (unpublished material).

The fully developed histologic appearance resembles a microinfarct of the skin. A wedge or v-shaped area of upper dermal and epidermal necrosis is surrounded by chronic inflammatory cells with occasional giant cells but lacking well-formed granulomas. There are many points of similarity between acute septic vasculitis and papulonecrotic tuberculid.

The lesions heal spontaneously over weeks to months, and more rapidly on anti-tuberculous therapy, which also prevents the appearance of new lesions.

Lichenoid tuberculid

Lichenoid tuberculid is a less common tuberculid. Eruptions of asymptomatic small lichenoid papules 0,5 to 3 mm in size occur chiefly on the abdomen, chest and back. They are usually follicular and grouped and show granulomatous perifollicular inflammation on histologic examination. The tuberculin test is often positive.[10, 31] A lichenoid tuberculid has also been described with a negative tuberculin test and there may be caseous necrosis on histologic examination.[25] Two patients developed lesions of lichen nitidus associated with tuberculosis (lichen nitidus is a papular eruption with a characteristic histology not usually associated with tuberculosis). The first patient developed lichen nitidus after a BCG vaccination,[4] but histology was not discussed. The second patient presented with lesions of lichen nitidus together with lupus vulgaris. The lichen nitidus was confirmed histologically and both the lichen nitidus and co-existent lupus vulgaris responded rapidly to anti-tuberculous therapy.[29]

Erythema induratum (Bazin's disease)

The lesions of erythema induratum are persistent or recurrent painful erythematous nodules on the back of the calves (usually of women, rarely of men). These nodules characteristically break down to ulcerate and discharge pus (Figure 8.7), in contrast to erythema nodosum which does not ulcerate. Past or active tuberculosis is usually present and the tuberculin test is almost invariably positive.[8, 27, 28]

Histologically it may be possible to demonstrate a necrotizing leucocytoclastic vasculitis in the deep vessels of the panniculus in association with features of lobular granulomatous panniculitis. Necrotizing vasculitis and panniculitis have a number of causes. In areas with a high incidence of tuberculosis, the latter should be considered and excluded. As *Mycobacterium tuberculosis* is seldom recovered from the lesion, a rapid response to anti-tuberculous therapy may be the only way of confirming the diagnosis.[8]

As with papulonecrotic tuberculid, doubt has been expressed as to the tuberculous nature of erythema induratum. Forstrom and Hannuksela[8] discuss the conflicting views regarding the relationship of tuberculosis to redness and nodularity on the skin of the leg. These authors studied 72 such patients (nine men and 63 women) whose nodules resolved on antituberculous therapy in all but four cases, regardless of whether or not they had evidence of past or present tuberculosis.

UNUSUAL MANIFESTATIONS OF TUBERCULOSIS OF THE SKIN

Acral gangrene in blacks, associated with tuberculosis, was described by Findlay and Morrison.[5] Seven of the 91 cases of papulonecrotic tuberculid described by Morrison and Fourie had associated gangrene of the extremities due to arteritis.[23]

It is also important to remember that an association has been described between tuberculosis and Takayasu's arteritis,[19] and it is possible that tuberculosis may play a role in the pathogenesis of this disease.

Iden *et al.*[14] reported a patient originally treated for temporal arteritis who developed papulonecrotic tuberculid following steroid therapy, emphasizing the complex relationship between tuberculosis immunity and inflammatory disease of vessels.

Another extremely rare form of tuberculosis occurred in four of the 91 cases of papulonecrotic tuberculid in Morrison and Fourie's series[23] — lupus vulgaris developed from papulonecrotic tuberculid lesions, evidently due to the local multiplication of tubercle bacillus. The resulting lesions were in all degrees of transition from papulonecrotic tuberculid to multiple annular small and large plaques of lupus vulgaris.

Some unusual forms of skin tuberculosis are difficult to classify, such as those cases which resemble lupus vulgaris in histology and morphology, though not in site or behaviour.[3]

THE DIAGNOSIS OF TUBERCULOSIS OF THE SKIN

Two of the specific criteria for the diagnosis of skin tuberculosis are absolute: the positive culture of *Mycobacterium tuberculosis* from the lesion, and successful guinea pig inoculation. Six relative but individually unreliable criteria include the clinical history and signs; the presence of active proven tuberculosis elsewhere in the body; the presence of acid-fast bacilli in the lesion; the histopathology; a positive

reaction to tuberculin; and the effect of specific therapy.[28] Details of the histopathology have been discussed, but it is worth emphasizing that the absence of tuberculoid granulomas is not uncommon and does not exclude the diagnosis, while the presence of granulomas facilitates the diagnosis but many other causes for granulomatous histology have to be excluded.

TREATMENT OF SKIN TUBERCULOSIS

Attention to the patient as a whole is of course an essential part of the management of skin tuberculosis and includes a careful search for an underlying focus of tuberculosis. This may be obvious on a careful history and clinical examination. Therapy will then depend on which organs are involved, the extent and type of lesions, the state of the patient's immunity and the stage of the disease.

When there is evidence of tuberculosis elsewhere a full anti-tuberculous regimen should be followed.

The standard drug regimens are discussed elsewhere. The recommended treatment of skin tuberculosis in the United Kingdom[28] is for the initial phase of eight weeks to include daily isoniazid (adults up to 300 mg daily; children 6 mg per kg daily) and rifampicin (adults 450–600 mg daily; children 20 mg per kg daily up to a maximum of 600 mg), supplemented by ethambutol (adults 15 mg per kg daily; children 25 mg per kg daily). The continuation phase of treatment with isoniazid and rifampicin lasts until the total length of therapy has been nine months. Ethambutol in a lower dose or streptomycin may be used in the continuation phase instead of rifampicin, but then treatment should be for longer than nine months.

REFERENCES

1 Beyt B F Jr, Ortbals D W, Santa Cruz D J, Kobayashi G S, Eisen A Z & Medoff G, 1981. Cutaneous mycobacteriosis: analysis of 34 cases with a new classification of the disease. *Medicine (Baltimore).* 60, 95–109.

2 Breatnach S M & Black M M, 1981. Atypical tuberculide (acne scrofulosorum) secondary to tuberculous lymphadenitis. *Clinical Experimental Dermatology.* 6, 339–44.

3 Brown F S, Anderson R H & Burnett J W, 1982. Cutaneous tuberculosis. *Journal of American Academy Dermatology.* 6, 101-6.

4 Dostrovsky A & Sagher F, 1963. Dermatological complications of BCG vaccination. *British Journal of Dermatology.* 75, 181–92.

5 Findlay G H & Morrison J G L, 1973. Idiopathic gangrene in African adults. *British Medical Journal.* l, 173.

6 Fisher I & Orkin M, 1966. Primary tuberculosis of the skin. Primary complex. *Journal of the American Medical Association.* 195, 314–6.

7 Förström L, 1969. Carcinomatous changes in lupus vulgaris. *Annals of Clinical Research.* l, 213–9.

8 Förström L & Hannuksela M, 1970. Antituberculous treatment of erythema induratum Bazin. *Acta Dermatovener (Stockholm).* 50, 143–7.

9 Goette D K, Jacobson K W & Doty R D, 1978. Primary inoculation tuberculosis of the skin. Prosector's paronychia. *Archives of Dermatology.* 114, 567–9.

10 Graham-Brown R A C & Sarkany I, 1980. Lichen scrofulosorum with tuberculosis dactylitis. *British Journal of Dermatology.* 103, 561–4.

11 Heilman K M & Muschenheim C, 1965. Primary cutaneous tuberculosis resulting from mouth-to-mouth respiration. *New England Journal of Medicine.* 273, 1035–6.

12 Heycock J B & Noble T C, 1961. Four cases of syringe-transmitted tuberculosis. *Tubercle.* 42, 25–7.

13 Holt L E, 1913. Tuberculosis acquired through ritual circumcision. *Journal of the American Medical Association.* 61, 99–102.

14 Iden D L, Rogers R S & Schroeter A L, 1978. Papulonecrotic tuberculid secondary to *Mycobacterium bovis. Archives of Dermatology.* 114, 564–6.

15 Kanan M W & Ryan T J, 1975. Endonasal localization of blood borne viable and non viable particulate matter. *British Journal of Dermatology.* 92, 475–8.

16 Kanan M W & Ryan T J, 1976. The localisation of granulomatous diseases and vasculitis in the nasal mucosa. In: Ryan T J (ed.). *Microvascular Injury.* London: W B Saunders.

17 Kennedy C & Knowles G F, 1975. Miliary tuberculosis presenting with skin lesions. *British Medical Journal.* 3, 356.

18 Lipper S, Watkins D L & Kahn L B, 1980. Nongranulomatous septic vasculitis due to miliary tuberculosis: a pitfall in diagnosis for the pathologist. *American Journal of Dermatopathology.* 2, 71–4.

19 Lupi-Herrera E, Sanchez-Torres G & Marcushamer J, 1977. Takayasu's arteritis: clinical study of 107 cases. *American Heart Journal.* 93, 94–103.

20 Michelson H E, 1948. Criteria for the diagnosis of certain tuberculoderms. *Journal of the American Medical Association.* 138, 721–6.

21 Miller F J W, 1953. Recognition of primary tuberculous infection of skin and mucosae. *Lancet.* l, 5.

22 Mitchell P C, 1954. Tuberculosis verrucosa cutis among Chinese in Hong Kong. *British Journal of Dermatology.* 66, 444–8.

23 Morrison J G L & Fourie E D, 1974. The papulonecrotic tuberculide — from Arthus' reaction to lupus vulgaris. *British Journal of Dermatology.* 91, 263–70.

24 Moschella S L, 1985. Diseases of the mononuclear phagocytic system. In: Moschella S & Hurley H (eds). *Dermatology.* 2nd ed. Philadelphia: W B Saunders.

25 Ockuly O E & Montgomery H, 1950. Lichenoid tuberculide: a clinical and histopathologic study. *Journal of Investigative Dermatology.* 14, 415-26.

26 O'Leary P A, Harrison M W, 1941. Inoculation tuberculosis. *Archives of Dermatology.* 44, 371–90.

27 Ryan T J, 1976. Infection, food and drugs as triggers of vasculitis: mycobacterial infections. In: Ryan T J (ed.) *Microvascular Injury.* London, W B Saunders.

28 Savin J A & Wilkinson D S, 1986. Mycobacterial infections including tuberculosis. In: Rook A, Wilkinson D S, Ebling F J G *et al.* (eds). *Textbook of Dermatology.* 4th ed. Oxford: Blackwell Scientific Publications.

29 Saxe N, 1985. Mycobacterial skin infections. *Journal of Cutaneous Pathology.* 12, 300–12.

30 Shermer D R, Simpson C G, Haserick J R & Van Ordstrand H S, 1969. Tuberculosis cutis miliaris acuta generalisata. *Archives of Dermatology.* 99, 64–9.

31 Smith N P, Ryan T J, Sanderson K V & Sarkany I, 1976. Lichen scrofulosorum. *British Journal of Dermatology.* 94, 319–25.

32 Warin A P & Wilson-Jones E, 1977. Cutaneous tuberculosis of the nose with unusual clinical and histological features leading to a delay in the diagnosis. *Clinical Experimental Dermatology.* 2, 235–42.

33 Wilson-Jones E & Winkelmann R K, 1986. Papulonecrotic tuberculid, a neglected disease in western countries. *Journal of American Academy Dermatology.* 14, 815–26.

34 Wolff K & Tappeiner G, 1987. Mycobacterial diseases: tuberculosis and atypical mycobacterial infections. In: Fitzpatrick T B, Eisen A Z, Wolff K *et al.* (eds). *Dermatology in General Medicine.* 3rd ed. New York: McGraw-Hill Book Co.

35 Wong K O, Lee K P & Chiu S F, 1968. Tuberculosis of the skin in Hong Kong, (a review of 160 cases). *British Journal of Dermatology.* 80, 424–9.

CHAPTER 9

Neurological tuberculosis

M Moodley

MENINGEAL TUBERCULOSIS

Introduction

Meningeal tuberculosis (TBM), is the most serious complication, the most common neurological presentation, and the most common cause of death from tuberculosis in childhood.[38] TBM is a disease usually of infants, children and young adults, in whom it is generally regarded as being a complication of primary infection. In the elderly adult it is viewed not only as a reactivation of a dormant state but as an illness with a long prodrome.[21] In the pre-antibiotic era tuberculous meningitis was uniformly fatal, and in Lincoln and Sewell's study the average duration of meningitis from the first symptom to death in untreated children was shown to be only 19,5 days.[38] In general, if TBM is left untreated it leads to death within six to eight weeks of onset,[11] but with modern treatment almost 100 per cent recovery can be achieved without sequelae if therapy is commenced before the child loses consciousness.[40]

Tuberculous meningitis is a relatively uncommon illness in technologically advanced countries, but in developing countries like South Africa its incidence is still high (especially in black and coloured communities) and, despite the advent of effective chemotherapy, it remains a devastating illness in terms of mortality and permanent sequelae. This was very clearly shown in a Johannesburg study by Freiman and Geefhuysen in 1970. They treated 131 black children, two thirds of whom were unconscious prior to therapy. About 40 per cent of all the patients died within a year and more than 50 per cent of the survivors had serious neurological sequelae.[27] At the King Edward VIII Hospital in Durban TBM accounts for 15 per cent of all cases of TB in children and has a mortality rate of about 19 per cent. There has been a sustained increase in TBM in the western Cape, where the notification rate per 10 000 population in 1987 was 0 for whites, 2,88 for coloureds and Indians, and 4,28 for blacks. By contrast the incidence in the United Kingdom is about two per million population per annum, with a mortality rate of approximately 20 per cent and with as many as 36 per cent of patients developing some permanent neurological sequelae.[13]

In developing countries malnutrition, overcrowding, poor primary health care facilities and delay in consultation, singly or in combination, all predispose towards a more severe form of the disease which invariably carries a high morbidity and mortality rate. It is not unusual for most patients to be hospitalized in an advanced stage of the disease with loss of consciousness and major neurological signs.[27]

Pathogenesis

Knowledge of the pathogenesis of TBM helps considerably to understand the evolution of the varied clinical syndromes of the disease. About 20 to 40 per cent of children with severe tuberculosis have extension of the disease to the meninges.[11] Infection at this site occurs in one of three ways:

- dissemination of bacilli within two years of primary infection;
- as a complication of existing TB (miliary, tuberculoma, TB spine and TB mastoiditis);
- as a result of reactivation of a latent focus.

Tubercle bacilli usually spread from a primary focus in the lung via the regional

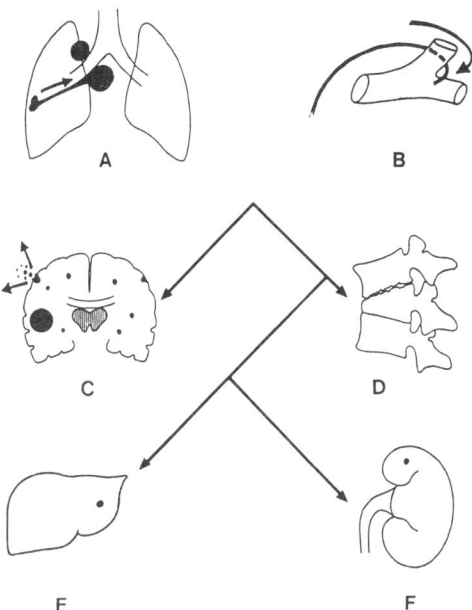

Figure 9.1. The pathogenesis of TBM. (A) Ghon focus; (B) thoracic duct; (C) miliary tubercles, tuberculoma, Rich's focus; (D) Pott's disease; (E) silent hepatic lesion; (F) silent renal lesion. (Adapted from Parsons M, 1988. *Tuberculous Meningitis*, 2nd ed. Oxford Medical Publications.)

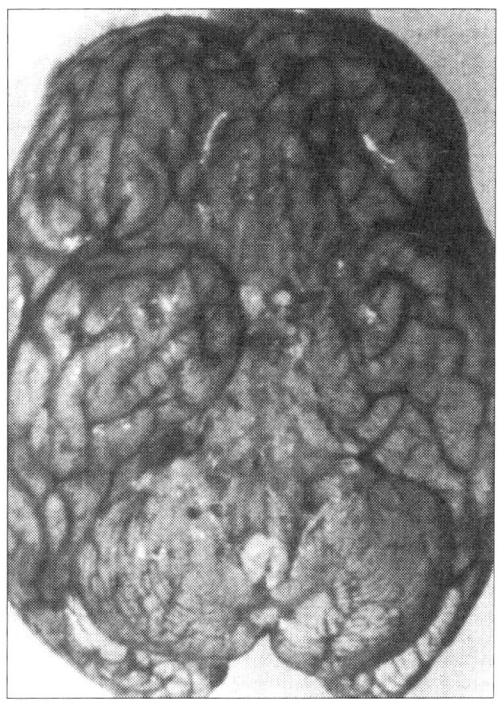

Figure 9.2. Thick exudate and fibrous adhesions covering brain stem of a two year old child who died from TBM.

lymph glands and thoracic duct to enter the circulation, from where they disseminate to the brain, meninges and various other organs.[48]

The dissemination may be massive, causing miliary TB which can lead to meningitis within months, but more commonly it is less severe, producing only one or two metastatic foci in the brain, meninges or spinal cord. These subsequently become encapsulated as host resistance is established. At a much later date the encapsulating tissue weakens and a caseating tubercle in the brain (Rich's focus) ruptures, releasing bacteria into the subarachnoid space (and on rare occasions into the ventricular fluid).[13, 48] The caseating tubercle is most commonly situated in the cerebral cortex or meninges. Foci in the bones (mastoid, spine) or in the substance of the spinal cord responsible for the occurrence of meningitis are much less common.[55] Prior to the landmark study of Rich and McCordock, there

was a strong belief that TBM was the direct result of the haematogenous dissemination of bacilli, but their numerous morphological and experimental studies have shown beyond doubt that TBM is caused by the intrathecal release of a mass of bacilli from a nearby cerebral or meningeal focus and not by direct haematogenous spread.[55]

Pathology

The release of tubercle bacilli into the subarachnoid space provokes an initial inflammatory response in the region of the ruptured tubercle, but later the brunt of the pathologic process falls on the basal meninges and ependyma. The inflammatory response which ensues is partly a result of hypersensitivity reactions to bacilliary components, especially tuberculoproteins.[38] The base of the brain becomes studded with tubercles while the convex surface remains relatively unaffected. The thick basal exudate covers cranial nerves, blood vessels

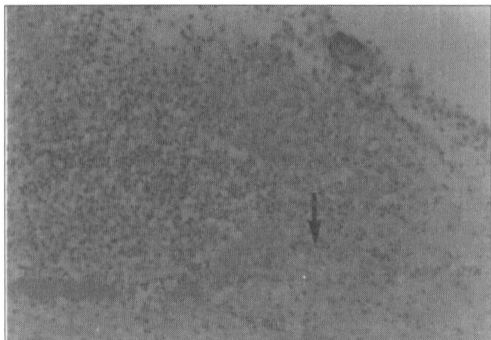
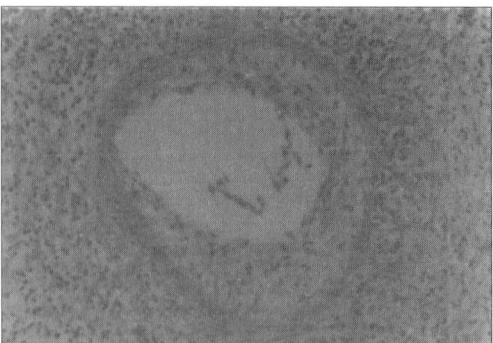

Figure 9.3. Histopathology slide of TBM and TB spinal cord. **Figure 9.3 (a)** Tuberculous meningitis (with lymphocytes, epitheloid histiocytes and giant cells) with extension of inflammation into cerebral cortex (arrow).

Figure 9.3 (b) Tuberculous endarteritis within meninges showing intimal fibrosis and surrounding tuberculous inflammation.

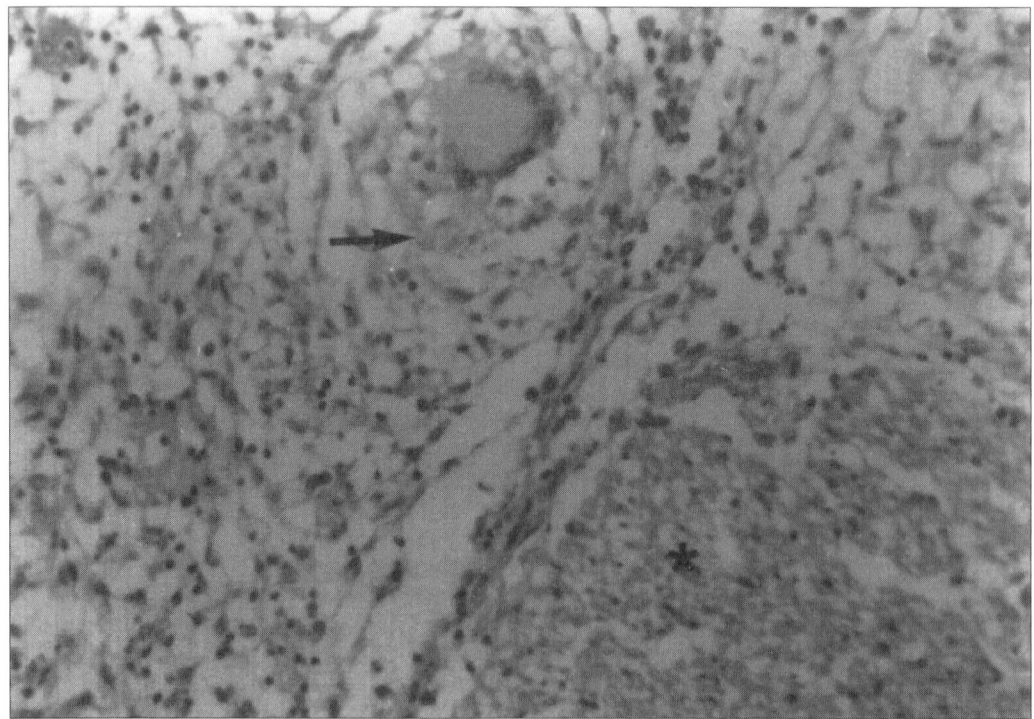

Figure 9.3 (c) Spinal nerve root (*) surrounded by tuberculous inflammation with granuloma formation (arrow).

and choroid plexus, and can lead to hydro-cephalus.

Vasculitis, which is secondary to inflam-mation around the blood vessels, affects vessels of all sizes, but endarteritic vascular occlusion appears to mainly involve the smaller perforating arteries arising from the Circle of Willis. In severely affected cases massive diencephalic and midbrain infarc-tion causes sequelae such as coma, hyper-tonicity and extensor rigidity; occasionally hypothalamopituitary dysfunction is pro-duced, with the syndrome of inappropriate antidiuretic hormone secretion. The ischae-mic or infarcted area becomes surrounded by local oedema which may give rise to focal convulsions, hemiplegia and brain stem syndromes. The inflammation can extend downwards to cause spinal arach-noiditis. The greater vascularity of the brain and incomplete myelinization may be fac-tors in the relatively poor prognosis of treated infants under one year of age.

Multiple cranial nerve palsies and myelo-pathy, often considered to be the result of entrapment by inflammatory exudate, may also be caused by infarction resulting from vasculitis.[16, 65]

Opto-chiasmatic arachnoiditis resulting in visual impairment or even blindness, with or without associated hydrocephalus, is a com-mon complication of TBM.[51] In this compli-cation, the basal exudate eventually becomes organized and forms adhesions which may result in further cranial nerve palsies, infarc-tion, and hydrocephalus. However, the hydrocephalus may in fact be due to defec-tive absorption of cerebrospinal fluid or to occlusion of the aqueduct, exit foramina, and especially the basal cisterns. Similar adhe-sions in the spinal canal can produce a spinal block and even a paraplegia.[48] Intracranial calcification occurs in 20 to 40 per cent of patients and usually becomes detectable two or three years after the onset of illness.[39]

Microscopically, the meningeal tubercles consist of a central zone of caseation, sur-rounded by epithelioid cells, lymphocytes, plasma cells, occasional giant cells and con-nective tissue. The exudate is made up of fibrin, lymphocytes, plasma cells, occa-sional polymorphonuclear leucocytes and areas of caseation necrosis.

Clinical features

Tuberculous meningitis may occur in patients of any age, sex or ethnic back-ground, though in developing countries like South Africa it occurs most commonly in children under six years of age, and pre-dominantly among blacks and coloureds. In children it is often a complication of pri-mary infection, usually developing within six months of the onset of infection, while in adults it may occur as an isolated form of TB. Of particular importance in children is that it may be precipitated by some inter-current illness (and especially by measles), occasionally by a mild head injury, or after anaesthesia for a surgical procedure.[36, 38]

Its clinical features may be divided into three main phases.[36] Initially the symptoms are non-specific with general malaise, low grade fever, apathy, irritability, intermittent headaches and muscle pains, while in some children vomiting, anorexia, behavioural problems, episodes of acute abdominal pain, diarrhoea and constipation or isolated fits may occur.[20, 33] The persistence and the combination of several of these symptoms should alert the clinician to the possibility of TBM before the classic clinical signs of meningitis make their appearance,[20] espe-cially as appropriate therapy at this early phase will ensure a 100 per cent cure rate.[2]

In adults, mental symptoms such as apa-thy, irritability and insidious change of per-sonality or fluctuating confusion may be the initial presenting features.[72]

The second phase starts after about two weeks with more definite neurological manifestations, including persistent head-aches, fluctuating levels of consciousness, neck stiffness, oculomotor nerve palsies, hemiparesis, tremulousness and involuntary movements. However, in infants a tense fontanelle may be the only evidence of meningitis.[36]

Progressively increasing drowsiness, mul-tiple cranial nerve palsies, hemiplegia, uri-nary retention, seizures and a state of decer-ebration ushers in the third and final phase of TBM. If left untreated, death will follow within four to eight weeks of the onset of symptoms.

Unusual presentations, especially in children, include onset with convulsions, focal neurological signs, and isolated cranial nerve palsies.[65] Occasionally both children and adults may present with features of raised intracranial pressure without any significant preceding illness.[36] In rare adult cases the presentation may be purely spinal, mimicking spinal cord compression, transverse myelitis or the Guillain-Barré Syndrome.[16, 48]

Clinico-pathological correlations are given in Table 9.1.

Presenting symptoms and signs observed in 47 children with TBM at King Edward VIII Hospital, Durban (1985–86) are shown in Tables 9.2 and 9.3.

Fever, cough and vomiting were the predominant presenting symptoms in children under two years of age, convulsions were noted in both young and old children, while headache was the initial complaint mainly in those over the age of five years.

The severity of the disease prior to treatment was classified into three stages by the British Medical Research Council in 1948.[44]

Stage 1
Patients with non-specific symptoms who have few or no signs of meningitis, who are fully conscious and who are in good general condition. The diagnosis is established mainly on cerebrospinal fluid findings.

Stage 2
Patients with mild mental confusion and/or who have neurological signs such as squints or hemiparesis.

Stage 3
Patients who are extremely ill, stuporose or comatose, and who will often have complete hemiplegia or paraplegia.

This classification of severity is of value in prognosis, especially in relation to

Table 9.1
Clinico-pathological features of TBM

UNDERLYING PATHOLOGY	SIGNS
Meningitis	Neck stiffness (infrequent under two years of age), Kernigs and Brudzinski's signs, opisthotonos
Raised intracranial pressure	Vomiting, increasing head size, bulging fontanelle, sutural separation and 'cracked-pot' note, bradycardia, mild hypertension and occasionally papilloedema, impaired consciousness, fits
Vascular complications (occlusions, infarction)	Convulsions, hemiplegia, quadriplegia, cranial nerve palsies (especially 3rd, 4th, 6th, 7th and occasionally 2nd) decerebrate rigidity
Encephalopathy	Abnormal behaviour, impaired alertness, dementia, spasticity, convulsions, coma
Basal ganglia involvement	Chorea, hemiballismus, athetosis, tremors, myoclonus, ataxia
Space-occupying lesion (Tuberculomas)	Asymptomatic, focal signs, raised intracranial pressure signs
Spinal arachnoiditis	Ascending or transverse myelitis: paraparesis, paraplegia, quadriplegia, sphincter disturbances, Guillain-Barré Syndrome
Adhesions	Cranial nerve palsies, infarctions, hydrocephalus, spinal block

treatment. The severity and outcome of the disease in the 47 children studied at the King Edward VIII Hospital in Durban is given in Table 9.4.

In an earlier South African study by Freiman and Geefhuysen of 131 patients treated for TBM, 44 were conscious and 87 unconscious at presentation. After six weeks of therapy, two of the conscious patients and 22 of the unconscious group died. One year after commencement of therapy, six of the conscious patients and 55 of those who were unconscious on presentation, had died. Furthermore, most of

Table 9.2
Symptoms in children with TBM*

SYMPTOMS	NUMBER OF CASES
Fever	19 (40%)
Cough	19 (40%)
Vomiting	19 (40%)
Convulsions	17 (36%)
Anorexia	9 (19%)
Headache	9 (19%)
Listlessness	8 (17%)
Lethargy	9 (19%)
Diarrhoea	7 (15%)
Loss of weight	3 (6%)

Table 9.3
Signs in children with TBM*

SIGNS	NUMBER OF CASES
Neck stiffness	37 (79%)
Fever	30 (64%)
Drowsiness	16 (34%)
Stupor/coma	15 (32%)
Cranial nerve palsies	
Facial nerve	16 (34%)
Oculomotor nerve	6 (13%)
Abducens nerve	5 (11%)
Hemiparesis	13 (28%)
Hydrocephalus	9 (20%)
Choroidal tubercles	5 (11%)
Ataxia/involuntary movements	4 (9%)
Papilloedema	2 (4%)
Quadriplegia	2 (4%)

* As seen in 47 children with TBM at the King Edward VIII Hospital, Durban in 1985–6

the survivors from the unconscious group had severe neurologic sequelae.[27] These studies highlight the point that the single most important factor influencing the outcome of treatment in TBM is the state of consciousness on admission to hospital.

Diagnosis

Clinicians in developing countries have to maintain a high index of suspicion about the possibility of TBM in children, as the disease often begins insidiously with non-specific symptoms and signs. Even in the fully developed case the diagnosis can present difficulties. If there is doubt about the cause of any meningitis, it is safer to treat for both TBM and acute bacterial meningitis until a definitive diagnosis can be made, as the outcome in TBM depends on the rapid institution of specific therapy. To ensure maximum recovery, therapy should begin within 10 days of the onset of illness.

History

A history of contact is important when a diagnosis of tuberculous meningitis is suggested, a fact which is reflected by several series of studies where sources were found in 30 to 80 per cent of cases.[48] In the series reported by Lincoln and Sewell contact history was available in 74 per cent,[38] while Kennedy and Fallon reported a figure of 56 per cent.[35] Unfortunately, this information is rarely volunteered and it is often obtained only after the diagnosis has been made. In the King Edward study a family history of tuberculosis was obtained in 32 per cent of children with TBM.

Physical examination

This will confirm the presence of meningitis, but will not establish the aetiology. Features which may provide a clue are extracranial evidence of tuberculosis (such as concomitant pulmonary tuberculosis or erythema nodosum). The finding of choroidal tubercles on fundoscopy may be helpful but in black children these are rarely seen (one study detected them in only 11 per cent of TBM patients). In the United Kingdom, however, choroidal tubercles are present at the onset in about half the cases[2, 34] and provide an immediate diagnostic clue.

Table 9.4
Stage of TBM at presentation and outcome

STAGES OF MENINGITIS	I	II	III	TOTAL
Patients	16	16	15	47 (100%)
Deaths	1	2	6	9 (19%)
Recovered without neurological sequelae	12	4	2	18 (38%)
Recovered with neurological sequelae	3	10	7	20 (43%)
Total recovered	15 (94%)	14 (88%)	9 (60%)	38 (81%)

Investigations

In most developing countries the diagnosis of TBM has to be based mainly on the results of the tuberculin test, chest roentgenogram and examination of the cerebrospinal fluid as the various biochemical and immunological tests shown in Table 9.6 may not be available. The various relevant tests are described here.

Simple routine investigations

These, such as the white cell count and erythrocyte sedimentation rate (ESR) are of limited value. A low serum sodium may reflect inappropriate anti-diuretic hormone secretion. In the King Edward VIII Hospital study the ESR was greater than 45 mm/hour in more than 60 per cent of cases in which this investigation was performed; a serum sodium of less than 130 mmol/l was present in 43 per cent of cases while in 17 per cent of cases it was under 120 mmol/l suggesting a diagnosis of inappropriate antidiuretic hormone secretion.

Tuberculin skin tests

The majority of patients with TBM will show a positive reaction, but a negative Mantoux reaction does not rule out the diagnosis as it may be falsely negative because of poor technique, malnutrition, overwhelming infection, the post-measles state or therapy with corticosteroids or immunosuppressants. Tuberculin testing of children should be routine in all hospitals as its omission may lead to delay in diagnosis. In the King Edward Hospital study a positive Mantoux reaction (greater than 14

mm) was obtained in 76 per cent (28 out of 37) of documented cases.

Chest roentgenogram

A radiograph of the chest may show enlarged glands, a primary complex or miliary TB in most children who develop TBM. During a 30 year period at one hospital in the United States only six per cent of patients with TBM had normal chest roentgenograms.[38] In the Durban study roentgenograms showed infiltrates in 81 per cent of cases; hilar, mediastinal or paratracheal adenopathy in 74 per cent; miliary shadowing in 19 per cent and pleural effusion in 11 per cent.

Cerebrospinal fluid (CSF)

Examination of the cerebrospinal fluid is central to the diagnosis of TBM. The fluid is usually under pressure, but herniation of the brain stem does not occur as cerebral oedema is uncommon; indeed lumbar puncture may provide some relief from intracranial tension. The characteristic cerebrospinal fluid in TBM is clear and forms a cobweb-like clot on standing. The cell counts range from 10 to 400 per mm^3 with lymphocytes predominating, but, during the early stages of the disease the cells in the CSF may be dominantly polymorphonuclear and the cell count may be as high as 1 000 per mm.[3] The protein content of the cerebrospinal fluid is almost always higher than normal and in more than half the cases is above 100 mg per cent — this is an important differentiating feature between the lymphocytic fluid of TBM and a viral meningitis.[44] With an impending spinal block it is elevated considerably and may give a xanthochromic appearance. The sugar is modestly decreased, but can be very low in advanced cases.

The CSF chloride is frequently low in the second or third stages of TBM but studies done in Durban have shown it to be unreliable when differentiating between TBM, acute bacterial meningitis and viral meningitis.[53] It has been suggested that the biochemical changes in the cerebrospinal fluid occur in a regular sequence — an increase in cells, rise in proteins, decrease in sugar and lastly a fall in chloride — but a cautionary note must be sounded about the so-called 'typical' changes of TBM: the CSF often does not follow this overall pattern and may in fact be normal when tubercle bacilli are present in the cerebrospinal fluid.[36] If it is remembered that the inflammatory reactions in the meninges may be likened to the tuberculin skin reaction, and that the latter may be negative in the presence of TB, then the variability of the CSF in TBM becomes understandable. If the CSF is normal but there is strong suspicion of TBM, the patient should be treated as such and a repeat lumbar puncture performed in 48 hours. This may reveal abnormalities even after the commencement of therapy. The CSF changes detected in the Durban study are given in Table 9.5.

In 42 per cent of cases there was an initial polymorph predominance. In 89 per cent of cases the CSF protein was greater than 0,5 g/l, in 56 per cent greater than 1 g/l, and in 29 per cent greater than 2 g/l. The cerebrospinal fluid sugar was normal in 18 per cent of cases, and in seven per cent the only abnormality was a raised protein level.

The ultimate proof of diagnosis of TBM is the demonstration of tubercle bacillus in the CSF. Acid-fast bacilli (AFB) may be seen on microscopy, but the success of this test depends on the amount of CSF, the number of samples scanned, the availability of skilled technicians and their determination to search for AFB. For these reasons the range of positivity is wide — 10–90 per cent, with the lower figures obtaining in the third world.[36] Culture of CSF is also not useful, as AFB are grown from only about

Table 9.5
Cerebrospinal fluid changes in black children with TBM

	RANGE	MEAN
Cells/mm³		
polymorphonuclears	0–2 020	150
lymphocytes	0–840	78
Protein (g/l)	0,1–47	3,35
Sugar (mmol/l)	0–6,2	2,0
Chloride (mmol/l)	84–140	110

10–20 per cent of samples and results take about four to six weeks. In the Durban study less than 10 per cent of cultures were positive for AFB.

If AFB are not found in the CSF, they should be looked for in the sputum or gastric aspirate, but in the author's experience the positivity rates are poor. Occasionally AFB may be isolated from an enlarged lymph node, liver or bone marrow biopsy. On treatment the CSF takes about three to four months to return to normal.

Miscellaneous tests

Recently a large number of different biochemical and serological tests have been described for the early and accurate diagnosis of TBM.[12, 41] These include *biochemical tests* (CSF adenosine deaminase activity, lactate dehydrogenase, lactate, tryptophan colour test and detection of AFB specific compounds such as tuberculostearic acid), *radio isotope studies* (bromide partition test — BPT); and *immunological tests* (for the detection of antigen, antibody or acute phase reactants). None of these tests have as yet gained widespread acceptance in clinical medicine or microbiological laboratories, either because they are non-specific or because they are too dependent on expensive technology for general use, especially in developing countries. In the author's experience the BPT and the inhibition of BCG–anti–BCG ELISA test were found to be the most useful tests in the early differentiation of tuberculosis from other causes of meningitis.[12, 54]

From successful experience, it is suggested that BPT be used in conjunction with bacterial and fungal antigen detection systems for the initial differentiation of clinically suspicious TBM from gram or culture negative bacterial and fungal meningitis. However, despite the availability of these various biochemical, radio isotope and immunological tests the difficulty in early and accurate diagnosis of TBM remains. New techniques that are associated with the molecular biology of micro-organisms are now being applied to the mycobacteria in modern mycobacteriology laboratories in the United States and Europe for early and accurate diagnosis of infections due to mycobacteria.[6, 29] The results of preliminary tests using polymerase chain reaction (PCR) are impressive.

Computer assisted tomography

CT scanning with contrast enhancement is a valuable aid to diagnosis and prognosis, and should be undertaken whenever such facilities are available. A CT scan is particularly useful when there are signs of raised intracranial pressure or focal neurological signs, as it has been suggested that basal oedema and ventricular enlargement, occurring together with basal enhancement are characteristic of advanced TBM.[10] The presence of basal and periventricular lucency carries a particularly poor prognosis in early tuberculous meningitis.[10]

Other findings on CT scan can include infarcts (especially in the territory of the middle cerebral artery and in the basal ganglia region); tuberculomas and occasionally an abscess.[5, 10]

In the Durban study at the King Edward VIII Hospital CT scans were obtained in 23 cases, with the following findings:

- basal enhancement in 14 (61 per cent);
- hydrocephalus in 11 (48 per cent);

Table 9.6
Investigations in suspected TBM

1. Tuberculin skin tests		
2. CSF:	• Routine examination	• WCC especially lymphocytes protein sugar
	• Ziehl Neelsen stain	• AFB
	• culture for myco-bacterium tuberculosis	
3. Radiology:	• chest roentgenogram	• hilar glands • primary complex • miliary TB
	• CT scan	• basal enhancement • basal lucency • periventricular lucency • hydrocephalus • basal ganglia/middle cerebral artery territory infarcts • tuberculoma
4. Miscellaneous: Biochemical tests		• CSF adenosine deaminase • CSF lactate dehydrogenase • CSF tuberculostearic acid (gas chromatography) • inhibition of BCG-anti-BCG ELISA
Radioisotope studies		• radioactive bromide partition test (blood: CSF ratio less than 1,6 = TBM)
Immunological tests		• detect mycobacterial antigen, antibody acute phase reactants
5. Molecular biology		• DNA probes (low sensitivity) • Polymerase chain reaction (high specificity and sensitivity)

- associated tuberculoma in four (17 per cent);
- infarction in three (13 per cent);
- focal calcification in three (13 per cent); and
- generalized cerebral atrophy in three (13 per cent).

In recent years computed tomography has become an important procedure for the monitoring of intracranial pressure in TBM as well as being an accurate method for detecting the presence of tuberculoma and then monitoring its disappearance under medical treatment.[60]

Differential diagnosis

When the cerebrospinal fluid shows a high cell count with predominance of lymphocytes, a raised protein concentration and a lowered glucose, a number of other conditions enter the differential diagnosis. These include partially treated pyogenic meningitis, viral meningo-encephalitis, fungal meningitis, brain abscess, typhoid, cerebral tumour, carcinomatous and leukemic meningitis, collagen vascular disease and sarcoidosis. In the black child neurocysticercosis should always be considered in the differential diagnosis. Other infections that can

cause aseptic meningitis with a low CSF glucose include syphilis, brucellosis and toxoplasmosis. If the clinical presentation is suggestive of any of the above, then appropriate tests should be carried out to confirm or exclude these possibilities. If a definitive diagnosis of TBM cannot be made and partially treated bacterial meningitis cannot be excluded, then it is mandatory to treat the ill patient with both antituberculous therapy and systemic antibiotics while continuing a thorough search for the aetiological agent.

The most important conditions to be differentiated from TBM according to CSF are given in Table 9.7.

If facilities for diagnosis are limited as they are in most third world countries, the following scheme can be adopted to manage suspected cases of TBM:

- take a careful history, especially noting contacts and duration of illness;
- detailed physical examination, especially for other sites of TB, foci of pyogenic infections, and exanthems due to viruses;
- do a Mantoux test and chest radiograph;
- CSF: microscopy for bacteria and cells; sugar with dextrostix (if very low treat for pyogenic meningitis and tuberculous meningitis (if normal likely to be viral);

Table 9.7
Differential diagnosis of CSF in TBM

CONDITION	DISTINGUISHING FEATURES
1. Pyogenic meningitis (meningococcus, pneumococcus, *Haemophilus influenzae*)	very low sugar, numerous polymorphonuclears, bacteria detected (smear, culture, antigens) normal in two weeks
2. Viral meningoencephalitis (coxsackie, echo, herpes, human immunodeficiency virus)	normal sugar, occasionally low slightly elevated proteins mostly lymphocytes no bacteria normal very rapidly
3. Fungal meningitis (cryptococcus, candida)	organism detected by special stains (especially India ink) or specific antisera
4. Brain abscesses	variable number of polymorphonuclears (closer abscess is to meninges higher the number) slightly raised protein normal or slightly lowered sugar

- treat for TBM if still in doubt and repeat CSF examination in two weeks; if CSF is then normal, it is unlikely to be TBM.

Treatment

The cornerstone of successful management of TBM is the early institution of chemotherapy, as there is a close correlation between the prognosis and the stage of the disease in which treatment is begun. Children treated during the first stage of meningitis almost invariably survive, often without significant sequelae, while children first treated after the occurrence of severe neurological changes are at great risk of a poor or fatal outcome.

Chemotherapy

In contrast to the rapid advances in the chemotherapy of pulmonary tuberculosis there is no agreement about the form of chemotherapy or the optimal duration of treatment for TBM.[49, 50] However, it is important to use drugs that cross the blood-brain barrier freely, and are relatively non-toxic, and are easily available. Of all drugs that are presently available, INH is the most important.

Drugs used in TBM

Most reputable units currently recommend the use of isoniazid (INH), rifampicin, pyrazinamide and streptomycin in the treatment of TBM. In adults pyridoxine 50 mg daily may be added as a prophylaxis against INH-induced peripheral neuritis. Parsons recommends a minimum of 18 months treatment with:

- INH and rifampicin for the full 18 months;
- intrathecal streptomycin for the first two weeks;
- pyrazinamide and intramuscular streptomycin for the first three months.[47]

The long duration of treatment may not be absolutely necessary — Phuapradit and Vejjajiva treated 24 adult patients with pyrazinamide, INH, rifampicin and intramuscular streptomycin daily during the first two months, followed by INH and rifampicin daily for seven months, with virtually complete recovery in all but two of the 24 patients who completed such a course. The two deaths occurred in patients who were comatose at the start of therapy and in whom post-mortem revealed minimal fibrosis but no evidence of residual infection.[50]

Therapy for TBM with streptomycin, isoniazid, rifampicin and pyrazinamide for a period as short as six months has also been shown to be successful in adult patients, but this form of therapy has not been tried in children. Visudhiphan and Chiemchanya recently treated 51 children with TBM with isoniazid and rifampicin for one year. Three of their patients died within the first week of admission and four patients were lost to follow up. Forty-four patients were followed for one and a half to seven years; of these 31 recovered completely. The 13 remaining patients recovered with neurologic sequelae ranging from mental retardation to motor weakness, seizures and hydrocephaly. However, although these two studies show apparent success with shorter regimens, present recommendations would favour treatment for at least 18 months.

At King Edward VIII Hospital, Durban a combination of INH, rifampicin, pyrazinamide and ethionamide is used. Pyrazinamide is stopped after six months and therapy is continued with INH, rifampicin and ethionamide for a period of one year. Thereafter INH and ethionamide are continued for another six months on an outpatient basis. If severe gastrointestinal tract side-effects ensue ethionamide is replaced by ethambutol, but this must be avoided in children under six years of age because it may be complicated by optic neuritis (which below this age may not be revealed by symptoms and therefore go undetected). INH (or neotizide) is given intramuscularly, until the patient is able to take it satisfactorily by mouth. The dose must be increased as the child gains weight. Hydronsan (detoxicated form of INH) can be given in the presence of other drug toxicities and may be life saving in TBM.

ACTH gel is used in all cases: 2 IU/kg 12 hourly; maximum 50 IU/day with added potassium. ACTH is continued until the CSF is normal and has remained so for two or three weeks (this may be a period of about three months). Prednisone in a dosage of 1–2 mg/kg/day may achieve a similar anti-inflammatory result. It is most important that once an adequate schedule has been introduced, it should not be modified except in accordance with weight gain or drug toxicity. Dosage should not be reduced for loss of weight, and patients should be regularly monitored for side effects of drugs and for hearing loss; and their CSF should be monitored until it returns to normal and has remained so for a few months.

Intrathecal therapy

Despite the controversy surrounding intrathecal therapy several authors favour this route, especially in the initial stages of illness.[25, 40, 48] Parsons advocates intrathecal streptomycin for the first two weeks of therapy.[47] The South African experience as reflected by Freiman and Geefhuysen's study is that while this form of therapy may reduce mortality, in so doing it actually increases the incidence and/or severity of sequelae.[27]

The practice of intrathecal therapy has long been abandoned at the King Edward VIII Hospital.

Adjuvant therapy

Adjuvant therapy is used in the hope that it will reduce the inflammatory basal exudate which is responsible for many of the serious neurological sequelae of TBM. Four substances (streptokinase, hyaluronidase, purified protein derivative and corticosteroids) have been used. Of these, only corticosteroids have found any significant place in the management of TBM.

The routine use of steroids in TBM is controversial, but nevertheless they have been strongly recommended by some authors while others are more cautious.[8, 23, 27, 32, 44] Steroids are given in the hope that they will reduce cerebral oedema and inflammatory exudate and so prevent the development of fibrous adhesions, especially about the base of the brain. They may also prevent spinal block, but their role in the prevention of arteritis is questionable. Treatment with steroids is commenced at a dosage of 1–2 mg/kg/day for a period of four to six weeks, or until the CSF has been normal for one or two months.

Treatment of complications

Hydrocephalus

Both obstructive and communicating hydrocephalus are common complications of TBM and may adversely affect the outcome of this disease. In young infants hydrocephalus should be suspected when the head enlarges, the sutures separate or the fontanelle bulges. In older children diagnosing raised intracranial pressure may be difficult as papilloedema is not a frequent finding. However, hydrocephalus should be suspected in any patient whose level of consciousness deteriorates on adequate therapy, or who develops further neurological signs, such as fits or increasing spasticity of the limbs. Schoeman *et al.* showed that continuous intracranial pressure monitoring plays an important role in the detection and management of raised intracranial pressure in TBM,[57] and in their experience a combination of CSF pressure monitoring and CT scanning provided the most useful information on the dynamics of obstructive hydrocephalus, and was the greatest help when making rational decisions on the need and time for CSF shunting.

Relief of hydrocephalus with a ventriculo-atrial or ventriculoperitoneal shunt, even in the active phase of the disease, has been shown to bring about a remarkable improvement in many patients.[9, 66] For communicating hydrocephalus, some authors have reported excellent results with the use of oral acetazolamide (to reduce CSF formation) and repeated lumbar punctures. Using this form of therapy Visudhiphan and Chiemchanya reduced raised intracranial pressure within two to three weeks in 22 of 24 patients studied.[66]

Syndrome of inappropriate antidiuretic hormone secretion

This is a not uncommon complication of TBM. In the King Edward VIII Hospital study 17 per cent of 47 patients with TBM had evidence of inappropriate antidiuretic hormone secretion. Simple fluid restriction seems to correct this disorder in most patients without recourse to hypertonic fluid infusion.

Convulsions

This is a common complication of TBM especially in infants. Diazepam or phenytoin can be used for the acute management of convulsions but for maintenance therapy, phenobarbitone, sodium valproate or carbamazepine are indicated. Phenytoin is not advocated for long term management as it interacts with isoniazid and rifampicin.

Spinal block

This is discussed in the section on myeloradiculopathy.

General measures

The general care and supervision of a patient with TBM is very important if the final outcome is expected to be satisfactory. Nutrition and hydration must be maintained, and this requires careful nursing, which may include nasogastric feeding. TBM is a chronic illness, often requiring intensive physiotherapy. Occupational therapy can be started when consciousness returns. A psychometric assessment may need to be obtained six months after the onset of TBM; ophthalmologic and audiometric assessments become necessary to detect visual and hearing disturbances which complicate TBM.

Prognosis

The outcome of TBM depends on many factors, but rapid diagnosis and early institution of appropriate therapy appear to be the most important.[24] Early diagnosis depends on clinical suspicion and laboratory competence. Many series have shown that if treatment commences in the first stage of the illness (before consciousness is affected) a 100 per cent cure rate, with or without minor sequelae, can be expected; if treatment is delayed until the third stage of the illness the mortality likelihood is more than 50 per cent.[48] Other factors affecting prognosis include the age of the patient (it is poor at the extremes of life) and severity of the disease (as when there is coexisting miliary tuberculosis).[20, 24, 35] Patients with hydrocephalus and decerebrate rigidity have low survival rates and severe sequelae.[20] Late sequelae of TBM include motor deficits, intellectual impairment, deafness, blindness and epilepsy, all of which appear to be more common in children.[20] Occasionally, hypothalamopituitary dysfunction manifesting as growth failure, diabetes insipidus, obesity and precocious puberty may occur.

SEROUS TUBERCULOUS MENINGITIS

This is a rare but well documented clinical entity occurring in children and adults with tuberculosis. The first cases were described by McGregor *et al.* (1934) and later by Lincoln (1947), who thought it was a hypersensitivity response rather than a true meningitis, and therefore called it 'serous meningitis'.[44] This entity was of great importance in the pre-antibiotic era because its favourable prognosis was in contrast to that of true tuberculosis meningitis which was invariably fatal. As it resolves spontaneously it has an excellent prognosis.[38, 44] All patients have illnesses indistinguishable from the early stage of tuberculous meningitis, all have low dose tuberculin hypersensitivity and frequently the cerebrospinal fluid shows a lymphocytic pleocytosis with a slight rise of protein. In some cases tubercle bacilli have been recovered from the cerebrospinal fluid.

TUBERCULOUS ENCEPHALOPATHY

This entity was first described in 1966 by workers from the Indian subcontinent.[15] The pathology is one of diffuse brain damage with oedema and occasionally perivascular myelin loss and, in rare cases, haemorrhagic leukoencephalopathy in the absence of overt tuberculous infection of the brain or meninges, and without infarction or hydrocephaly. The clinical presentation is with convulsions, increasing spasticity, decerebration and a rapid decline in consciousness to a state of coma. This condition was believed to be an exaggerated hypersensitivity reaction to the tubercle bacillus. It mainly affects younger children and is reversible in most cases with appropriate therapy. Therefore, in areas of increased prevalence of tuberculosis, a high index of suspicion must be maintained at all times in children who present with a rapid onset of coma, as this condition is eminently treatable.

TUBERCULOMAS
Introduction

Like tuberculo-meningitis, tuberculomas remain a significant problem in developing countries. In the Indian subcontinent the incidence ranges from about 20 to 30 per cent of all intracranial space-occupying lesions;[18, 52] while in Africa the figures are 12,5 per cent for Nigeria[46] and 14 per cent for Zimbabwe, Zambia and Malawi.[37] In Durban, 14 cases were reported over a three year period, 36 per cent occurring in children less than five years of age.[70] It is only 60 to 80 years since a similar situation existed in Europe and the United States,[1, 19, 28, 44] but with improved socio-economic conditions and the advent of effective antituberculous therapy, the incidence in these areas has progressively decreased. However, with the recent influx of Asian immigrants to the United Kingdom the possibility of tuberculoma once again arises when an Asian-born person presents with an intracranial space-occupying lesion.[44]

Pathogenesis and pathology

Tuberculomas develop as a result of the haematogenous spread of bacilli from a distant focus, usually the lung, to the brain. In children it is mostly a complication of primary infection, but in adults it results predominantly from reactivation of dormant disease.[61] Tuberculomas are for the most part solitary lesions, but some 15 to 34 per cent are multiple.[19] In children the majority of lesions are infratentorial, whereas in adults they are predominantly supratentorial.[14] These lesions are usually located in the frontal lobe in adults and in the cerebellar hemispheres in children;[48] an uncommon location is the brain stem.[62]

The majority of lesions are small ranging from about 2 to 40 mm in diameter, but lesions up to 8 cm in diameter have been reported.[48]

On macroscopic examination a tuberculoma is a well circumscribed, firm greyish-white mass with a central area of caseation. Histologically the necrotic centre is surrounded by epithelioid cells, lymphocytes and numerous Langhan's giant cells.

In contrast to tuberculomas elsewhere in the body, intracranial lesions do not readily heal by fibrosis and should therefore always be regarded as active, as tubercle bacilli can be found in at least 50 per cent of cases.[48]

Clinical features

In areas where tuberculosis is rife, intracranial tuberculomas are primarily a problem of children and young adults, although any age group may be affected. In India[18] and Rumania[4] 86 per cent of patients with tuberculomas were under the age of 25 years.

(a)

(b)

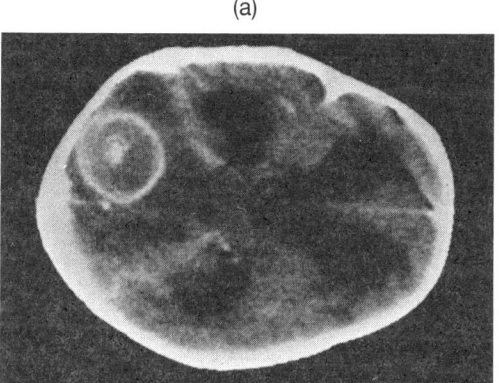 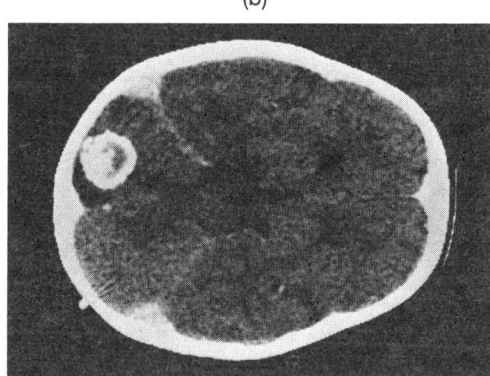

Figure 9.4. Post fossa tuberculoma with hydrocephalus. Typical target lesion **(a)** showing resolution with calcification after a one year course of antituberculous therapy **(b)**.

Clinical features are in no way specific. The initial symptoms and signs are those associated with increased intracranial pressure (headache, vomiting, papilloedema) and epileptic seizures.[4, 14, 22, 56, 64] Most tuberculomas are small and do not give rise to signs of increased intracranial pressure, but localizing signs can occur, such as a cerebral hemisphere lesion giving rise to a slowly developing contra-lateral hemiplegia, while a cerebellar lesion may present with ataxia. In the 28 patients reported in the United Kingdom since 1974, 39 per cent had focal motor and/or sensory symptoms, while a few complained of dysphasia,

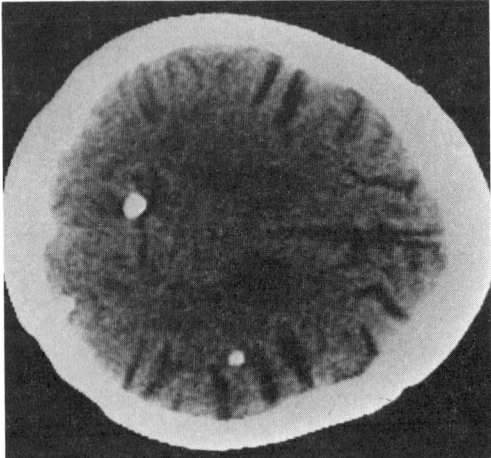

Figure 9.5. Calcified tuberculomata. Note focal atrophy in relation to larger calcification.

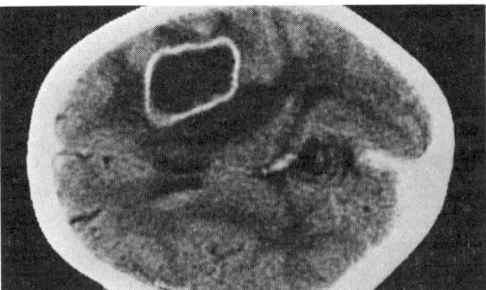

Figure 9.6. Tuberculous abscess. The left lateral ventricle is markedly compressed. There is displacement of supratentorial ventricle to the right. An extensive area of patchy decreased density is present in the left frontal and parietal region with ring like enhancement on intravenous conray administration consistent with abscess. AFB cultured from abscess fluid.

intellectual failure, anosmia, hemianopia, diplopia or ataxia.[48]

Fever and impairment of general health are uncommon features, but a past history or current evidence of TB is common, occurring in about 50 per cent of cases.[1, 18, 52]

Clinical manifestations of brain stem tuberculomas are varied. In the series reported by Talamas *et al.*, patients exhibited a constellation of focal brain stem signs,[62] among which oculomotor palsies predominated, and especially isolated dysfunction of the third and sixth cranial nerves. Motor deficits in the form of hemiparesis occurred in over 80 per cent of cases and limb ataxia in just under 30 per cent of cases.

Investigations

Routine haematological investigations (WCC, ESR) are not helpful. In some 25 to 50 per cent of cases, the ESR may be raised to more than 50 mm/hour,[18, 48] and a normal ESR in no way excludes the diagnosis. In most patients CSF examination yields normal findings, but an increased protein content and a mononuclear pleocytosis is sometimes found.[56, 64] In one series an isolated protein elevation was the most common abnormality, found in 88 per cent of sampled patients.[58]

Tuberculin skin reactions are also not very helpful as the positivity rate ranges from 25–75 per cent.[19] On diagnosis chest roentgenograms are usually normal, a minority of abnormal roentgenograms (about 25–50 per cent of cases) showing an old tuberculous infection[19] or active disease (about 40–50 per cent of cases).[1, 52]

The commonly held view that intracranial tuberculomas usually calcify has been shown to be untrue by several large series in which the incidence of calcification varied from 1,4 to 6 per cent.[1, 4, 18, 52] More often, evidence of raised intracranial pressure is seen on plain skull radiograph, with sutural separation being a common feature in children.

Isotope brain scans and angiograms reveal abnormalities in over 80 per cent of cases; but in recent years these investigations have been superseded by computerized tomography which has become the investigation of choice for tuberculomas. CT scans show either isodense or minimally hyperdense lesions, which enhance in a homogeneous or ring-like manner after the administration of contrast material.[70]

The 'target sign' (a central nidus of calcification or central enhancement, surrounded by a ring of enhancement) has not been seen in any other tumour and may be regarded as being characteristic of a tuberculoma.[70] Occasionally, it may be extremely difficult to differentiate a tuberculoma from an abscess or other granulomatous diseases, and, in the case of a pyogenic abscess the enhancement ring may resemble that of a tuberculoma. In the author's experience, however, all abscesses scanned so far have shown a markedly decreased density relative to brain substance within the enhancement ring.[70]

Magnetic resonance imaging is an important recent addition to presently available neurodiagnostic techniques, and is a sensitive method for detecting tuberculomas. Recent studies have shown it to be more sensitive than CT in demonstrating the full extent of the lesion, especially in patients with brain stem tuberculomas which exhibit exophytic growth into the Pontine cisterns.[62] However, there is still doubt about its ability to differentiate tuberculomas from other brain stem lesions.[62]

Treatment

Prior to the advent of effective antituberculous therapy the mainstay of treatment for tuberculomas was biopsy and excision, and these invariably carried a high mortality rate.[19, 48]

The development of effective chemotherapy and the advent of computerized tomography have encouraged clinicians to rely entirely on medical therapy. On the application of antituberculous therapy, CT may show progressive resolution of the lesions within a few months.[56, 64]

Presently there seems to be no place for surgery in the management of tuberculomas, except for the shunting of patients with hydrocephalus and raised intracranial pressure, or for stereotactic biopsy of the lesion in cases where the diagnosis remains in doubt.[19, 62]

Current medical therapy includes INH, rifampicin, pyrazinamide and ethionamide or ethambutol. The optimal duration of treatment is uncertain. Mayers *et al.* recommend triple therapy (INH, rifampicin, ethambutol) for the first three months, followed by INH and rifampicin for the next 18 months,[43] but on the other hand, Harder *et al.* suggest a 12 month treatment, provided a three drug regimen is given for the full period.[30] The use of corticosteroids in the treatment of intracranial tuberculomas is controversial.[43]

Occasionally, a patient may present with fits, focal signs or evidence of raised intracranial pressure during the course of successful treatment of intracranial tuberculomas. This is usually caused by paradoxical expansion of the intracranial lesion.[31, 63] Such events occur some weeks or months after the commencement of antituberculous therapy and have been thought to be due to immunologic modulation.[31] It is a transient phenomenon and does not require alteration of therapy, but on rare occasions surgical decompression may be necessary to relieve the increased intracranial pressure.[48]

TUBERCULOUS ABSCESS

Tuberculous brain abscesses are rare intracranial complications of TB. Like tuberculomas they arise as a result of haematogenous dissemination from the lungs, but histologically and clinically they resemble pyogenic brain abscess. Why these lesions occur instead of the more common tuberculoma is unknown. One view is that they are due to an uneven balance between defence mechanisms and the size and virulence of the infecting inoculum.[48, 71]

Whitener reserves the term 'tuberculous abscess' for pus-filled cavities containing tubercle bacilli but lacking the granulomatous elements associated with TB.[71]

Tuberculous brain abscesses resemble tuberculomas in their demography, location and aspects of clinical presentation (fits, focal neurological signs and signs of raised intracranial pressure), but they differ in that they present acutely, are more aggressive and therefore produce more severe illness with fever and impairment of consciousness being more common. CSF abnormalities, in particular a persistently low glucose level, are more common than with tuberculomas.

In the pre-antibiotic era this condition was invariably fatal, but with appropriate antituberculous chemotherapy and surgical excision and drainage, the mortality and morbidity have been reduced remarkably.

Adequate chemotherapy of tuberculous brain abscess should include at least three of the drugs that cross the blood-brain barrier (INH, rifampicin, pyrazinamide and ethambutol). The optimal duration is uncertain but prolonged therapy for at least 18 to 24 months is advocated in order to avoid recurrence of the tuberculous process.

TUBERCULOUS MYELO-RADICULOPATHIES

Intraspinal tuberculosis, with the exception of the extradural lesions associated with Pott's disease, is rare in both developed and developing countries.[3, 48] Several pathogenetic mechanisms are known to cause lesions of the spinal cord and nerve roots, the most important of which are:

- vertebral tuberculosis (Pott's disease) (see Chapter 10);
- tuberculomas, both extra- and intradural (extra- and intramedullary);
- spinal meningitis (radiculomyelitis) — primary, secondary to basal meningitis, and secondary to vertebral disease.

Intraspinal granulomas (tuberculomas)

Intraspinal granulomas are about twenty times less frequent than the corresponding intracranial lesions,[3] and can be either extra- or intradural. The latter may be intra- or extramedullary. Of all the types of spinal tuberculomas the extradural variety is the most common, while the intradural extramedullary variety is the least common.[17, 42] To illustrate this point Dastur found, among 74 patients with paraplegia not due to overt Pott's disease, 48 with extradural granulomas, 19 with 'spinal meningitis', one with meningitis secondary to an extradural infection, and six with intramedullary tuberculomas.[17] Most patients with intraspinal

tuberculous granulomas are in the younger age group, 80 per cent being under 30 years of age.[3] Extradural tuberculomas (measuring about 5–7 mm) may form a cover around the dura mater from which they may be detached, whereas subdural tuberculomas are usually attached to the inner aspect of the dura mater and to the spinal cord from which they may be difficult to separate.[3] These granulomas can compress one aspect of the cord or they may completely cover the cord. This compression may be localized to one or two cord segments or may extend over a length of the subarachnoid space.[17]

Intramedullary tuberculomas (measuring about 7–10 mm) are embedded in the substance of the spinal cord from where they can be easily enucleated. In most reported series of tuberculous spinal granulomas, the thoracic region is the most common site involved.[3, 17]

Patients with intraspinal tuberculous granulomas commonly present with a history of root pains followed within weeks or months by paraplegia and sphincter incontinence. A history of tuberculosis meningitis may not be forthcoming but often there is evidence of active or healed tuberculosis elsewhere.[48] The ESR, white cell count and x-rays of the spine are unhelpful, while the CSF may be xanthochromic with a very high CSF protein (Froin's Syndrome). CT-myelography is the investigation of choice and this may reveal a complete block. Magnetic resonance imaging may be a useful additional investigative technique as it has been shown to be helpful in differentiating epidural sepsis from other intraspinal tuberculous lesions.[59]

In contrast to cerebral tuberculomas, the treatment of choice for intraspinal tuberculomas includes surgical resection and antituberculous chemotherapy. The prognosis for complete recovery is good if the lesion is localized and can be totally excised.

Spinal meningitis (radiculomyelitis)

Tuberculous lesions of the spinal cord and nerve roots (radiculomyelitis) are rare in the western world, in contrast to the incidence in certain Asian countries.

As the various forms of spinal tuberculosis with paraplegia have very similar clinical and pathological features, Wadia has suggested that the designation 'radiculomyelitis' be used as a generic term and has proposed the following classification:[68]

1. primary tuberculous radiculomyelitis;
2. radiculomyelitis secondary to intracranial tuberculous meningitis;
3. radiculomyelitis secondary to vertebral tuberculosis.

Tuberculous radiculomyelitis or arachnoiditis is usually secondary to the downward extension of intracranial (basal) tuberculous meningitis,[7] but occasionally the spinal meninges may be affected by direct extension from a primary tuberculous focus in the vertebrae, producing spinal block and paraplegia.

Primary tuberculous radiculomyelitis is an uncommon but well-documented entity, with the largest series emanating from the Indian subcontinent where Wadia and Dastur have described 38 cases of this condition out of 70 cases from all causes.[69]

As in intracranial tuberculous meningitis, radiculomyelitis is thought to arise as a localized arachnoiditis from a primary Rich's focus in the spinal meninges or cord. The tissue at the site of lesion and beyond is covered in a thick exudate which contains tubercles, and in which the cord and nerve roots are compressed; vasculitis involving the spinal arteries and veins ensues with subsequent cord infarction.

The clinical features of this syndrome are principally those of a radiculomyelopathy that is acute, subacute or chronic; ascending or transverse, and detected at single or multiple levels. It affects both children and adults. In the acute form there is fever and stiffness of the neck and back with superficial tenderness, spinal root pains, paraplegia, sphincter disturbance, areflexia and extensor plantar responses. If left untreated radiculomyelitis often leads to the development of tuberculous meningitis.

Investigations

Most patients prove to have tuberculosis elsewhere and nearly all have marked tuberculin sensitivity.[45] X-ray of the spine is normal, while chest roentgenograms may show evidence of tuberculosis. The CSF is usually xanthochromic with a high CSF protein suggesting a spinal block (Froin's Syndrome). Tubercle bacilli may not be found in smears and cultures, but a positive bromide partition test may support the diagnosis.[48]

Myelography by either the lumbar or the cisternal route reveals multiple irregular filling defects, cyst formation or spinal block.[26] Myelography is essential as a localized spinal block has to be surgically decompressed. At surgery a biopsy may be taken which may help confirm the diagnosis.

Differential diagnosis

The differential diagnosis includes conditions that cause spinal cord compression, ascending or transverse myelitis, and the Guillain-Barré Syndrome. Other causes include syphilis, cryptococcal infection and carcinomatous meningitis.

Treatment

Antituberculous treatment with INH, rifampicin, pyrazinamide and ethambutol should commence immediately the diagnosis of tuberculous radiculomyelitis is considered. Surgery has little to offer in the management of this condition except in the case of a localized spinal block. The role of steroids is uncertain, but Wadia, who has considerable experience in this area, recommends a three month course of oral prednisolone (60 mg/day for one month and then in a smaller dose for a further two months) and 50 mg of hydrocortisone intrathecally twice daily as soon as spinal block is suspected.[68]

As with tuberculous meningitis the hope of complete resolution is related to the duration of symptoms prior to the commencement of the appropriate antituberculous chemotherapy.

REFERENCES

1 Anderson J M & Macmillan J J, 1975. Intracranial tuberculoma — an increasing problem in Britain. *JNNP.* 38, 194–201.

2 Anonymous, 1971. Tuberculous meningitis in Children. *British Medical Journal.* 5739, 1–2.

3 Arseni C & Samitca D C. Intraspinal tuberculous granuloma. *Brain.* 83, 285–92.

4 Arseni C, 1958. Two hundred and one cases of intracranial tuberculoma treated surgically. *JNNP.* 21, 308–11.

5 Bhargava S & Tandon P N, 1980. Intracranial tuberculomas: a CT study. *British Journal of Radiography.* 53, 935–45.

6 Brisson-Noel A *et al.*, 1989. Rapid diagnosis of tuberculosis by amplification of mycobacterial DNA in clinical samples. *Lancet.* 1069–71.

7 Brooks W D W, Fletcher A P & Wilson R R, 1954.Tuberculous radiculomyelitis. *Quarterly Journal of Medicine.* 23, 275.

8 Bulkeley W C M, 1953. Tuberculous meningitis treated with A C T H and isoniazid. A comparison with intrathecal streptomycin. *British Medical Journal.* 11, 1127–29.

9 Bullock M R R & Van Dellen J R, 1982. The role of cerebrospinal fluid shunting in tuberculous meningitis. *Surgical Neurology.* 18, 274–7.

10 Bullock M R R & Welchman J M, 1982. Diagnostic and prognostic features of tuberculous meningitis on CT scanning. *Journal of Neurology and Neurological Psychiatry.* 45, 1098–101.

11 Coovadia H M & Loening W E K, 1988. *Paediatrics and Child Health.* 2nd ed. Cape Town: Oxford University Press.

12 Coovadia Y M *et al.*, 1986. Evaluation of adenosine deaminase activity and antibody to mycobacterium tuberculosis antigen 5 in CSF and the radioactive bromide partition test for the early diagnosis of TBM. *Archives of the Diseases of Childhood.* 61, 428–35.

13 Cybulska E, 1988. Tuberculous meningitis. *British Journal of Hospital Medicine.* 1, 63–6.

14 Dastur D K, Lalitha V S & Prabhakar V, 1968. Pathological analysis of intracranial space-occupying lesions in 1 000 cases including children. *Journal of Neurological Science.* 6, 575–92.

15 Dastur D K & Udani P M, 1966. Pathology and pathogenesis of tuberculous encephalopathy. *Acta Neuropathologica (Berlin).* 6, 311–9.

16 Dastur D K & Wadia N H, 1969. Spinal meningitides with radiculomyelopathy. Pathology and pathogenesis. *Journal of Neurological Science.* 8, 261–97.

17 Dastur H M, 1972. A tuberculoma review with some personal experiences. (Part 2: Spinal cord and its coverings). *Neurology, India.* 20, 127–31.

18 Dastur H M & Desai A D, 1965. A comparative study of brain tuberculomas and gliomas. *Brain.* 88, 375–96.

19 De Angelis L M, 1981. Intracranial tuberculoma: Case report and review of the literature. *Neurology* 31, 1133–6.

20 Delage G & Dusseault M, 1979. Tuberculous meningitis in children. *Canadian Medical Association Journal* 120, 305–9.

21 Dixon P E & Hoey C, 1984. Tuberculous meningitis in the elderly. *Postgraduate Medical Journal.* 60, 586–8.

22 Elshibly E M & Ellidir A R, 1986. Intracranial tuberculoma in a Sudanese child: response to medical treatment. *Annals of Tropical Pediatrics.* 6, 183–5.

23 Escobar J A, *et al.*, 1975. Mortality from tuberculous meningitis reduced by steroid therapy. *Pediatrics.* 56, (6), 1050–55.

24 Fallon R J & Kennedy D H, 1981. Treatment and prognosis in tuberculous meningitis. *Journal of Infection.* 3, (1), 39–44.

25 Fitzsimons J M, & Smith H.V, 1963. Tuberculous meningitis: special features of treatment. *Tubercle.* 44, 103–11.

26 Freilich D & Swash M, 1979. Diagnosis and management of tuberculous paraplegia with special reference to tuberculous radiculomyelitis. *Journal of Neurology, Neurosurgery and Psychiatry.* 42, 12–8.

27 Freiman I & Geefhuysen J, 1970. Evaluation of intrathecal therapy with streptomycin and hydrocortisone in tuberculous meningitis. *Pediatrics.* 76, (6), 895–901.

28 Garland H G & Armitage G, 1933. Intracranial tuberculoma. *Journal of Pathology and Bacteriology.* 37, 461–71.

29 Good R C & Mastro T, 1989. The modern mycobacteriology laboratory. How it can help the clinician. *Clinical Chest Medicine.* 10, (3), 315–22.

30 Harder E, Al-Kawi M Z & Carney P, 1983. Intracranial tuberculoma. Conservative management. *American Journal of Medicine*. 74, 570–6.

31 Hendrickse W A, 1984. Paradoxical expansion of intracranial tuberculomas during chemotherapy. *Lancet*. 2, 749–50.

32 Hockaday J M & Smith H M V, 1966. Corticosteroids as an adjuvant to the chemotherapy of tuberculous meningitis. *Tubercle*. 47, 75–91.

33 Idris Z H *et al.*, 1976. Tuberculous meningitis in childhood. *American Journal of the Diseases of Childhood*. 130, 364–7.

34 Illingworth R S & Lorber J, 1956. Tubercles of the choroid. *Archives of the Diseases of Children*. 31, 467–9.

35 Kennedy D H & Fallon R J, 1979. Tuberculous meningitis. *Journal of the American Medical Association*. 241, (3), 264–8.

36 Kocen R S, 1977. Tuberculous meningitis. *British Journal of Hospital Medicine*. 18, 436–4.

37 Levy L F, 1973. Tuberculoma of brain in Malawi, Rhodesia and Zambia. *African Journal of Medical Science*. 4, 399.

38 Lincoln E M & Sewell E M, 1963. *Tuberculosis in Children*. New York: Mcgraw Hill Book Company Inc.

39 Lorber J, 1958. Intracranial calcification following tuberculous meningitis in children. *American Review of Tuberculosis*. 78, 38–61.

40 Lorber J, 1960. Treatment of tuberculous meningitis. *British Medical Journal*. 1, 1309–12.

41 Mann M D, MacFarlane C M, Verburg C J *et al.*, 1982. The bromide partition test and CSF adenosine deaminase activity in the diagnosis of tuberculous meningitis in children. *South African Medical Journal*. 62, 431–2.

42 Mathuriya S N, Khosla V K & Banerjee A K, 1988. Intradural extramedullary tuberculous spinal granulomas. *Clinical Neurology and Neurosurgery*. 90, 2, 155–8.

43 Mayers M M, Kaufman D M & Miller M H, 1978. Recent cases of intracranial tuberculomas. *Neurology, (Minneapolis)*. 28, 256–60.

44 Miller F J W, 1982. *Tuberculosis in Children*. Edinburgh: Churchill Livingstone.

45 Miller F J W, 1982. Tuberculous arachnoiditis and radiculitis. In: Miller F J W (ed.) *Tuberculosis in Children*. Edinburgh: Churchill Livingstone.

46 Odeku E L & Adeloye A, 1969. Cerebral tuberculomas in Nigerian patients. *Tropical and Geographical Medicine*. 21, 293–304.

47 Parsons M, 1989. The treatment of tuberculous meningitis. *Tubercle*. 70, 79–82.

48 Parsons M, 1988. *Tuberculous Meningitis. A Handbook for Clinicians*. 2nd ed. Oxford: Oxford Medical Publications.

49 Perez-Stable E J & Hopewell P C, 1989. Current tuberculosis treatment regimens. *Clinical Chest Medicine*. 10, (3), 323–39.

50 Phuapradit P & Vejjajiva A, 1987. Treatment of tuberculous meningitis: role of short-course chemotherapy. *Quarterly Journal of Medicine*. 62, (239), 249–58.

51 Ramachandran P *et al.*, 1986. Three chemotherapy studies of tuberculous meningitis in children. *Tubercle*. 67, 17–29.

52 Ramamurthi B & Varadarajan M G, 1961. Diagnosis of tuberculomas of the brain. *Journal of Neurosurgery*. 18, 1–7.

53 Ramkissoon A & Coovadia H M, 1988. Chloride levels in meningitis. *South African Medical Journal*. 73, 522–3.

54 Ramkissoon A, Coovadia Y M & Coovadia H M, 1988. A competition ELISA for the detection of mycobacterial antigen in tuberculous exudates. *Tubercle*. 69, 209–12.

55 Rich A R & McCordock H A, 1933. The pathogenesis of tuberculous meningitis. *Bulletin of the Johns Hopkins Hospital*. 52, 5–37.

56 Rossi L N & Duzioni N, 1985. Intracranial tuberculomas in a child: regression on the CT scan under conservative therapy. *Neuropediatrics*. 16, 228–30.

57 Schoeman J F *et al.*, 1985. Intracranial pressure monitoring in tuberculous meningitis. Clinical and computerized tomographic correlation. *Developmental Medicine and Child Neurology*. 27, 644–54.

58 Sibley W A & O'Brien J L, 1956. Intracranial tuberculomas: A review of clinical features and treatment. *Neurology (Minneapolis)*. 6, 156–65.

59 Smith D F, Smith F W, & Douglas J G, 1989. Tuberculous polyradiculopathy: The value of magnetic resonance imaging of the neck. *Tubercle*. 70, 213–6.

60 Smith M H D, 1989. Tuberculosis in children and adolescents. *Clinical Chest Medicine*. 10 (3), 381–95.

61 Stead W W, 1967. Pathogenesis of the sporadic case of tuberculosis. *New England Journal of Medicine.* 277, 1008–12.

62 Talamas O, Del Brutto O H & Garcia-Ramos G, 1989. Brainstem tuberculoma. An analysis of 11 patients. *Archives of Neurology.* 46, 529–35.

63 Teoh R, Humphries M J, & O'Mahoney G, 1987. Symptomatic intracranial tuberculomas developing during treatment of tuberculosis: a report of 10 patients and a review of the literature. *Quarterly Journal of Medicine.* 1987, 63, 449–60.

64 Tyler B, Bennett H & Kim J, 1983. Intracranial tuberculomas in a child: computed tomographic scan diagnosis and non surgical management. *Pediatrics.* 71, 952–4.

65 Udani P M, Parekh U C & Dastur D K, 1971. Neurological and related syndromes in CNS tuberculosis. *Journal of Neurological Science.* 14, 341–57.

66 Visudhiphan P & Chiemchanya S, 1979. Hydrocephalus in TBM in children. Treatment with acetazolamide and repeated lumbar puncture. *Journal of Pediatrics.* 95, (4), 657–60.

67 Visudhiphan P & Chiemchanya S, 1989. Tuberculous meningitis in children: Treatment with isoniazid and rifampicin for twelve months. *Journal of pediatrics.* 114, 875–9.

68 Wadia N H, 1973. Radiculomyelopathy associated with spinal meningitis. In: Spillane, J D (ed). *Tropical Neurology.* Oxford: Oxford University Press.

69 Wadia N H & Dastur D K, 1969. Spinal meningitis with radiculomyelopathy. Pathology and pathogenesis. *Journal of the Neurological Sciences.* 8, 261–97.

70 Welchman J M, 1979. Computerized tomography of intracranial tuberculomata. *Clinical Radiology.* 30, 567–73.

71 Whitener D R, 1978. Tuberculous brain abscess. Report of a case and review of literature. *Archives of Neurology.* 35, 148–55.

72 Williams M & Smith H V, 1954. Mental disturbance in tuberculous meningitis. *Journal of Neurology and Neurological Psychiatry.* 17, 173–82.

CHAPTER 10

Tuberculosis of bones and joints

T L Sarkin

Locomotor manifestations of tuberculosis are found predominantly in the bones, joints and the spine. However, tuberculosis of *bone*, which is not close to or within the capsule of a synovial joint, is not common. Involvement of the *joints* is the most common skeletal manifestation of a tuberculous infection. *Spinal* tuberculosis,[1] or Pott's disease, with it's grave complication, Pott's paraplegia, is a disease which is so serious and so different from the other tuberculoses that it will be considered separately.

TUBERCULOSIS OF BONES

This form of tuberculosis is uncommon, but when it does occur, it involves the sternum, the short bones of the hands and feet (such as the metacarpals, the metatarsals, and the phalanges) and, (on rare occasions) the shafts of the long bones such as the radius and ulna, or a rib. The skull, apart from the mastoid, is rarely involved.

Clinical features

The possibility of a tuberculous infection should be considered in any unusual bone swelling or erosion. There is often some pyrexia present; the ESR is raised and the leucocyte count is essentially normal. The Mantoux test is nearly always positive. Aspiration of pus or biopsy is essential if a positive tissue diagnosis and organism identification is to be obtained. Characteristic radiological findings are rare; factioun and pseudo-cyst formation; periosteal reaction is uncommon but may however be seen in the bones of the heads and feet.

Treatment

These days bedrest is only necessary if there is widespread infection, or it is likely that there will be imminent spread to a joint. Selection of the correct anti-tuberculous regimen is essential.

TUBERCULOSIS OF JOINTS

'Acute' and 'chronic' arthritis

Twenty years ago joint infections were still being divided into 'acute' and 'chronic' forms, according to tradition. An 'acute' arthritis was synonymous with a pyogenic infection, while a chronic arthritis usually indicated a tuberculous cause.

This division was further emphasized by differences in management as well as by the results of treatment. Pyogenic infections were traditionally managed in general hospitals by standard surgical principles, which included joint drainage. If the treatment was early enough, the outcome of pyogenic infections was often a functionally good joint.

Tuberculous infections, on the other hand, did not heal well. Joint tuberculosis was traditionally treated in a sanatorium by long periods (often years) of immobilization. Joint drainage was not performed for fear of secondary infection and sinus formation, and in a tuberculous joint infection the loss of function was accepted as inevitable. Treatment was aimed at the best possible result — a stiff, ankylosed joint in a functional position.

Today, with successful drug therapy in the treatment of tuberculosis, these differences have largely disappeared and the principles of treatment for all joint infections are now essentially similar. The difference in clinical presentations of pyogenic and tuberculous joint infections is seldom clear-cut. A pyogenic arthritis with organisms of low-virulence can closely resemble a tuberculous infection, while a tuberculous arthritis can have a relatively acute and rapid course. Therefore, the terms 'acute' and 'chronic', as applied to joint infections, are no longer as useful as they used to be. It follows that the clinical suspicion of the underlying organism in a joint infection is no longer an acceptable basis on which to plan therapy. Every attempt must be made to identify positively the causative organism in an infective arthritis, and until this has been achieved the clinician must maintain an open mind.

Pathology

Mycobacterium tuberculosis may, in theory, reach the joint by four possible routes. These are: continuity; contiguity; blood; and the lymphatics.[2]

- *Continuity* of infection occurs when a primary osteitis of the femoral neck, which is intra-articular in a child, spreads to involve the hip joint. This is the most common route.
- *Contiguity* of infection may occur with a penetrating wound, a surgical incision or an injection into a joint. This is seldom tuberculous in origin, being much more commonly due to *Staphylococcus aureus*.

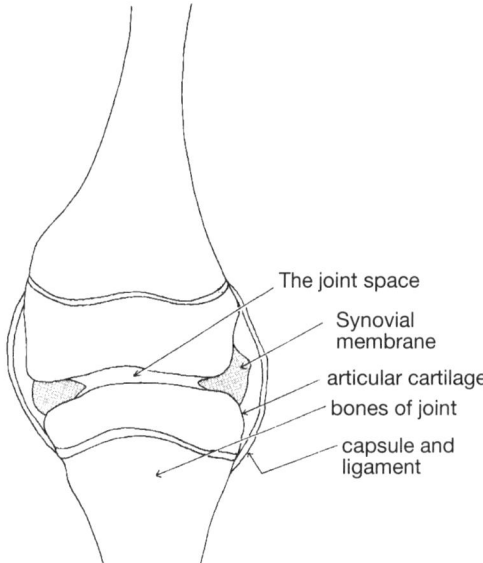

Figure 10.1. Sites of pathology in tuberculous infection of a joint.

The joint space
Synovial membrane
articular cartilage
bones of joint
capsule and ligament

- *Blood*-borne infection of a joint occurs in association with a bacteraemia or a septicaemia. In South Africa co-existent lung or bowel infection is rare.
- *Lymphatic* dissemination may occasionally occur by, for example, the spread of organisms from the mesenteric glands to the spine.

Once the organism becomes established in the joint, the pathological changes which occur may be considered as occurring in the following five 'areas' (see Figure 10.1):

- *the joint space*. At first a clear sticky exudate collects, which rapidly becomes thick, opaque and purulent;
- *the synovial membrane*. This becomes hyperaemic and swollen and forms granulation tissue which spreads over the articular surfaces, causing them to erode. Fibrosis takes place when healing occurs, leading to joint stiffness (fibrous ankylosis). Later, ossification leads to joint fusion (bony ankylosis);
- *the articular cartilage*. The articular cartilage loses its hard glass-like texture to become soft, yellow and fibrillar. Small fragments are dislodged into the joint where they contribute to the pus, leaving bare haemorrhagic bone;
- *the bones of the joint*. Osteoporosis occurs in the early stages as a result of hyperaemia and disuse. Later, direct bone infection and erosion take place as the cartilage is eroded;
- *the soft tissues, capsule and ligaments*. These become oedematous and lax, allowing the joint to subluxate and dislocate. The enlarging collection of pus in the joint bursts through the capsule into the surrounding soft tissues to form a cold abscess, and eventually discharges through the skin as a sinus from a dislocated and destroyed joint.

Clinical features

The clinical features depend on the pathological processes noted above. The most characteristic *symptom* in a joint infection is joint pain which is made worse by any attempt to move the joint. In low grade infections such as tuberculosis, some degree of movement may be tolerated. 'Night cries' are a characteristic feature of joint tuberculosis — the joint moves causing pain whenever the child relaxes during sleep, causing the child to cry. The child awakens and immobilizes the joint, but the cycle repeats itself as the child falls asleep again.

The patient may be of any age, but tuberculous infections are more common in children, and especially those from a poor socio-economic background. The general condition of a patient with a tuberculous arthritis depends on the dynamic interaction between the organism and the relative immunity of the patient, and can vary from very few clinical manifestations to signs of toxaemia, malaise, pyrexia and anaemia.

In the early stages, the joint is noted on *inspection* and *palpation* to be held flexed in the most comfortable position. Later, sinuses may be present and the joint may be drawn into a more severe deformity by reflex muscle spasms. At more advanced stages, subluxation and dislocation may be present.

Both the active and passive *movements* of a joint are characteristically reduced in all directions.

Measurement of the lower limb is useful. When the hip is involved, examination may reveal an 'apparent' shortening early in the infection as a result of the adduction deformity which develops. Later, 'true' shortening may also be present because of bone erosion or joint dislocation.

Investigations

The most useful investigations are blood tests, joint aspiration, radiograph, Mantoux test, and biopsies.

Blood tests

The ESR is raised in a patient with tuberculous joint infection.

Aspiration of the joint fluid

This procedure together with examination of the joint fluid is important. Macroscopically the fluid is seen to be thick, yellow and sticky, while microscopically the

organisms can rarely be identified on direct smear. However, they can more commonly be identified on culture.

Radiographs

Radiographs of tuberculous joint infections may initially show no abnormality. However, osteoporosis soon develops, as evidenced by a pale washed out appearance of the bone. This is followed by a loss of muscle planes. The joint outline becomes obscured and obvious bone erosions are seen. Later, if the infection is allowed to progress, subluxation and dislocation of the joint take place.

Mantoux test

If the test is negative, tuberculosis is unlikely, unless the patient is immunologically suppressed as may occur after measles etc.

Biopsy

If organisms are not cultured on aspiration, a synovial biopsy may be necessary to establish the diagnosis.

Treatment

Treatment may be considered under a number of headings.

General treatment and antibiotics

Essential to the management of a tuberculous joint infection is the general care of the patient. Bedrest is advisable and an antituberculous drug regimen must be instituted.

Joint immobilization and prevention of deformity

The infected joint must be immobilized and splinted in its 'position of optimum fixation', which is the position in which the joint, if it should become soundly ankylosed, is at its greatest efficiency. Immobilization is also an important part of the treatment of the inflammatory process itself. Splintage also prevents joint deformity which may result from the reflex muscle spasm which occurs with joint erosion. The method of splintage depends both on the joint involved and on the final anticipated function of the joint itself.

If there is a reasonable expectation that the infection will be controlled before significant joint destruction has occurred, immobilization with traction is advisable. By preventing contact between the apposing joint surfaces, the likelihood of ankylosis and erosion are reduced. In the lower limb, combined traction and immobilization are most satisfactorily provided by a Thomas splint with light skin traction.

If, on the other hand, joint destruction is anticipated, a solid bony ankylosis in the optimum position of function should be aimed at. This requires contact between the joint surfaces, and traction should then not be applied, as this delays bone fusion by separating the apposing joint surfaces.

Drainage

Aspiration is an essential step in the management of any joint infection. Its value is both in obtaining a sample of synovial fluid for the positive identification of the infecting organisms and their sensitivity, and in providing drainage of the joint to reduce tension, thereby promoting local blood circulation.

The aspiration should always be as complete as possible and should be repeated as often as is necessary to keep the joint empty. Open drainage of the joint is sometimes indicated under cover of an established anti-tuberculous regimen.

In the hip joint of infants, open drainage is more effective than aspiration in reducing joint tension, and is therefore nearly always indicated. It is performed as follows: the joint is opened through a short anterior incision and a segment of capsule removed to ensure continuing drainage. The joint is washed out and a drain inserted down to the capsule. If the infection is severe, drainage will be inadequate unless the drain is inserted into the joint. The eventual functional result is, however, likely to be worse.

Rehabilitation to activity

After the infection has become quiescent, as judged by the disappearance of all signs of an effusion or local tenderness, and if the joint surfaces have not been significantly eroded so that a functioning joint can be anticipated, a staged and controlled rehabilitation programme may be commenced.

The rigid immobilization of the joint should be discontinued and gentle active exercises commenced. If, after a week, this causes no exacerbation of local symptoms or signs, limited weightbearing is commenced and activity gradually increased. If, at any stage, symptoms or signs of activity re-appear, the programme is slowed or halted until the joint is again quiescent. Rehabilitation is then allowed to proceed once again, but more cautiously.

Surgical reconstruction

There are three surgical procedures which, for different indications, may be required after a joint infection.

• An *osteotomy* is the simplest method of correcting a fixed joint deformity.
• An *arthrodesis* of the joint is indicated for an unsound ankylosis which is painful; or because of the probability that a focus of residual infection remains within the fibrous tissue of the joint, and this may flare up and become active in the future. The arthrodesis may, at the same time, be used to correct any fixed deformity which is present.
• A *joint replacement* has recently been suggested in very special circumstances such as: (a) where both hips have been destroyed by infection and are ankylosed; (b) where sufficient time has elapsed, usually many years; and (c) where no evidence of any active infection can be detected either clinically or on full laboratory investigation.

DIFFERENCES BETWEEN ADULTS AND CHILDREN WITH BONE AND JOINT TUBERCULOSIS

Bone and joint tuberculosis in children and adults differ in three main ways.

Firstly the differences between 'human' and 'bovine' bacilli on which so much emphasis was placed in the earlier days of the management of bone and joint tuberculosis have largely disappeared. These organisms were of similar appearance, but exhibited differences in both culture and animal inoculation. Traditionally the majority of cases of infection in children under 10 years of age were due to 'bovine' organisms, while adults were nearly always infected with 'human' organisms. This emphasis, however, has largely vanished, and with better inoculation and care of cattle and milk herds, little emphasis is now placed on this difference.

A second difference in tuberculous infection of children and adults was that in young children the 'bovine' bacilli often gained entrance to the body through the alimentary tract. In adults, infection usually occurred as a result of droplet inhalation of *Mycobacterium tuberculosis.* Traumatic implantation, by a needle or a surgical incision, may occur in both children and adults, but is today very rare in both.

Thirdly, children are much more responsive to treatment than are adults. Even in cases of severe spinal tuberculosis with cord compression, children will nearly always respond successfully to non-surgical anti-tuberculous treatment. Unfortunately, this is not the case in adults, in whom, even with surgical decompression of spinal cord compression, the prognosis is much worse than in children. This is true for all forms of bone and joint tuberculosis.

INDIVIDUAL JOINT INVOLVEMENT

Of the individual joints affected by tuberculosis, the spinal joints, (especially those in the thoracic region) are the most commonly

Table 10.1
Incidence of individual joint involvement

FREQUENCY OF INVOLVEMENT*		
Spine	48	%
Hip	29	%
Knee	12	%
Elbow	8	%
Ankle		2,5%
Shoulder		0,4%
Other		0,1%
Total	100	%

* As noted at the King Edward VIII Hospital, Durban

involved, the other large joints in the body having a decreasing incidence of involvement. The relative incidence of the large joints involved in the body is well illustrated in Table 10.1, which is taken from a very large series of unpublished cases recorded at King Edward VIII Hospital in Durban.

Hip

The hip is affected by tuberculosis more often than any other single joint outside the spine. In children, the most common complaint is a limp, although, in an early case, this may disappear after rest. In adults, there is pain which is often referred to the thigh or knee.

Examination reveals a positive Thomas Hip Flexion Test and limitation of the extremes of all movements, even in the early phase.

A radiograph of the pelvis and both hips usually reveals the diagnosis. Widespread local osteoporosis, even in the early case, is usually present around the affected hip by the time the patient presents for treatment. Later, localized erosions will occur with a fading and fuzziness of bone outline. The radiograph must always include an anteroposterior view of both hips for comparison, and if doubt still persists, a series of radiographs taken at intervals of a few weeks will usually establish the diagnosis.

The differential diagnosis usually includes sprains or Perthes' disease. A sprain should recover fully after 7 to 10 days rest in bed. Perthes' disease characteristically has minimal physical signs, but there are gross and obvious radiological changes which are usually present even on first presentation. These changes include:

- flattening of the femoral head;
- widening of the joint space;
- fragmentation of the femoral head;
- widening of the femoral neck.

Differentiation between tuberculosis and Perthes' disease of the hip

There are usually overt clinical signs in tuberculosis, including very marked limitation of joint movement. Radiographs of the joint in tuberculosis of the hip (certainly in the early presenting case) are, on the other hand, virtually normal except for

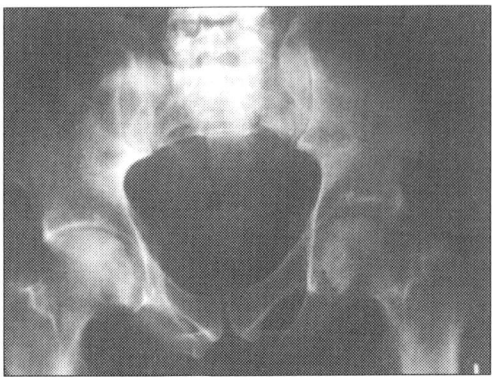

Figure 10.2. An early tuberculous infection of the left hip. Note the early osteoporosis of the left hip and slight area of erosion of the femoral head, but not much else. In tuberculosis the x-ray features are far less than the clinical signs would suggest.

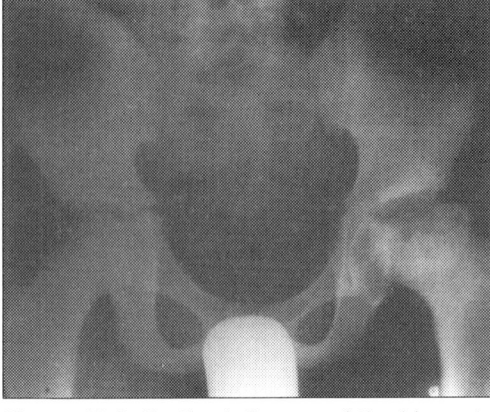

Figure 10.3. Perthes' disease of the hip: note the flattening of the femoral head; the widening of the hip joint space; the fragmentation of the femoral head; the widening of the femoral neck. In Perthes' disease the x-ray signs are gross, obvious and much exceed the clinical findings.

generalized osteoporosis around the joint (Figure 10.2).

In Perthes' disease the emphasis is exactly the opposite. There are usually obvious, gross and marked radiological signs as listed above (Figure 10.3), but clinically the hip movements are nearly always minimally limited, and there is only a minimal limp on walking (Figure 10.3).

In tuberculosis bed rest and traction, to keep the affected joint surfaces apart and to prevent deformity, are helpful. This is especially useful during the early stages of the disease when a functional joint is still achievable. A full anti-tuberculous regime by drugs for 18 months is necessary.

Knee

In the early stages of tuberculosis of the knee, a purely synovial infection without bone involvement may supervene, especially in children. Eventually, unless treatment is instituted, bone involvement and erosion occur.

In the knee onset tends to be insidious, with loss of normal function, swelling and reduced movement.

Radiographs should always be taken of both knees on the same antero-posterior radiograph plate with the same exposure (to compare bone density). Generalized

osteoporosis and loss of bone outline of the joint are the earliest features. Treatment is standard, and similar to the management of tuberculosis of the hip or spine.

Wrist

Tuberculosis of the wrist occurs almost solely in adults. Clinically and radiologically, the infection closely resembles rheumatoid arthritis, but whereas the pathology in rheumatoid arthritis is often bilaterally symmetrical, it is rarely so in tuberculosis.

Ankle, shoulder and elbow

Any of these joints may be involved. The clinical features and radiological findings are similar to the more commonly affected joints, such as the hip and knee, and treatment is similar.

Spinal tuberculosis

Tuberculosis of the spine may occur at any age. The dorsal and lumbar regions are most commonly involved, while tuberculosis of the cervical spine is less common.

Pathogenesis

Usually, as a result of a bacteraemia, *Mycobacterium tuberculosis* organisms are seeded out into the body of a vertebra

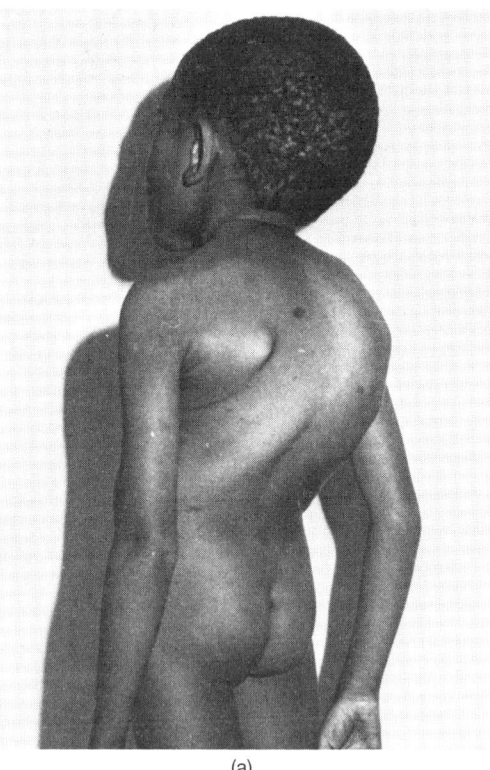
(a)

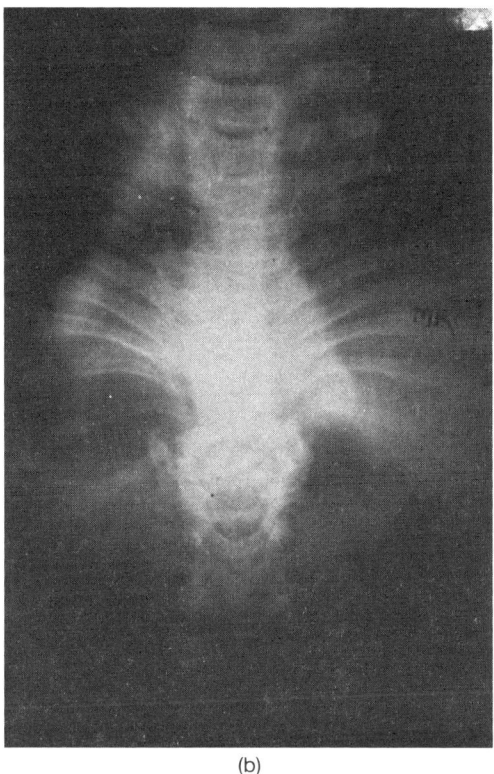
(b)

Figure 10.4. Clinical **(a)**, and radiological **(b)** features of a typical tuberculous infection of the thoracic spine. A gibbus is clearly seen. The tuberculous infection nearly always affects two adjacent vertebrae. As the bones of the vertebrae soften, the disc 'collapses' into the vertebrae, so that 'narrowing' of the disc space is seen on radiographs of the spine. Tuberculous pus forms a 'cold' abscess. This cold abscess may produce pressure on the spinal cord causing a 'Potts' paraplegia' of the early-onset type, or track into the psoas muscle or retropharyngeal space, forming abscesses at these sites.

(Figure 10.4). Less commonly the spread is from abdominal para-aortic lymph glands via the lymphatics to the vertebral body.

The infection typically affects the bodies of two adjacent vertebrae. As bone destruction, softening and erosion occur, so the intervening disc sinks into the bodies so that, on radiograph, a decreasing disc space becomes apparent. As further destruction of the vertebrae progresses, the vertebral bodies become compressed and a kyphosis, known as a 'gibbus', develops. A tuberculous cold abscess then collects.

The cold abscess can spread in various directions. It can compress the spinal cord and result in paraplegia (Pott's paraplegia), or it can spread along the sheath of the psoas muscle to produce a 'psoas abscess'.

In the cervical region a cold abscess can present as a retropharyngeal abscess.

Clinical features

In addition to evidence of poor general health, low-grade pyrexia, raised ESR, and positive Mantoux, patients with spinal tuberculosis show three characteristic local features: pain, limitation of movement and deformity (Figure 10.5). The prominence of these features varies, however, depending on which region of the spine is affected.

In those areas of the spine where there is normally a free range of movement, as in the cervical and lumbar regions, pain and limitation of movement are prominent. The patient resists turning the head or bending forward at the waist, and does so slowly

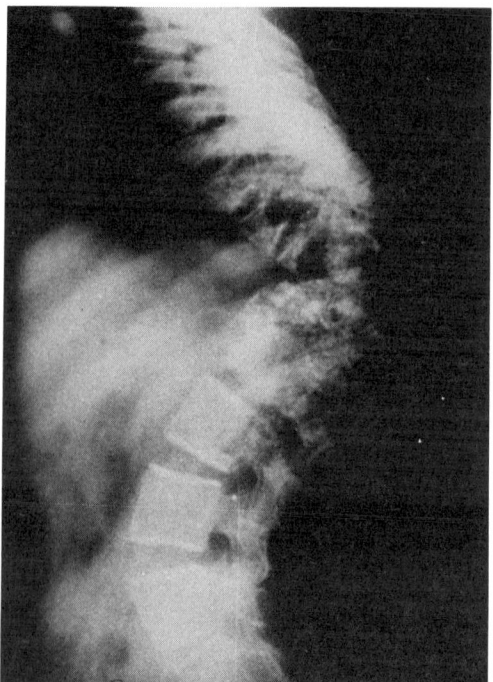

Figure 10.5. An old healed tuberculous infection of the spine with gross bony collapse and gibbus formation. Paraplegia at this stage is due either to vascular changes or bone pressure on the spinal cord. This is 'late' onset paraplegia. The prognosis is poor and surgical decompression is usually unsuccessful.

and stiffly, keeping the painful area in one piece. Deformity in these areas is not a prominent feature, the bone destruction being masked by 'adaptation' of the joints.

On the other hand, in the thoracic spine, where there is normally very little, if any, movement, deformity (in the form of a 'gibbus') is an early and prominent feature, while pain and limitation of movement are clinically much less obvious.

These features are summarized in Table 10.2.

Radiographic features

The classical radiological features of spinal tuberculosis are as follows:

- narrowing of the disc space is often the earliest sign. Later the disc space disappears and the vertebral bodies fuse;
- 'two body disease' of adjacent vertebrae is a characteristic feature of infection. Osteoporosis occurs early. Later, erosion and wedge compression of the bodies is seen;
- paravertebral soft tissue swelling due to cold abscess is seen especially clearly in the thoracic region.

Biopsy

Where facilities are available, it is advisable to establish the diagnosis with certainty by performing a needle biopsy under general anaesthesia with x-ray control. The bone core and pus which is aspirated should be examined histologically and microbiologically (stain and culture).

Treatment

The treatment of spinal tuberculosis includes a combination of rest, good nutrition, anti-tuberculous chemotherapy, and a splint in the form of a back support (which is not always used, however).

In the more radical management of spinal tuberculosis that is practised in some countries, the accepted principles of surgical drainage are applied.[3] General treatment, anti-tuberculous therapy and local rest are employed as discussed, but in addition early surgery is performed in the active stages of the infection to treat and halt the progress of the disease. Where pus is present, it is drained, and where sequestra are present, they are removed. Early fusion is carried out to prevent deformity and to hasten healing.

Table 10.2
Features of spinal tuberculosis

	CERVICAL SPINE	THORACIC SPINE	LUMBAR SPINE
Pain	Prominent	—	Prominent
Deformity	—	Prominent	—
Limitation of movement	Prominent	—	Prominent

Although tuberculous disease of the spine can undoubtedly be controlled by using adequate anti-tuberculous chemotherapy alone, it seems that, if the facilities exist, the final spinal deformity will be less severe if early radical surgery is practised.[4] The morbidity of surgery is also a factor to be considered if such interventions are made. However, this whole field is still somewhat controversial. Surgery has little place in most underdeveloped environments where the disease is most commonly seen and resources are scarce.[5]

The management of spinal tuberculosis with paraplegia (Pott's paraplegia)

Paraplegia, resulting from vertebral compression, is a complication of spinal tuberculosis. Typical features of upper motor neurone weakness occur with increased muscle tone, brisk reflexes, muscle clonus, extensor plantar responses, and hypoaesthesia below a sensory level. Loss of bladder control is common. Two forms of Pott's paraplegia are commonly described.

Early onset paraplegia occurs during the active stage of infection. The cord compression is then due to pus and sequestra, and the majority recover. In children, especially, treatment by anti-tuberculous chemotherapy is usually all that is required, and recovery is rapid. In all adults, and in children where recovery is delayed, or if the paraplegia becomes complete, surgical decompression is advisable.

Late onset paraplegia occurs many years after healing of the infection has occurred (Figure 10.5). The spinal cord compression is then either due to an increasing bony deformity (as a result of fibrous 'sagging' or osteoporosis), or it is due to vascular insufficiency of the cord. The prognosis in late onset paraplegia is generally worse than if the onset had been early.

All cases of paraplegia due to spinal tuberculosis should be actively investigated and treated. Many so-called late onset paraplegias are really due to reactivation of the disease; even late bony compression of the cord can sometimes be successfully decompressed.

A myelogram and computerized scan are indicated in all cases. Operative decompression should always be attempted if a block exists, even in late onset paraplegia.

THE OVERALL MANAGEMENT OF LOCOMOTOR TUBERCULOSIS

Although there is little absolute evidence of the extra value of surgery over conservative treatment in the modern management of tuberculosis of the bones, joints and tendons, there are various facts that have emerged from wide-ranging surveys and reports.

Open surgical drainage of a Pott's paraplegia

There is an absolute indication for open surgical drainage of a Pott's paraplegia in an adult. In these cases, if trained personnel are available and facilities of the hospital are adequate, a transthoracic decompression of the spine allows the best approach. In this procedure a rib is resected on the left side of the chest, and an extra-pleural approach made to the spine. The cold abscess is drained; any sequestra are removed, and the excised rib is used to bone graft the defect and act as a support. Visualization of the pathology is excellent, but training and sophistication of surgery are needed. This clears the cord compression.

Posterior costo-transversectomy

Where transthoracic surgery is inadvisable (due to inadequate surgical experience, poor theatre facilities or poor ICU facilities) a posterior costo-transversectomy allows simple decompression of a fluid cold abscess. In this procedure an approach is made posteriorly. Since a marked 'gibbus' is often present, the affected vertebra is thrown into prominence. A section of rib, with an attached piece of transverse process, is resected and the fluid cold abscess sucked out. The approach does not allow as excellent a clearance of the bone disease, but it is a relatively simple, fast and safe procedure where neither the surgeon's training nor the theatre need be sophisticated.

Non-surgical treatment of bone and joint tuberculosis

Where surgical facilities are not ideal, or where a large number of cases prevents widespread introduction of surgical techniques, conservative non-surgical treatment of bone and joint tuberculosis is, in general quite satisfactory. Anti-tuberculous drugs should be continued for at least 18 months.

Bedrest

Although bedrest is advantageous in the treatment of tuberculosis, it is not cost-effective (from a public health point of view) to achieve this by building tuberculosis hospitals. The money is better spent on education, better nutrition of the whole population, home-based care and use of rapidly effective drugs such as rifampicin.

REFERENCES

1 Editorial, 1974. Tuberculosis of the spine. *British Medical Journal.* 4, 613–4.
2 Girdlestone G R & Somerville E W, 1952. *Tuberculosis of Bone and Joint.* 2nd ed. Oxford: Oxford University Press.
3 Medical Research Council Working Party on Tuberculosis of the Spine, 1973. First report — a controlled trial of ambulant out-patient treatment and in-patient rest in bed in the management of tuberculosis of the spine. *Journal of Bone and Joint Surgery.* 55B (4), 678–97.
4 Medical Research Council Working Party on Tuberculosis of the Spine, 1978. Sixth report — five-year assessment of controlled trials of ambulatory treatment, debridement and anterior spinal fusion in the management of tuberculosis of the spine. *Journal of Bone and Joint Surgery.* 60B (2), 163–77.
5 Tuli S M, 1975. Results of treatment of spinal tuberculosis by 'middle-path' regime. *Journal of Bone and Joint Surgery.* 57B (1), 13–23.

CHAPTER 11

Tuberculosis, workers and occupations in South Africa

U G Lalloo and J T Mets

INTRODUCTION

Pulmonary tuberculosis (PTB) is the most common non-occupational lung disease in South African industry, and there are three likely explanations for this:

- the high background incidence of tuberculosis in South Africa;
- the predominantly poor socio-economic living conditions of the majority of the work force, about 65 per cent of whom are black; and
- adverse working conditions such as excessive exposure to dust, extremes of temperature, shift work, long hours away from home, and other stresses which predispose to the development and spread of tuberculosis.

Tuberculous disease in workers, with its attendant morbidity and loss of time from work, has a negative impact on industry. Industry in turn has a potentially critical role to play in the strategies of control, which can also contribute to the social upliftment of deprived communities by providing occupational health services and suitable employment conditions. In general, information on tuberculosis in industry in South Africa and on the risk of developing it in different occupational groups, including health workers, is scanty. Considerably more data on the association with silica exposure in the mining industry are available. The relationship of silicosis with tuberculosis is covered in a separate chapter. Tuberculosis among the work force, both occupational and work-related, its impact on workers and industry, and methods of management and control, are the subject of this chapter.

HISTORICAL PERSPECTIVES

The association of silicosis and tuberculosis was recognized by Agricola as early as the sixteenth century in miners in the Carpathian mountains.

Thackrah (1795–1833), a physician who practised general and occupational medicine in England and who himself died of tuberculosis at the age of 37, observed a high prevalence of pulmonary consumption in miners of sandstone, dry grinders of metal and in tailors.[22]

The history of tuberculosis in industry might have been buried within the history of silicosis were it not for the pioneering work of Dr E L Collis from England who published his seminal observations in 1925.[43] He published the results of a detailed analysis of the Registrar-General's mortality statistics of England for 1891, 1901 and 1911. He found 15 occupational groups (some with a known silica dust hazard) in which mortality for tuberculosis was above the standard rates for all males. During the second half of the nineteenth century Sir John Simon, also of England, had considered the possibility that occupational factors other than dust might be responsible for the development of phthisis. Collis identified barmen, costermongers, dock labourers, messengers and porters as being at the highest risk. He concluded that working conditions might affect tuberculosis incidence in three ways:

- by undermining general resistance to disease (poverty and alcoholism);
- by direct damage to lung tissue (silicosis); and
- by increasing the risk of infection (overcrowding at work).

Table 11.1
Economically active population of South Africa and the
self-governing territories by industry – 1985 *

	REPUBLIC OF SOUTH AFRICA	SELF GOVERNING TERRITORIES
Forestry, fishing agriculture and hunting	1 179 590	133 887
Mining and quarrying	743 065	33 033
Manufacturing	1 379 518	188 332
Electricity, gas and water	92 720	9 528
Construction	556 339	107 130
Commerce, catering and accommodation services	941 876	131 582
Transport and communication	418 156	57 911
Financing, insurance and real estate	339 204	13 488
Community, social and personal services	1 965 040	279 047
Unspecified**	1 076 855	312 794
TOTAL	8 692 363	1 266 730

* Data not available for TBVC States. **See text.
Source: South African Central Statistical Services, Pretoria.

Table 11.2
Distribution of employees over industrial classes (Workmen's Compensation Act)
(1986 report of the Workmen's Compensation Commissioner)

CLASS	INDUSTRY	EMPLOYEES (ALL RACES) x1 000 (%)	PROPORTION WHO ARE BLACK WORKERS
1	Agriculture/forestry	716 (16)	82%
15	Trade and commerce	664 (15)	46%
13	Iron and steel	525 (12)	59%
5	Building/construction	291 (7)	75%
18	Local authorities	284 (6)	69%
7	Textiles	256 (6)	46%
6	Food/drinks/tobacco	246 (5,5)	63%
10	Chemical	183 (4)	61%
17	Transport	152 (3,5)	64%
8	Wood	117 (2,5)	66%
11	Mining * (Acc. Fund)	89 (2)	80%
12	Bricks/tiles/glass	84 (2)	76%
9	Paper/printing	64 (1,5)	36%
11	Leather	42 (1)	36%
3	Fishing	4 (0,1)	16%
	Other	781 (16)	38%
	TOTAL	4 458 (100)	60%

* The total number of employees in mines and quarries was reported to be 756 637 for midyear 1986, of which at least one third came from outside the South African borders.

Donald Hunter[22] regarded pulmonary tuberculosis as a work-related disease in publicans, cellarmen, barmen, wine waiters, brewers and others who had ready access to alcohol and he stated that overcrowding, bad ventilation and lighting, overfatigue and excessive hours of labour all played their part in 'spreading tuberculosis'.

Stewart and Hughes (quoted in Hunter)[22] found that the overall incidence of tuberculosis was three times higher in factories with more than 600 workers than it was in small factories with less than 100 operatives (1949, 1951). They attributed this to overcrowding in the workrooms.

According to Collins,[10] the beginning of the present tuberculosis epidemic in southern Africa is intimately linked with the rapid industrialization that occurred at the beginning of this century after the discovery of gold and other minerals on the Reef. Tuberculosis was imported to this country by white miners who came mainly from Cornwall in England but also from other European countries. The disease spread like wildfire among the native population which was immunologically 'virgin' in relation to tuberculosis. The poor working conditions, particularly underground in the mines, the slum-like living conditions, and the migrant labour system all provided ideal circumstances for the rapid spread of the disease across the country. The epidemic of tuberculosis in South Africa began in the gold mining industry and then spread throughout the country's disadvantaged communities to become a major public health problem. The history of the spread of tuberculosis, poverty and disease during the Industrial Revolution in England over more than a century appears to repeat itself much more rapidly in developing countries in present times.[26] The advent of the AIDS epidemic with its potential for reducing resistance to other diseases threatens to escalate this problem to colossal proportions (see Chapter 6).

POPULATION STATISTICS AND OCCUPATIONAL CATEGORIES

In order to provide a perspective on tuberculosis in industry an overview of population statistics and the distribution of the work force are given in Tables 11.1 and 11.2.

South Africa had been politically divided by the Nationalist government into the Republic, the six self-governing territories and the four so-called independent homelands (TBVC states). The labour force is made up of workers from these artificial divisions and migrant labourers, mainly miners, from the neighbouring countries of Lesotho, Mozambique, Botswana and Zimbabwe. Of the total population within South Africa, 30,9 per cent was economically active in 1985, and 36 per cent in 1988. Blacks had the lowest proportion of economically active persons, the figures being worst for the self-governing territories and the TBVC states. By comparison, 48,2 per cent of the United States population and 47,4 per cent of the United Kingdom population were economically active in 1981. In Malawi the figure was 41,2 per cent in 1977 while it was 47,2 per cent in Ethiopia in 1978.[6] In June 1988 there were 10,7 million economically active persons in South Africa, representing a compound growth rate of 1,9 per cent between 1970 and 1988 compared with 2,17 per cent for the total population (excluding the TBVC states).[8] It is notable that the number of workers in the mining sector dropped by 7,4 per cent from 724 587 in 1985 to 670 671 in 1988. The work force in construction and building fell by 22 per cent while in manufacturing it dropped by only 0,5 per cent. There was an increase in the trade, catering and accommodation sector (by 3,3 per cent) and in transport and communications (by 17 per cent), while in government and civil services and local authorities it decreased by 1,3 per cent.[8]

Table 11.1 shows the distribution of the work force in 1985 over industrial sectors according to the 10 major divisions used in the Standard Industrial Classification of All Economic Activities (SIC) (3rd edition 1981). The category 'unspecified' incorporates activities not adequately defined, unemployed persons and persons not economically active.

According to A P T du Toit, Head of Central Statistical Services (personal communication, 16 March 1987), the estimated labour force in 1985 amounted to about 10 million people, of whom 8,4 million were employed in the formal sector, 0,5 million in the informal sector, and 1,1 million were unemployed.

The urban/non-urban ratio of the black population during the 1985 census was 53:47. Since then urbanization has increased. The percentage of 'employable' people in the age group 15 to 65 years in 1988 was 56,5 per cent for blacks, 63,8 per cent for coloureds, 68,5 per cent for Indians and 65,2 per cent for whites.[17]

By mid-year 1988 there were 1,05 million registered unemployed people of whom 83 per cent were black and 12 per cent were coloured, representing respectively 12,3 per cent and 10,2 per cent of the economically active population estimates for each racial group.[8] It should be stressed that these figures reflect only the registered unemployed — the actual numbers are likely to be higher!

Unemployment should be regarded as a serious health risk, not only for the worker himself, but also for his dependants!

While the data provided by the Central Statistical Services are useful for sketching an overall picture, those reported by the Workmen's Compensation Commissioner are likely to be more accurate in respect of the employees insured under the Workmen's Compensation Act. The latest available report (for 1986) reflects the proportional distribution over industrial categories in a way that is different to the Standard Industrial Classification but is useful for the discussion of health risk in relation to pulmonary tuberculosis.

Table 11.2 shows the distribution of employees over industrial classes ranked in order of numbers employed, as well as the proportion of black employees in each class and of the total number insured. About 60 per cent of these were black.

As socio-economic status and level of labour often correlate with racial group, this is relevant when risks of contracting tuberculosis are considered.

OCCUPATION RELATED DISEASE

The risk of contracting or developing pulmonary tuberculosis at work is not restricted to those employees who are actually exposed to infection with the tubercle bacillus by virtue of their job. Although in the past it was thought that exposure to coal and asbestos dust was associated with an increased risk of PTB the current view is that this is not the case unless silica exposure is present as well.[22] Other adverse factors, which may be grouped under the heading 'working conditions', are in turn influenced by background factors such as prevalence in the community, socio-economic status, living conditions, and life styles. There is a paucity of information on the incidence of tuberculosis in industry other than that in association with silicosis in foundries, brick, tile, and glass factories in South Africa.[36]

The World Health Organization (Technical Report Series No. 714 of 1985) draws a distinction between 'occupational' and 'work-related disease'. 'Occupational tuberculosis' is defined as tuberculous disease contracted in the course of a specific employment and which results from contact with the tubercle bacillus present as an inherent factor in such employment. 'Work-related tuberculosis' would be contracted in the course of employment where the infecting agent is not inherently present. For example, a nurse at a tuberculosis hospital and a farm worker on a farm with infected and contagious cattle are at risk for 'occupational tuberculosis', but a brick worker who works under stressful, poor environmental conditions and who lives at a low socio-economic level might contract 'work-related' pulmonary tuberculosis.

In the case of 'occupational tuberculosis' there is a direct cause-effect relationship between hazard and disease, even if it is influenced by other factors. In work-related tuberculosis a host of factors, including working environment, prevailing conditions in the community, and individual factors are involved.

Occupational tuberculosis

It is well documented[47] that medical laboratory workers, dentists, doctors and nurses in contact with contagious material or patients are at risk of developing tuberculosis and passing the infection on to patients, particularly the immuno-compromised. Veterinarians and people involved in some animal husbandry and abattoirs are also at increased risk.

In 1984 in England and Wales the risk to all National Health Service staff combined was calculated as 14,5 per 100 000 compared with the national incidence of tuberculosis of 12 per 100 000 in the general population in that year.[28] However, medical laboratory staff had been shown to have nine times the risk in 1957 and five times the risk in 1976, while mortuary attendants had seven times the risk in 1984.

The risk to medical personnel in countries like South Africa, where the prevalence in the general population is so much higher, must be much greater. Unpublished data quoted by Kistnasamy and Yach[23] claim an incidence of 470 per 100 000 employees in the Tygerberg Hospital in the Cape in 1985. This is about the same rate as was found, on average, among the industrial worker population they also investigated.

Krarup *et al.* evaluated the role of the chest radiograph in health service employees in the Leicestershire health authority in the United Kingdom.[25] No signs of PTB were found in 1 994 radiographs taken over a two-year period. A chest radiographic survey of 48 radiographers at King Edward VIII Hospital in Durban in March 1990 yielded two cases of active PTB. Although the numbers were small, this represented a very high risk in this category of health workers. Upon review of the two radiographers with active tuberculosis it was discovered that one had had symptoms of weight loss, night sweats and swelling of the cervical lymph nodes for approximately three months prior to the survey, but had not sought medical attention. She had been employed as a radiographer at the hospital for six years. The second radiographer, employed for 15 years at the hospital, admitted to a non-productive cough for three weeks prior to the survey. The risk for tuberculosis in the different categories of employees in the health industry needs further evaluation. The greatest risk to the health worker is the patient with unsuspected tuberculosis, rather than the patient on therapy for tuberculosis.

Pathologists, autopsy room technicians and medical students are at great risk for tuberculosis. Five out of 22 pathologists in the Department of Anatomical Pathology of King Edward VIII Hospital in Durban developed active tuberculosis between 1985 and 1989 (personal communication, Dr K Cooper). This figure represents an alarmingly high risk, especially as none were diagnosed at routine chest radiographic screening. As in the case of the radiographers with tuberculosis this finding militates against the value of radiographic screening (see below).

Another matter of concern is the high rate of non-compliance with tuberculosis control measures by physicians as noted in a recent study from the University of Illinois, Chicago.[21] Graduates from this university were studied regarding their compliance with tuberculosis control measures, such as regular chest radiography, tuberculin skin testing, isoniazid preventive therapy and BCG vaccination. Of the respondents, only 31 per cent had received BCG and only 48 per cent of the unvaccinated individuals had periodic chest radiographs. Only 112 out of the 1 460 tuberculin positive unvaccinated physicians took isoniazid preventive therapy as recommended by the American Thoracic Society. These findings are disturbing both in terms of physician non-compliance, and of the physician's capacity to promote preventive action among their patients. It also raises concern about compliance of health workers with screening procedures.

In South Africa silicosis, tuberculosis, and the combination of the two diseases in workers have qualified for compensation in mines and quarries since 1925.[4]

Under certain conditions, it may be accepted by the Workmen's Compensation Commissioner that active tuberculosis has resulted from an 'accidental' occurrence (such as a health worker having been infected by an 'open' tuberculosis patient), and compensation is then payable under the Workmens' Compensation Act.

In the United Kingdom, the National Insurance Act, Prescribed Diseases

Regulations of 1967 (amended from 1948), allows compensation to a worker who contracts tuberculosis as a result of 'close and frequent contact with a source or sources of tuberculosis infection by reason of employment'. A specification then follows which includes nursing, administration of medicines, laboratory and research work and 'attendance' upon persons suffering from tuberculosis as high risk activities.

The list of prescribed diseases under the Social Security Act of 1975 presently in force in the United Kingdom simply specifies: 'contact with a source of tuberculosis'.

It is imperative that pulmonary tuberculosis be included under the scheduled diseases of the Workmen's Compensation Act in South Africa under a similar prescription, providing cover for health workers at risk.

Work-related tuberculosis

'Multifactorial work-related' diseases (such as pulmonary tuberculosis) are often more common than occupational diseases and therefore deserve appropriate attention by the health service infrastructure, which incorporates occupational health services. This concept of work-relatedness is of substantial importance to health care workers for protecting and promoting the health of workers in any occupation, and is discussed at length in the World Health Organization Technical Report Series No. 714 mentioned above.

Levi[26] observed that: 'if the fit between the worker and his job is bad, if the worker is unable to control his work conditions, if he copes ineffectively and lacks social

Table 11.3
Observed TB incidence in various occupational categories by race

FIRST AUTHOR YEAR (REF)	REGION	OCCUPATIONAL CATEGORIES AND RACE		INCIDENCE RATES /100 000
Cowie 1989[13]	All mines	Black gold miners		500
Meyers 1986[36]	Western Cape	Black foundry workers		3700
Meyers 1985[34]	Western Cape	Black brick workers		1800
London 1987[27]	Boland	Canning workers (a) Coloureds		706 (751)*
		(b) Blacks		1288 (1070)*
Mets 1984[31]	Eastern Cape	Motor manufacturing workers		
		Coloureds and blacks		989 (508)*
Mets 1984[31]	Western Cape	A. All sectors combined		
		Coloureds		496 (334)*
		Blacks		1001 (1393)*
		B. By sector:	Food	770
			Textile	440
			Engineering	400
			Paper/printing	370
			Others	260
Kistnasamy 1987[23]	Western Cape	A. All industries: Asians		438
		Blacks		899
		Coloureds		537
		Whites		19
		B. By sector:	Textile	829 ⎤
			Iron and steel	766 ⎟
			Food and canning	611 ⎟
			Building and construction	521 ⎟ Overall
			Chemical	418 ⎟ 472
			Paper/printing	371 ⎟
			Transport	292 ⎟
			Trade and commerce	229 ⎦

*Incidence in general population of the region during time of study where data were available.

support, potentially pathogenic reactions occur'. He points out that unemployment or underemployment are also health risks of some magnitude but are rarely considered as such.

The potentially aggravating factors which play a role in causing work-related disease are discussed in some detail by Abrams.[1] These are:

- work conditions (environmental hazards, hours of work, excessive physical and psychological stresses);
- host susceptibility (genetic and by virtue of socio-economic factors that influence nutritional status, educational level, cultural aspects and fatigue);
- community conditions (such as environmental pollution, housing, urbanization and industrialization);
- lifestyle behavioural factors such as smoking and alcohol abuse.

It is clear that excessive psychological job stress, malnutrition, socio-economic gradients and destructive lifestyles, together with adverse environmental and work conditions, are all factors which increase the risk of tuberculosis as a work-related disease for certain categories of workers in South Africa.

It would be useful to be able to quantify such risk, e.g. by class or category of industry and by type and level of occupation.

Local studies on tuberculosis in non-mining workers,[23, 27, 31] are summarized in Table 11.3. The results support incidental findings of other studies by Myers *et al.*[34, 36] which were aimed at evaluating general respiratory health in a foundry and in brickworkers in the western Cape area. In 1986 they found a prevalence of past and present tuberculosis of 15 per cent in 107 black workers in a foundry, while 3,7 per cent had active tuberculosis requiring treatment.[36]

In a series of four papers on the respiratory health of brickworkers they reported a 1985 prevalence rate of 9,3 per cent (on radiographic grounds) among 268 mainly migrant black manual brickworkers.[34]

In an earlier study of stevedores exposed to asbestos in the eastern Cape in 1982 they had found a radiographic prevalence rate of past and present tuberculosis of 13,7 per cent.[35] Exposure to asbestos was not associated with tuberculosis in this study.

The study by Mets[31] in Cape Town covered about seven per cent of the work force in the area (24 471 people in 29 enterprises) and investigated *inter alia* the occurrence of active tuberculosis found during 1981 and 1982 among that worker population. For the population surveyed, the incidence rate for black workers was 1 001 per 100 000 per annum, and for coloured workers 496 per 100 000 per annum. These rates were similar to those found by the same author over the period 1971 to 1980 in a population of 4 750 black and coloured, unskilled and semi-skilled workers in a motor manufacturing plant in the eastern Cape, an incidence rate of 989 per 100 000.

London[27] described the incidence rates of notified active tuberculosis in canning workers in the Boland, Paarl area during 1987 (Table 11.3). He found an incidence of 706 per 100 000 for the coloured canning workers of both sexes and of 1 288 per 100 000 for the black workers, adjusted for seasonal employment.

The calculated relative risk ratio for black males was 2,1 compared with the other workers. When compared with the general local rate in Paarl the coloured canning workers showed an overall lower incidence and the black canning workers a higher one. Kistnasamy and Yach[23] found an overall tuberculosis incidence rate of 472 per 100 000 with varying rates in different categories of industry and occupations (from 829 in the textile industry to 229 in trade and commerce).

Rates (per 100 000) differed markedly between racial categories, 899 for black, 537 for coloured, 438 for Indian, and 19 for white workers. For coloured workers the highest rates were found in the building industry (920) followed by the textile industry (804). The highest rates were found in companies which had higher proportions of 'labourers', thus demonstrating the possible influence of socio-economic class (5 and 4 in the Schlemmer and Stopforths categorization).[39] Overall it would appear that tuberculosis prevalence among worker populations in South Africa may vary between about 10 and 15 per cent, and annual incidence rates between 0,5 and 3 per cent.

The Tuberculosis Research Institute has been quoted as stating that there may be under-reporting of up to 50 per cent of actual cases. Denominators for the general population are inaccurate and no age-standardized rates are available. Most of the data refer to adult populations in the age group from 15 to 60 years. However, the available data do give some indication of the potential risk of contracting PTB when employed in a particular occupation and industrial category, but it must be stressed that such 'occupational' influence does not take into account other determining factors, such as socio-economic class *per se*, host susceptibility, community conditions and lifestyles as already discussed above.

Table 11.4 has been drawn up on the basis of the scanty data available to the authors, and shows the estimated incidence rates of tuberculosis for particular industries and rates for general populations in the area. The figures shown under 'Risk Ratio' are no more than crude estimates and are subject to a variety of errors of estimation. It would appear that gold miners, black foundry, brick and canning workers, are at higher risk of contracting tuberculosis than are their counterparts in the community, while workers in the food industry, textile and iron and steel categories are also at a somewhat higher risk. Other categories show a lower incidence and risk ratio when compared with the general population in their area.

It may be concluded that for the foreseeable future one may expect to find between

Table 11.4
Crude risk ratios for tuberculosis by occupational/industrial category for black and coloured workers in South Africa

YEAR	INDUSTRIAL CATEGORY	REGION	TB RATES/ 100 000†	RISK RATIO
1987	Gold miners	S.Tvl	500:(281)*	1,8
		O.F.S	500:(205)*	2,4
1986	Black foundry workers	Cape	3 700:(976)*	3,8
1985	Black brick workers	Cape	1 800:(840)*	2,1
1987	Coloured canning workers	Boland	706:(751)	0,94
	Black canning workers	Boland	1 288:(1 070)	1,2
	Food/canning workers	Cape	611:(681)	0,9
1981	Food industry	Cape	770:(443)**	1,7
	Textile		440:(443)	0,99
1982	Engineering		400:(443)	0,9
	Paper/printing		370:(443)	0,83
1987	Textile	W.Cape	829:(718)***	1,15
	Iron and steel		766:(754)	1,02
	Local authority		643:(790)	0,81
	Food/canning		611:(778)	0,79
	Building/construction		521:(695)	0,75
	Chemical		418:(754)	0,55
	Printing/paper		317:(693)	0,46
	Transport		292:(768)	0,38
	Trade and commerce		229:(717)	0,32
	Overall		472:(609)	0,78

†Rates in brackets are for, as far as possible, comparable groups of the general population in the local area

Sources: * Epidemiological Comments, 1987. 14, 8.
National Health and Population Development
** Medical Officer of Health, Cape Divisional Council annual reports
*** Based on racial distribution data, National Health and Population Development and Workmen's Compensation Commissioner's reports.

one and three cases of active pulmonary tuberculosis per annum for every two hundred black and coloured persons employed as unskilled or semi-skilled labourers, or perhaps even at the skilled level. In addition one would expect to find active cases on pre-employment medical examination, of which a chest x-ray is an essential component.

That would mean an annual case load in the order of about 25 000 for workers insured under the Workmen's Compensation Act and of about 45 000 for the estimated 8,4 million people employed in the formal sector in South Africa.

IMPACT OF TUBERCULOSIS ON WORKERS AND INDUSTRY

During the early decades of this century when tuberculosis was becoming an increasing problem on the mines, it became the policy to send any mine worker who was diagnosed as having PTB home as soon as he was fit enough to travel.[45] In those early years of the century there was no effective cure and there was little hope of recovery. Collins,[10] describing the spread of tuberculosis in South African workers and their communities, shows how the epidemic gained momentum from the industrial revolution which occurred during and after the Second World War, with its attendant urbanization, overcrowding and slum conditions.

Collins also mentions that as far back as 1953, Dormer was treating patients with active tuberculosis at work in South Africa. Ambulant treatment was practised by one of the authors in the late 1950s in Indonesia, where it was shown that the adverse impact on workers and their families was lessened by keeping the patients employed and earning their living. South Africa has features of both developed and developing countries. While health problems may be the cause of unemployment, unemployment may also be a factor in causing health problems such as tuberculosis.

Impact on workers

The most serious and feared impact on workers when they contract PTB is loss of employment. The South African National Tuberculosis Association in June 1985 made a plea to employers not to dismiss a worker on the grounds of tuberculosis alone, stating:

The patient who is diagnosed reasonably early and who is under correct treatment will be rendered non-infectious almost at once. He is usually fit for work, and should be allowed to continue working and earn a wage to support his family, who are obviously at special risk because they were exposed to infection before he was diagnosed.

In some cases it may be necessary to hospitalize the worker-patient for a period of a few weeks. Then sick pay, special grants or, when appropriate, support from the Unemployment Insurance Fund may alleviate the economic loss to the worker. It is vital that workers should be allowed to return to work under supervised treatment as soon as they are fit enough to perform their tasks. As recently as 1982 it was found that nine out of 168 workers (5,4 per cent) had been dismissed solely because they had open tuberculosis.[31] This occurred in firms which were providing health services. The position must be considerably worse elsewhere.

The risk of being dismissed is the most serious problem for the worker-patient who contracts tuberculosis. There is also the social stigma, which varies according to the patient's community and culture and the knowledge or ignorance of family, relatives, friends and other contacts. The social implications may be grave.

Moloantoa[32] discusses not only the loss of job, interference with work, disruption of family life and the practical problems of an economic nature resulting from PTB, but also the expectations, attitudes and traditional beliefs of patients. Unsophisticated systems of beliefs about the attitudes to tuberculosis were also found to prevail in urbanized black populations. Perceived causes of diseases were sorcery (65 per cent), poisoning of food (60 per cent), infidelity (five per cent) and 'inheritance' (20 per cent). These perceptions can affect patients in their social life. Sixty-five per cent of patients interviewed indicated the need to consult a traditional healer for prevention or cure of tuberculosis, often in addition to visiting a clinic, doctor or hospital.

Impact on industry

Dismissing worker patients 'just because they have tuberculosis' would be counter productive. Such a policy results in a loss of trained employees, and requires hiring and training of new labour with a potential loss of production in the interim. Amounts payable as sick pay and special grants, and the indirect costs of unemployment insurance all affect production costs.

However, treating employees who have contracted PTB and who are medically fit while continuing to work would be in the best interest of industry as well as being cost effective.

If a factory employing a work force of 500 and an occupational health nurse to look after them has five cases of lung tuberculosis a year, this would result in a loss of only about 120 workdays, assuming that they would all have to be booked off for a few weeks as being unfit for work. This is negligible compared to the approximately 3 750 days that would be lost through the expected absenteeism of the whole work force at even a low absenteeism rate of three per cent.

It has been noted that workers on closely supervised tuberculosis treatment at a motorcar manufacturing plant in fact showed a better absenteeism record than their non-tuberculosis counterparts: 3,6 workdays lost per person per annum against eight for the latter.

In economic terms the negative impact on industry of treating the expected 45 000 cases per annum in South Africa at the workplace would be slight and the benefits of so doing enormous.

The cost of medicines is borne by the State (estimated as R1 192 per patient for the year 1987 under the Tuberculosis Control Programme)[16] and these are administered by Local Authority clinics as a free service.

MANAGEMENT AND CONTROL OF TUBERCULOSIS AT WORK

Under the title *Controlling Tuberculosis in Africa* published by the World Health Organization magazine *World Health* of January 1982, S J Nkinda stated that: 'case finding plus chemotherapy is the most potent weapon for tuberculosis control'. Mass radiography was once popular but it is not recommended today. Passive case-finding whereby patients with chest symptoms present themselves to health facilities is the approach recommended. For control purposes the main disseminators of infection are those patients with pulmonary tuberculosis whose sputum shows the presence of bacilli. Of these patients 80 per cent are found to have had a persistent cough and the majority of them are discovered as self-reporting patients rather than through active case finding by mass miniature radiography. The essence of control is the early identification of patients, effective and adequate treatment, and follow up of patients and contacts. This requires creating awareness by (health) education, determining high risk populations, developing facilities for diagnosis, treatment, primary and secondary prevention, and for the monitoring of the whole process.

This raises the question of who should be responsible for all this, apart from the State's Department of Health and the medical departments of local authorities. For worker populations the answer of course would be that the responsibility lies with employers who have the health of their work forces at heart, shared by the workers themselves. One of the ways employers could discharge this responsibility is by providing occupational health services at work, with untold benefits to both workers and themselves in addition to the contribution it would make to society through good tuberculosis control. Occupational health services are by their nature prevention-orientated but should, in an underdeveloped country like South Africa, also provide an infrastructure for basic primary and curative health care as part of an integrated health service.

Prevention

Prevention of pulmonary tuberculosis in an adult working population would firstly need to address the known risk factors for endogenous reactivation of dormant infection, widely prevalent if not present in all workers. These have already been discussed.

Secondly, although not all medical authorities agree that adult to adult contact often leads to subsequent tuberculosis disease, prevention would be promoted by early diagnosis of tuberculosis cases and the prompt commencement of chemotherapy. Providing an occupational health service would cover these aspects effectively.

Case finding

Over the years there have been many debates about the merits of the different methods of case finding. 'Active case finding' involves regular chest radiography of all employees (or even a sputum examination) while 'passive case finding' involves waiting for the worker to present him- or herself for examination.

Screening (active case finding)

There now appears to be a reasonable consensus that mass screening of general populations, even when there is a fairly high prevalence of tuberculosis, is not really worthwhile. In the Netherlands in 1981 the yield was only six active cases per 100 000 adult males examined (down from 43 cases in 1961), and this led to general population screening being abandoned in 1983.[2] However, migrant and immigrant labourers (such as those from Spain and Turkey) are regularly subjected to chest radiography.

The United States Center for Diseases Control (United States Department of Health and Human Services) advocates in its Tuberculosis Policy Manual of August 1986 that: 'health departments should identify appropriate groups for screening (e.g. … immigrants from Central and South America, South East Asia etc. …)'.

In 1985, Seager[40] stated that (as reported by the medical officers of health of the larger municipalities in South Africa) the mean case yields for indiscriminate mass radiography was 0,25 per cent, 'not much higher than the national incidence in blacks of 0,23 per cent'. Seager was of the opinion that:

there is no selection in favour of finding cases when screening work seekers and factory employees and it is therefore wrong to screen these as opposed to high risk groups such as the unemployed and hostel residents (3,6 per cent yield) and contacts (4,8 per cent yield).

Myers[33] cogently argued against generalizing Seager's results to work force situations. In Cape Town reported yields for the general population in 1981 varied between 0,2 per cent (Langa) and 0,89 per cent (Guguletu).[31] For pre-employment tests in blacks it was 0,24 per cent (1988) up to 0,7 per cent in some municipal and divisional council clinics in the Cape.

In contrast to these the yield for passive case finding after self-presentation, as reported by Seager, was 7,8 per cent. Myers argued that this high rate may result from the way cases are being detected at present, the emphasis being on passive case finding.

The Department of Health's policy on tuberculosis control allows for selective radiography of 'high risk' groups under certain conditions. Facilities must be available for diagnosis, treatment, follow up, information and education, contact tracing and continuous case finding. The authors suggest that the black and coloured labour force, especially those in socio-economic classes 4 and 5 and selected occupations which are regarded as at high risk, should be screened on a regular basis, over and above programmes of passive case finding. Screening of work seekers as part of a pre-employment examination is also recommended.

This view is supported by the South African Society of Occupational Medicine which published guidelines for the management of PTB in their newsletter No. 10 of May 1986.

Passive case finding

Passive case finding, which is case finding based on the prompt investigation and diagnosis of tuberculosis in people presenting themselves, was shown by Seager[40] to have a mean yield of 7,8 per cent, higher than any other method. Similar findings are reported for industry.

Over a period of seven years, 16 861 pre-employment and routine periodic chest radiographs of a worker population in the

Table 11.5
Summary of medical control guidelines

1. Pre-employment medical examination chest x-ray
   Periodic chest x-rays (high risk groups).

2. Early detection
   Health monitoring (e.g. weight checks)
   High clinical suspicion level
   Awareness of workers, supervisors, and management
   Health education to encourage self-presentation.

3. Diagnosis
   Liaison with clinics/hospitals
   Contact screening.

4. Ambulant treatment
   Supervision (attendance record)
   Support, maintain at work.

5. Follow up after completion of treatment
   Routine chest x-rays (2 to 5 years)
   Clinical (quarterly for two years)
   Check weight regularly
   Support

eastern Cape yielded 52 active tuberculosis cases (0,3 per cent), while 143 new patients (nearly three times as many) were discovered over a period of eight years by passive case finding among the work force of about 5 000 workers. Even more striking is the fact that in Cape Town, occupational health nurses in 1981–2 found a total of 137 cases of PTB among a work force of 24 471, which represented 81 per cent of all the cases diagnosed during the two years. Routine periodic radiography identified only 32 cases (19 per cent).[31]

This resulted from an active programme of passive case finding in which occupational health service staff were encouraged to look for early symptoms and signs in all workers who came to the medical department for any reason at all. Even higher yields might be produced by sustained efforts to educate workers, supervisors and medical staff about the importance of persistent cough, apparent loss of weight, tiredness, feeling unwell, poor appetite, nightsweats, raised body temperature, vague pains in the chest, and haemoptysis.

Contact screening is of great importance. Not only do close family, relatives, and people living in the same house need to be evaluated, but also workers in close daily contact with colleagues with open PTB, particularly when working under crowded conditions. Saunders *et al.*[38] reported that five per cent of the contacts investigated in Soweto were subsequently notified as having PTB. Atwell and Pearson[3] found a reinfection rate of two per cent in spouses of proven contagious partners.

In the workplace the decision regarding which 'contacts' must be screened is determined by the environmental conditions at work of the sentinel case found.

Diagnosis

For adults in countries which have a high prevalence of tuberculosis the tuberculin test is of little value. The diagnosis of pulmonary tuberculosis ultimately rests upon demonstrating the bacillus in secretions, serous fluids or tissues, and sputum by direct smear or culture testing. Chest radiographs alone are often used for diagnostic decisions but should generally serve only as supporting evidence. Histological examination may be used in more sophisticated health centres. For occupational health services there is considerable merit in using a scoring system based on diagnostic criteria such as those advocated by Cowie and Escreet at the Oppenheimer Hospital in Welkom.[15]

Treatment

The current policy of ambulant, so called 'supervised', therapy appears still to be associated with a high default and non-compliance rate. The Cape Divisional and City Councils reported an overall non-compliance rate of between 30 and 40 per cent. Non-compliance is generally defined as being the intake of less than 80 per cent of prescribed doses of chemotherapy, which implies that cure can be effected with a minimum of 80 per cent of doses. Others use a cut-off point of 75 per cent of prescribed doses. Saunders *et al.*[38] found that in Soweto in 1978, (when chemotherapy was still prescribed for more than a year), only 28 per cent of patients actually received a minimum of 80 per cent of doses. Fisher[20] reported that in the Cape area in 1981, when an 'extra-short' course of 25 weeks of chemotherapy was prescribed, 75 per cent of patients received more than 80 per cent of doses while they had been on 'supervised' ambulant treatment.

More favourable compliance rates are noted when patients are treated at work. Escreet *et al.*,[19] reporting in 1984 on a group of 282 patients on the mines (where patients are treated under conditions which are favourable for supervised therapy), noted that 85 per cent of patients were adequately treated.

A penetrating study in 1984 by Bell and Yach[5] on tuberculosis patient compliance in the western Cape, found an overall compliance (defined as having received 75 per cent of the prescribed doses) of 82,5 per cent. The highest compliance rates were found among the full-time employed (up to 89 per cent); the lowest in the unemployed and in blacks. The average compliance for age group 20 to 50 years was about 83,5 per cent and compliance increased with age.

An in-house survey by one of the authors of 200 worker-patients treated at a motorcar manufacturing plant in the 1970s found that 110 of these had defaulted for less than 14 per cent of their treatment days (doses) and 90 others between 14 and 25 per cent. All 200 patients had received at least 75 per cent of the prescribed doses while remaining at work, at a time when one to two years' treatment was still the norm.

In Cape Town, in a favourable setting where there was an occupational health nurse at the workplace[31] he found that on average the attendance rate for treatment was 94 per cent for the 97 patients who had completed treatment and also for another 64 who were still on treatment at the end of the survey. Only two of the 161 patients had taken less than 75 per cent of doses prescribed.

The more favourable rate of compliance with tuberculosis treatment at work appears to be dependent on the motivation of the patient, the supervising medical staff and on the employer, while also being influenced by factors related to the treatment regimes, such as short or long term, intermittent or continuous, their acceptability, side effects, and accessibility.

It may well be that administering rifater (which combines rifampicin, isoniazid and pyrazinamide in one tablet) up to a maximum of five tablets a day, will appreciably improve compliance with ambulant treatment.

In the Cape area rifater was made available by the Regional Director of the Department of National Health and Population Development in January 1988, and was recommended for use in working populations by Cowie and Brink.[14]

Outcome of chemotherapy

It is important to take into account the relapse rate in patients who have completed their treatment. The World Health Organization has reported a relapse rate of between 3 and 10 per cent in developed countries. Atwell and Pearson[3] in 1980 reported a 20–30 per cent relapse rate on the then-standard two years' therapy, but of only two per cent on four-drug therapy. Shennan,[41] in the Transkei, found a relapse rate of 9,2 per cent over a period of 30 months after treatment and expects eight per cent of patients to re-appear with a relapse within three years after their index attack. Collie and Kuestner reported for 1985 and 1986 a relapse rate of about 10 per cent of all treated cases under the Tuberculosis Control Programme in South Africa.[9] Mets found that 27 of the 520 worker patients treated by him at work over a period of seven years (1973–9) relapsed within five years (5,2 per cent), eight during the first two years after completing treatment, 12 during the third and seven during the fourth and fifth years. For most of these, notable factors were excessive usage of alcohol and concomitant malnutrition in addition to the stresses of working life; endogenous reactivation was the most likely mechanism involved.

The AIDS epidemic is predicted to lead to an escalation of the tuberculosis incidence.[11] Active tuberculosis is likely to develop in individuals who are harbouring the tuberculosis bacillus as a result of the suppression of their cell-mediated immunity following infection with the human immunodeficiency virus infection.

Costs of treatment

The cost of drugs used in treatment is seldom more than 16 per cent of the total cost of the services provided. Pearson,[37] discussing the cost of rifampicin in 1980, calculated the individual drug bill for patients treated for a total of 100 days in that year to be R93,74 per person (about R18,75 per month), and concluded that the savings achieved by short-course ambulant treatment using rifampicin (as opposed to long-term regimens involving hospitalization) would not only defray the cost of an outpatient service but would allow an expansion of services such as domiciliary therapy. In 1982 Tibbit[44] discussed the important economic implications of the use of rifampicin containing short-course therapy as advocated by Pearson. He emphasized that drug costs were between 2,4 and 7,25 per cent of the total costs per patient.

Collie and Kuestner[9] estimated that the annual cost per case in the Tuberculosis Control Programme was R414 for clinic cases and R2 818 for hospital cases in 1986.[18] While it is important to be aware of the costs, it must be noted that they are met by the health authorities because tuberculosis treatment is provided free of charge to patients, including treatment administered at work in cooperation with the clinics.

Facilities

Facilities for examining suspected cases, the screening of high risk groups and contacts, and treatment are made available by health authorities. Reliable and sympathetic supervision of the treatment of tuberculosis cases by employers would improve compliance. The provision of health services at work, not only for tuberculosis but also for preventive medicine and primary health care in an integrated service co-operating with the services outside the workplace would certainly improve the effectiveness of the Tuberculosis Control Programme.

The presence of in-house health services in industry varies widely. Cornell[12] reported in 1983 that only 12,9 per cent of all the companies she surveyed in the Cape area provided a health service, while 43 per cent of the larger companies with more than 500 employees did not provide a health service.

Overall, 8,5 per cent employed a full-time nurse (qualified sister), 3,7 per cent a part-time nurse and 11,4 per cent a part-time doctor.

In 1984 Sitas *et al.*[42] found that an 'in-house health service' was provided in the Germiston area by only 11 per cent of all those factories which responded to their questionnaire. These employed at least a part-time nurse (qualified sister) or else full-time nurses, some with a doctor. Again, as expected, larger factories were more likely to provide such a service. The National Centre of Occupational Health Report of Johannesburg and Randburg Industries (No. 17/89 on Occupational Health Services in 1987) showed that 18 per cent (316 factories with 64 129 employees) provided a medical service on the premises by at least a registered part-time nurse or doctor.

A health service survey in the Port Natal and New Germany/Pinetown area undertaken in 1987 by one of the members of the South African Society of Occupational Medicine found that 46 per cent (of 149) factories provided an 'in house' health service.

Based on the results of a survey by Kocks of a total of 233 occupational health services distributed over a wide range of economic activities,[24] the cost of providing a professional in-house service was on average about R10,50 per month per employee in October 1989. These were all staffed by a medical practitioner and a registered nurse.

Medical control and guidelines

A tuberculosis control programme has the long term goal of reducing the incidence of infection, the prevalence of disease and mortality. The workplace is not only the best place to treat a worker patient but also the best place to find him or her if there is an occupational health nurse on site. Here the emphasis lies on reducing the prevalence of disease and its effects by early detection and adequate treatment.

One requirement for these objectives is the awareness that tuberculosis in adults need not be a dangerous disease for the employees themselves and is certainly not a danger for other people in their working environment if the diagnosis is made early and treatment at work is well supervised. Another is that management, health staff and workers must be aware of the potential threat of the disease and be prepared to cope with the problems arising out of this, primarily by preventive measures and early case finding.

CONCLUSION

Pulmonary tuberculosis is perhaps the most common important non-occupational disease to be found in industrial populations in South Africa. Providing in-house occupational health services will not only promote the Tuberculosis Control Programme but also serve workers as well as employers in other ways and contribute to the upliftment of workers, their families and communities.

Such services can be provided in a cost-effective manner and would cater for the needs of high risk groups of workers as far as tuberculosis is concerned. Passive case finding appears to be the most appropriate method for early detection in industry, but it should be supplemented by selective mass screening by means of chest radiography for those worker populations regarded as being high risk groups. The impending AIDS epidemic is expected to lead to an increase in the already high incidence of tuberculosis among the worker population.

Greater awareness and close cooperation between industry (and in particular their occupational health services) and State Health authorities will help to alleviate the problem.

REFERENCES

1 Abrams H K, 1984. Aggravation of lung disease. *Scandinavian Journal of Work Environmental Health.* 10, 487–93.

2 Anon., 1983. Actueel bevolkingsonderzoek op tuberculose kan worden gemist. *Tijdschrift van Sociale Geneeskunde.* 61, 68.

3 Atwell A G & Pearson J O, 1980. Routine outpatient short-course chemotherapy for pulmonary tuberculosis: a radiographic presentation. *South African Medical Journal.* 58, 1041–6.

4 Bachmann O M, 1990. Compensating for occupational lung disease. *South African Medical Journal.* 77, 202–7

5 Bell J & Yach D, 1988. Tuberculosis patient compliance in the western Cape 1984. *South African Medical Journal.* 73, 31–3.

6 Central Statistical Services, 1985. *South African Statistics.* Pretoria: Government Printer.

7 Central Statistical Services, 1987. *R S A Statistics in Brief 1987.* Pretoria: Government Printer.

8 Central Statistical Services, 1989. *South African Labour Statistics 1989* and *R S A Statistics in Brief 1989.* Pretoria: Government Printer.

9 Collie A & Kuestner H G V, 1989. The Tuberculosis Control Programme 1985–6. *South African Medical Journal.* 76, 676–80.

10 Collins T F B, 1982. The history of southern Africa's first tuberculosis epidemic. *South African Medical Journal.* 62, 780–8.

11 Collins T F B, 1989. Tuberculosis in South Africa. *South African Society of Occupational Medicine Newsletter No. 24.* Nov. 1989.

12 Cornell J, 1984. Workplace health services and employment in manufacturing industry in Greater Cape Town. Carnegie conference paper 289. *South African Labour Bulletin.* 9, 42–58.

13 Cowie R L, 1989. The five ages of pulmonary tuberculosis and the S.A. goldminer. *South African Medical Journal.* 76, 566–7.

14 Cowie R L & Brink B A, 1989. Short-course chemotherapy for pulmonary tuberculosis with a rifampicin-isoniazid-pyrazinamide combination tablet. *South African Medical Journal.* 77, 390–1.

15 Cowie R L & Escreet B C, 1980. The diagnosis of pulmonary tuberculosis. *South African Medical Journal.* 57, 75–7.

16 Department of National Health and Population Development, 1988. *Epidemiological Comments. Vol.15, No. 11.* Pretoria: Government Printer.

17 Department of National Health and Population Development, 1989. *Epidemiological Comments. Vol.16, No. 11.* Pretoria: Government Printer.

18 Department of National Health and Population Development, 1990. *Epidemiological Comments. Vol.17, No. 1.* Pretoria: Government Printer.

19 Escreet B C, Langton M E & Cowie R L, 1984. Short-course chemotherapy for silico tuberculosis. *South African Medical Journal.* 66, 327–9.

20 Fisher S A, 1986. Experiences with extra-short course tuberculosis chemotherapy in the Divisional Council of the Cape. *South African Journal of Science.* 82, 393.

21 Geiseler P J, Nelson K E & Crispen R G, 1987. Tuberculosis in physicians, compliance with preventive measures. *American Review of Respiratory Diseases.* 135, 3–9.

22 Hunter D, 1969. *The Diseases of Occupations.* 5th ed. London; English Universities Press.

23 Kistnasamy B & Yach D (in press). Tuberculosis in commerce and industry in a western Cape suburb, South Africa, 1987. *American Journal of Industrial Medicine, 18, 87–93.*

24 Kocks D J, 1988. The cost of occupational health service in South Africa. *South African Society of Occupational Medicine Newsletter No. 22,* May 1988.

25 Krarup K C & Scarisbrick D A, 1989. Control of tuberculosis in health service workers: the role of the chest radiograph. *Journal of the Society for Occupational Medicine.* 39, 128–30.

26 Levi L, 1984. Work, stress and health. *Scandinavian Journal of Work Environmental Health.* 10, 495–500.

27 London L, 1989. Incidence of tuberculosis among canning workers in the Boland. *South African Medical Journal.* 76, 554–7.

28 Lunn J A & Mayho V, 1989. Incidence of pulmonary tuberculosis by occupation in the National Health Service in England and Wales 1980–1984. *Journal of the Society for Occupational Medicine.* 39, 30–2.

29 Meiklejohn A, 1949. Silicosis in potteries. *British Journal of Industrial Medicine.* 6, 230

30 Mets J T, 1980. The diagnosis of pulmonary tuberculosis. *South African Medical Journal.* 57, 669.

31 Mets J T, 1984. TB control and occupational health services. *Curationis.* 37, 19–22.

32 Moloantoa K E M, 1982. Traditional attitudes towards tuberculosis. *South African Medical Journal.* Special issue 'Tuberculosis in the Eighties', 29–31.

33 Myers J E, 1986. Tuberculosis screening in industry. *South African Medical Journal.* 70, 251–2.

34 Myers J E & Cornell J, 1989. Respiratory health of brickworkers in Cape Town, South Africa. *Scandinavian Journal of Work Environmental Health.* 15, 188–94.

35 Myers J E *et al.*, 1985. A respiratory epidemiological study of stevedores intermittently exposed to asbestos in a South African port. *American Journal of Industrial Medicine.* 7, 273–83.

36 Myers J E *et al.*, 1987. A respiratory epidemiological survey of workers in a small South African foundry. *American Journal of Industrial Medicine.* 12, 1–9.

37 Pearson J O, 1980. False economy in tuberculosis treatment. *South African Medical Journal.* 57, 588–9.

38 Saunders L D, Irwig L M, Wilson T D, Kahn A & Groeneveld H, 1984. Tuberculosis management in Soweto. *South African Medical Journal.* 66, 330–3.

39 Schlemmer L & Stopforth P, 1979. *A Guide to the Coding of Occupations in South Africa. Fact Paper No. 4.* Durban: University of Natal Centre for Applied Social Studies.

40 Seager J R, 1986. Is active case-finding an effective TB control measure? *South African Journal of Science.* 82, 389.

41 Shennan D H, 1989. Results from three years' operation of the Transkei Tuberculosis Register. *South African Journal of Epidemiology and Infection.* 4, 33–6.

42 Sitas F, Davies J C A, Kielkowski D and Becklake M R (NCOH Johannesburg), 1986. *South African Society of Occupational Medicine Newsletter No. 11,* August 1986.

43 Stewart A, 1957. Tuberculosis in industry. *Symposium on Tuberculosis, Bristol.* Bristol: J W Arrowsmith Ltd.

44 Tibbit L R, 1982. The economics of short-course therapy for tuberculosis in the Cape Divisional Council area. *South African Medical Journal.* Special issue, 'Tuberculosis in the Eighties', 31-3.

45 Webster D, 1982. A social history of tuberculosis in South Africa. *Medical Students Conference 1982 — 'Consumption in the Land of Plenty — TB in South Africa,* University of Cape Town Medical Students Council.

46 White N, 1982. TB as an occupational illness. *Medical Students Conference 1982 — 'Consumption in the Land of Plenty — TB in South Africa,* University of Cape Town Medical Students Council.

47 World Health Organization, 1986. *Early Detection of Occupational Disease.* Geneva: World Health Organization.

CHAPTER 12

Silicosis and tuberculosis

R L Cowie

INTRODUCTION

Historically, pulmonary tuberculosis has been viewed as being the coup de grâce in men who had acquired silicosis through their work. Since the 'terrible consumption' was first described by Agricola in the sixteenth century, the two diseases have been difficult to separate.[1] Tuberculosis and silicosis were lumped together as phthisis, infective silicosis, silico-tuberculosis and tuberculo-silicosis and it was only in 1935 that Simson and Strachan[34] made clear distinctions between silicosis alone and silicosis with tuberculosis. The significance of factors such as the type of silicosis, the prevalence of tuberculosis in the general population and the role of mycobacteria other than tuberculosis (MOTT) has become clear in the last five decades.

DEFINITIONS

Silicosis is not a single disease. It is a range of disorders which are determined by the intensity of exposure to respirable particles of silica-containing dust.[42]

Acute silicosis is the most severe form of the disease and arises in response to intense exposure to quartz or to the more fibrogenic forms of crystalline silicon oxide, cristobalite or tridymite. The intensity of the exposure is such that lung disease has been known to develop after only six months of such exposure. Nodule formation in acute silicosis is poor, and the gas-exchanging portions of the lung are involved by the disease. The radiological appearance of acute silicosis is non-specific and it may resemble the ground-glass opacification seen in several other interstitial lung diseases. Acute silicosis is rare and is usually the result of failure to recognize or control silica dust production in small *ad hoc* operations and new industries. The most striking examples in modern times of acute silicosis have occurred during tunnelling through quartz in the construction of the Johannesburg Post Office tunnel and the Gaulley Bridge tunnel.[36] Other reported cases have followed exposure in silica-flour (abrasive powder) production.[23] Mycobacterial disease almost invariably complicates acute silicosis.

Accelerated silicosis follows four to 14 years of high to moderate intensity silica-containing dust exposure. At the one end of its spectrum it is similar to acute silicosis and at the other to chronic silicosis. Nodules are generally well developed but they tend to be more widely distributed than in chronic silicosis and may impinge upon alveolar walls. On the chest radiograph, the nodules are usually distributed uniformly through the lung fields. Accelerated silicosis is not uncommon and has recently been reported in the men who remove rust from deep sea oil rigs by sandblasting,[43] in silica-flour mill workers[6] and those employed in the manufacture of slate pencils.[32] Mycobacterial disease often complicates accelerated silicosis.

Chronic silicosis is the most common form of the disease and is generally associated with the established, controlled, silica-dust-producing industries, including mining. The disease develops after many years of exposure to a low intensity of respirable silica-containing dust, and it is unusual to detect chronic silicosis before at least 15 years of exposure. Indeed, it is commonly only apparent after 30 years of working in a low dust or low silica-content dusty environment. Nodule formation is well developed in chronic silicosis and the nodules are remote from the areas of the lung where gas exchange occurs. Nodules tend to predominate in the upper lung zones. Mycobacterial disease occurs more commonly in chronic silicosis than in the general population.

Pulmonary tuberculosis should be broadened in the context of silicosis to include, not only the more common disease of *Mycobacterium tuberculosis*, but also diseases caused by MOTT. In general, the diagnostic criteria, including the radiological appearance, the presence of acid- and alcohol-fast bacilli on sputum smear examination, or the finding of mycobacteria on sputum culture, a positive tuberculin skin test and, when necessary, histological examination of involved tissue, should be applied to establish a diagnosis of pulmonary tuberculosis.[15] The criteria required to distinguish MOTT disease from *Mycobacterium tuberculosis* disease in which MOTT have colonized, have been defined and require that strong cultures of only the MOTT be obtained from several separate specimens of sputum.[3]

HISTORY

Agricola[1] reported in the sixteenth century that he had found women in mining areas who had been widowed as often as seven times when their successive miner husbands succumbed prematurely to 'consumption'. When gunpowder was invented in 1627 and drilling machines were introduced to the mines in 1636, the potential to produce respirable particles of quartz dust was greatly increased. The risks of silicosis progressively increased as mechanization resulted in the production of more and more small-particle dust. The industrial revolution produced the European epidemic of tuberculosis, and so miners who survived the heat, the accidents, hookworm infestation and mercury or arsenic poisoning, became disabled with silicosis and died of tuberculosis.[18] From the mines of Europe, men with silicosis and tuberculosis came to South Africa to dig for gold on the Witwatersrand. Men from rural southern Africa

flocked to the gold mines to find work. These men had not previously encountered tuberculosis and were, as a result, highly susceptible to infection with *Mycobacterium tuberculosis*. Their susceptibility was heightened as they were massively exposed to silica dust in the poorly ventilated early Witwatersrand mines. Men working with drilling machines developed silicosis after as little as two years,[21] and usually within five years of exposure. Within seven years of the diagnosis of silicosis, the majority of these men had developed pulmonary tuberculosis and, in the absence of any effective therapy, the majority were then dead within a year.[37] As dust control was improved, silicosis took longer to develop, acute silicosis gave way to accelerated silicosis and accelerated to chronic silicosis. The miners' susceptibility to tuberculosis decreased as the silicosis became more chronic and the risks of becoming infected decreased as the prevalence of tuberculosis in the general, white, population declined. Similar changes occurred elsewhere in the developed world except in the black population of southern Africa where the prevalence of tuberculosis remained high and black miners with silicosis, albeit chronic silicosis, still retain a high risk of developing pulmonary tuberculosis.[11]

MECHANISM

Men and women with silicosis are more susceptible to mycobacterial disease than are those without silicosis. This association is not a simple one. The risks of tuberculosis for those with silicosis depend upon the nature of their silicosis and upon the prevalence of tuberculosis in their community. Mycobacterial infection and disease appear to be an almost inevitable outcome in those with acute silicosis — a disease which was common in the early days of gold mining in South Africa and elsewhere, but which is rare today. The risk of tuberculosis in men with accelerated silicosis is extremely high and where the prevalence of tuberculosis in the community is low, men with accelerated silicosis often develop MOTT disease.[5, 42] Under modern working conditions, it is unusual to find any form of silicosis other than the chronic variety: in chronic silicosis, the risks of developing tuberculosis are low in low tuberculosis prevalence communities.[42] Nevertheless, the greater risk persists for those with silicosis[28, 39, 40] and increases as the severity of the chronic silicosis increases.[11, 39]

The mechanism which renders those with silicosis more susceptible to mycobacterial infection and disease is thought to involve the incompetence of the lung macrophage induced by crystalline silica. Experimental studies have demonstrated the inability of macrophages dusted with silica to overpower *Mycobacterium tuberculosis*[2, 14] and even usually non-pathogenic mycobacteria.[42] But the relevance of these studies to the human situation has been disputed,[42] and macrophages obtained from men with silicosis have been found to have normal viability and function.[13] It is also noteworthy that no investigator has been able to demonstrate an increased susceptibility to mycobacterial infection in men with exposure to silica dust who do not have silicosis. Watkins-Pitchford believed that the smallest amount of exposure to silica-containing dust was sufficient to increase the risk of developing pulmonary tuberculosis but this view has not been confirmed. The role of dust exposure in the risk of pulmonary tuberculosis in South African gold miners is almost impossible to assess. Although a working population of gold miners has a greater incidence of pulmonary tuberculosis than that found in the general population from which they originate, it is not possible to attribute this difference to their occupation. The increased incidence may be explained by the several ways in which such a working population differs from the general population. The incidence of pulmonary tuberculosis in men increases with age:[10, 25] a working population excludes children and, as this age group dominates in a third world population, the average age of the working population is usually at least 10 years older than that of the general population. Pulmonary tuberculosis may be at least twice as common in men than in women[10] and the incidence of the disease would thus be expected to be higher in an all-male

working population. A study in Scandinavia has shown that single men in an urban environment have an incidence of pulmonary tuberculosis that is as much as eight times greater than their married, rural counterparts;[19] this observation could well apply to the migrant southern African worker who becomes, in effect, a single man in an urban environment and might thus have an increased risk of developing pulmonary tuberculosis whether or not his work exposes him to silica-dust. Lastly, the intense radiological surveillance programme which exists on the mines[31] ensures that no case of pulmonary tuberculosis goes undetected — a far cry from the situation which applies to the general black southern African population with whom these miners have been compared.

It is also not possible to compare gold miners with other working groups: the strongest and healthiest men select themselves for the rigorous but rewarding work on the mines, leaving the less strong and healthy to fill positions in other industries. Thus the incidence of pulmonary tuberculosis in other working populations might be expected to be higher than that of the gold miner,[27] but to confound matters this healthy worker effect is further complicated by the increased incidence of the disease in mine workers with silicosis, including those whose silicosis is not yet visible on their chest radiographs.[35] Thus, in the absence of proof that silica-dust exposure without silicosis can predispose to pulmonary tuberculosis, it must be concluded that, while there is indisputable evidence of the susceptibility of those with silicosis to mycobacterial infection and disease, the precise mechanism of this susceptibility is not clear.

EPIDEMIOLOGY OF SILICOSIS AND PULMONARY TUBERCULOSIS

A study of black South African gold miners (Cowie, unpublished data) has examined the incidence of pulmonary tuberculosis in men without silicosis and in men with chronic, simple silicosis. The men with and without silicosis were of similar age (46,7 and 44,7 years, respectively) and there was no difference in ages of the silicotic men in the three different categories of radiographic nodule profusion. A total of 340 men had no evidence of silicosis, 432 men had category 1 nodule profusion[20] on their chest radiographs, 376 had category 2, and 49 had category 3. The incidence of pulmonary tuberculosis in these men has been examined over a four and a half year period and the annual incidence of tuberculosis increased from one per cent in men without silicosis to 8,6 per cent in men with silicosis with category 3 nodule profusion (see Figure 12.1). This study has confirmed that the risk of developing pulmonary tuberculosis is increased in men with chronic silicosis and that the risk increases progressively with the extent of the silicosis.

MOTT disease is relatively rare in those developing countries which have a high prevalence of tuberculosis. However, a study of black South African gold miners with first episode pulmonary tuberculosis revealed that only MOTT were cultured from 16,9 per cent of the men with silicosis

and 5,7 per cent of those without silicosis (Cowie[44]). The MOTT cultured were *Mycobacterium kansasii* in 67 per cent of the cases (including 144 cultures from men with relapsed pulmonary tuberculosis) and *Mycobacterium scrofulaceum* in 26 per cent. These two MOTT are known to be associated with dusty occupations, including mining, and to be more prevalent in men with occupational and other lung diseases.[30, 41] Not all of the cases from whom MOTT were cultured fulfilled the criteria for the diagnosis of MOTT disease[41] but the findings do, at least, show that the MOTT in the mining environment differ from those in the general community[24] and that they are found significantly more often in men with silicosis.

DIAGNOSIS

The diagnosis of pulmonary tuberculosis in men with silicosis has been said to be extremely difficult, but this difficulty is more apparent than real and has arisen from the

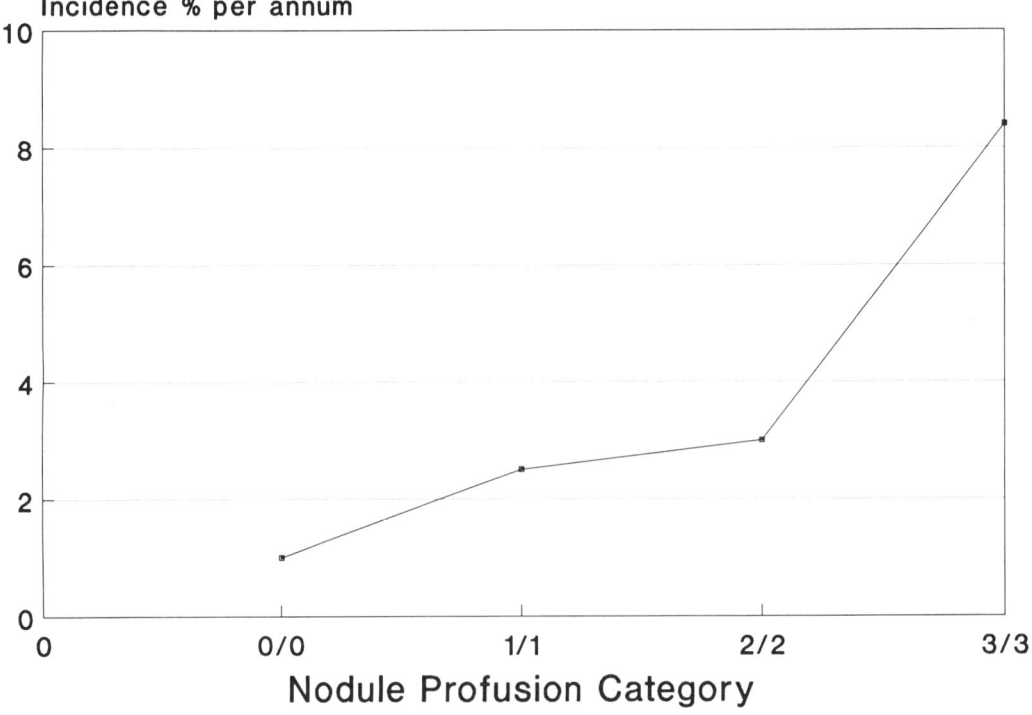

Figure 12.1. Annual incidence of pulmonary tuberculosis in 340 black South African gold miners without evidence of silicosis and in 860 with silicosis over a four and a half year period.

too-liberal assumption that men with progressive silicosis have tuberculosis.[37] In order to accommodate the conventional wisdom that men with silicosis die from tuberculosis, the criteria for tuberculosis at post-mortem were stretched to include the presence of an area of necrosis in a single silicotic nodule[34] or a calcified granuloma in a hilar node.[38] In chronic silicosis, the diagnosis of pulmonary tuberculosis in men with suggestive changes on their chest radiographs is usually readily established in the usual manner with sputum smear examination and culture.[15] In the few instances when sputum bacteriology is negative, notwithstanding sputum induction,[17] and the suspicion of tuberculous disease remains high, a fibre-optic bronchoscopy with bronchial washings and a transbronchial lung biopsy might establish the diagnosis. If the investigations are negative and the risks of observation are considered to be too great, a full course of anti-tuberculosis therapy should be considered, especially in men with advanced chronic, or accelerated, silicosis who have a positive tuberculin test. Unfortunately, the therapeutic trial is seldom diagnostic as bacteriologically-negative tuberculosis is often indolent and the lesions consist largely of scar tissue.

While establishing a diagnosis of pulmonary tuberculosis in a man with silicosis, it should not be presumed that the disease is caused by *Mycobacterium tuberculosis*. At least three sputum specimens should be sent for culture to a laboratory capable of doing drug sensitivity testing and mycobacterial identification.

TREATMENT

The treatment of pulmonary tuberculosis in men with silicosis has been revolutionized by the inclusion of rifampicin.[12, 16, 22, 26] Previously, it had been believed that tuberculosis could never be cured[33] and that men with silicosis and tuberculosis should remain on treatment for the rest of their lives.[29]

Treatment of pulmonary tuberculosis in men with chronic silicosis should whenever possible include rifampicin, pyrazinamide and isoniazid. The inclusion of other drugs will depend upon the local prevalence of

resistant strains of *Mycobacterium tuberculosis*. Therapy with an established short-course chemotherapy regimen can then be applied without further modification.[12, 16, 26]

When MOTT are consistently cultured from the sputum, treatment will need to be modified according to the type of mycobacterium grown. Treatment with conventional therapy should be completed unless there is overwhelming evidence that the MOTT is the cause of the disease and not simply colonizing the lesion. *Mycobacterium kansasii*, the most common of the MOTT found in South African gold miners,[12, 30] is generally responsive to therapy. A recent study has shown that rifampicin and ethambutol given for a period of nine months is sufficient therapy,[9] but the standard recommendation has been for a rifampicin- and ethambutol-containing regimen given for a period of 18 months.[41] In practice, a report that a MOTT has been cultured usually precedes information concerning its identification and its *in vitro* drug sensitivities. Ethambutol and ethionamide should then be added to the regimen and once it is confirmed that the MOTT is *Mycobacterium kansasii*, ethionamide can be stopped. The other components of the regimen should continue to the end of the usual treatment period, in case *Mycobacterium tuberculosis* and not the MOTT is the cause of the disease. Thereafter, rifampicin and ethambutol should continue to complete 18 months of treatment. The other MOTT which occur in miners are of the MAIS (avium, intracellulare and scrofulaceum) group, *Mycobacterium scrofulaceum* being the most common. These MOTT are characterized by being poorly responsive to therapy (although this view has recently been challenged),[7] but treatment with combinations of two or more of ethionamide, ethambutol, cotrimoxazole, clofazamine or amikacin may be of value. Another approach has been to ignore the results of *in vitro* testing of individual drugs and to give combinations of rifampicin, isoniazid and ethambutol.[8] Treatment with the selected regimen should continue for at least two years. Surgical excision of the lesion should be considered in every case where one of the MAIS complex MOTT is *known* to be the cause of the disease, if the lesion is localized, and if the patient's general pulmonary status is compatible with surgery.[4]

PREVENTION

The risk of developing pulmonary tuberculosis is so great in men with advanced chronic silicosis and in those with acute or accelerated silicosis that preventive chemotherapy should be considered in those men who are tuberculin positive. Whilst isoniazid given for 12 months is the only form of 'chemoprophylaxis' which has been formally evaluated, it has a doubtful role in developing countries where isoniazid resistant mycobacteria are prevalent. Multi-drug chemoprophylaxis given for three months is currently being studied in men with silicosis, but its effectiveness has yet to be evaluated.

PROGNOSIS

When pulmonary tuberculosis in men with chronic silicosis is treated with an effective rifampicin-containing short-course regimen, the results are similar to those of the treatment of pulmonary tuberculosis without silicosis.[12, 16, 26] Treatment failure may occur when the disease is caused by a multi-resistant strain of *Mycobacterium tuberculosis* or by MOTT, but is usually due to non-compliance. Relapse rates will depend upon the efficacy of the regimen used and the degree of supervision of therapy which has been provided.

In general, the lesions of pulmonary tuberculosis resolve to the same extent in men with silicosis as they do in the absence of silicosis. There is some theoretical evidence that tuberculosis might cause progression of silicosis,[42] and whilst an occasional patient might have rapid progression of lung nodularity which persists after treatment of pulmonary tuberculosis, this is an infrequent development. In a prevalence study of men with silicosis, those who had been treated for pulmonary tuberculosis did have a small but statistically significant reduction in lung function when compared with similar men who had not had tuberculosis.[11] However, in general men with pulmonary tuberculosis that has been diagnosed timeously and effectively treated, with or without silicosis, have little or no permanent residuum of that disease.

CONCLUSION

Men with silicosis will always be more susceptible to mycobacterial infection and disease than is the general population, but this susceptibility can be decreased by improved dust control in the workplace. Although the large controlled industries such as mining are responsible for most of the cases of silicosis, their employees are less susceptible to mycobacterial disease because they tend to have a modest degree of chronic silicosis. In the gold mines on the Orange Free State gold fields, severe (category 3) chronic silicosis occurs in approximately 0,1 per cent of the total work force and in about 0,85 per cent of men who have worked underground for more than 30 years.[11] Attention needs to be paid to smaller industries such as small foundries, slate pencil manufacturers, sandblasters, abrasive powder manufacturers, tunnelers and quarries where workers are at risk of developing accelerated, and even acute, silicosis.

More important, but more difficult than silica-containing dust exposure control, is the general need to reduce the prevalence of tuberculosis in the community. The reduction of tuberculous disease in industrialized countries has had a dramatic influence on the risk of tuberculosis in men and women with silicosis.

Prevention of tuberculosis in those who already have silicosis might well be achieved with multi-drug chemoprophylaxis, but the most important measure is close surveillance to ensure that tuberculous disease is detected and treated at the earliest possible stage.

REFERENCES

1 Agricola G, 1912. De Re Metallica (Basel, 1556), translated by Hoover H C & Hoover L H. *The Mining Magazine*.

2 Allison A C & Hart D A P, 1968. Potentiation by silica of the growth of *Mycobacterium tuberculosis* in macrophage cultures. *British Journal of Experimental Pathology*. 49, 465–76.

3 American Thoracic Society, 1981. Diagnostic standards and classification of tuberculosis and other mycobacterial diseases (14th ed). *American Review of Respiratory Diseases*. 123, 343–58.

4 American Thoracic Society, 1983. Treatment of tuberculosis and other mycobacterial diseases. *American Review of Respiratory Diseases*. 127, 790–6.

5 Bailey W C, Brown M, Buechner H A, Weill H, Ichinose I F & Ziskind M, 1974. Silico-mycobacterial disease in sandblasters. *American Review of Respiratory Diseases*. 110, 115–25.

6 Banks D E, Morring K L, Boehlecke B A, Althouse R B & Merchant J A, 1981. Silicosis in silica flour workers. *American Review of Respiratory Diseases*. 124, 445–50.

7 Banks J, 1989. Treatment of pulmonary disease caused by opportunist mycobacteria. *Thorax*. 44, 449–54.

8 Banks J & Jenkins P A, 1987. Combined versus single antituberculosis drugs on the *in vitro* sensitivity patterns of non-tuberculous mycobacteria. *Thorax*. 42, 838–42.

9 British Thoracic Society Research Committee, 1986. British Thoracic Society study of nine months' treatment with rifampicin and ethambutol in *Mycobacterium kansasii* pulmonary infection (abstract). *Thorax*. 41, 709.

10 Comstock G W, 1982. Epidemiology of tuberculosis. *American Review of Respiratory Diseases*. 125 (suppl), 8–15.

11 Cowie R L, 1988. *Silicosis, Pulmonary Dysfunction and Respiratory Symptoms in South African Gold Miners*. MD Thesis, University of Cape Town.

12 Cowie R L, Langton M E & Becklake M R, 1989. Pulmonary tuberculosis in South African gold miners. *American Review of Respiratory Diseases*. 139, 1086–9.

13 Davis G S, 1986. Pathogenesis of silicosis, current concepts and hypotheses. *Lung*. 164, 139–54.

14 Ebina T, Takahashi Y & Hasuike T, 1960. Effects of quartz powder on tubercle bacilli and phagocytes. *American Review of Respiratory Diseases*. 82, 516–27.

15 Escreet B C & Cowie R L, 1983. Criteria for the diagnosis of pulmonary tuberculosis. *South African Medical Journal*. 63, 850–4.

16 Escreet B C, Langton M E & Cowie R L, 1984. Short-course chemotherapy for silico-tuberculosis. *South African Medical Journal*. 66, 327–30.

17 Gatner E M S, Gärtig D & Kleeberg H H, 1977. Sputum induction by saline aerosol. *South African Medical Journal*. 51, 279–80.

18 Gordon D, 1954. Dust and history. *Medical Journal of Australia*. 2, 161–6.

19 Horwitz O, 1971. Tuberculosis risk and marital status. *American Review of Respiratory Diseases*. 104, 22–31.

20 International Labour Office, 1980. *Guidelines for the Use of ILO International Classification of Radiographs of Pneumoconioses*. Geneva: International Labour Office.

21 Irvine L G & Watt A H, 1912. Miners' phthisis. *Transvaal Medical Journal*. 8, 30–9.

22 Jones F L, 1982. Rifampin-containing chemotherapy for pulmonary tuberculosis associated with coal workers pneumoconiosis. *American Review of Respiratory Diseases*. 125, 681–3.

23 Kilgore E S, 1932. Pneumoconiosis — an unusually acute form. *Journal of the American Medical Association*. 99, 1414–6.

24 Kleeberg H H, 1981. Epidemiology of mycobacteria other than tubercle bacilli in South Africa. *Review of Infectious Diseases*. 3, 1008–12.

25 Kästner H G V, 1979. Trends in four major communicable diseases. *South African Medical Journal*. 55, 460–73.

26 Lin T-P, Suo J, Lee C-N & Yang S-P, 1987. Short-course chemotherapy for pulmonary tuberculosis in pneumoconiotic patients. *American Review of Respiratory Diseases*. 136, 808–10.

27 McMichael A J, Spirtas R & Kupper L L, 1974. An epidemiologic study of mortality within a cohort of rubber workers, 1964–72. *Journal of Occupational Medicine*. 16, 458–64.

28 Monaco A, 1964. Antituberculosis chemoprophylaxis in silicotics. *Bulletin of the International Union Against Tuberculosis*. 35, 51–6.

29 Morgan E J, 1979. Silicosis and tuberculosis. *Chest*. 75, 202–3.

30 Nel E E, Linton W S, van der Merwe W, Berson S D & Kleeberg H H, 1977. Pulmonary disease associated with mycobacteria other than tubercle bacilli in miners. *South African Medical Journal.* 51, 779–83.

31 *Occupational Diseases in Mines and Works Act, No. 78 of 1973.* Government Gazette 6th July, 1973, No 3970.

32 Sayed H N & Chatterjee B B, 1985. Rapid progression of silicosis in slate pencil workers, II. A follow-up study. *American Journal of Industrial Medicine.* 8, 135–42.

33 Schepers G W H, 1964. Silicosis and tuberculosis. *Industrial Medicine and Surgery.* 33, 381–99.

34 Simson F W & Strachan A S, 1935. Silicosis and tuberculosis: observations on the origin and character of silicotic lesions. *Publication XXXVI of the South African Institute of Mining Research.* 6, 367–406.

35 Sluis-Cremer G K, 1980. Active pulmonary tuberculosis discovered at post-mortem examination of the lungs of black miners. *British Journal of Disorders of the Chest.* 74, 374–8.

36 Smith C S & Wikoff H L, 1933. The silica content of the lungs of a group of tunnel workers. *American Journal of Public Health.* 23, 1250–4.

37 Watkins-Pitchford W, 1927. The silicosis of the South African gold mines and the changes produced in it by legislative and administrative effort. *Journal of Industrial Hygiene.* 9, 109–39.

38 Webster I, 1959. Some aspects of the pathology of silicosis found in miners from the South African gold mines. In: Orenstein A J (ed.). *Proceedings of the Pneumoconiosis Conference Johannesburg 1959.* London: Churchill.

39 Westerholm P, 1980. Silicosis, observations on a case register. *Scandinavian Journal of Environmental Health.* 2 (Suppl), 5–86.

40 Westerholm P, Ahlmark A, Maasinig R & Segelberg I, 1986. Silicosis and risk of lung cancer or lung tuberculosis, a cohort study. *Environmental Research.* 41, 339–50.

41 Wolinsky E, 1979. Nontuberculous mycobacteria and associated diseases. *American Review of Respiratory Diseases.* 119, 107–59.

42 Ziskind M, Jones R N & Weill H, 1976. Silicosis (state of the art). *American Review of Respiratory Diseases.* 113, 643–65.

43 Ziskind M, Weill H, Anderson A E, Sammi B, Neilson A & Waggenspack C, 1976. Silicosis in shipyard sandblasters. *Environmental Research.* 11, 237–43.

44 Cowie R L, 1990. The mycobacteria of pulmonary tuberculosis in South African gold mines. *Tubercle.* 71, 39–42.

CHAPTER 13

Radiographic manifestations

J A Beyers

INTRODUCTION

Conventional radiography is of paramount importance in the diagnosis of pulmonary tuberculosis, as this diagnosis is usually suggested for the first time as a result of changes detected on radiographs of the lungs.

However, the inherent limitations of radiography in its ability to demonstrate minimal pulmonary changes and to differentiate between widely different pathological processes, and the lack of agreement between and within readers in their identification and evaluation of radiographic changes must constantly be borne in mind. To maintain a healthy balance between over- and under-diagnosis the following points are emphasized:

- full size radiographs of excellent technical quality in postero-anterior and lateral projections must be available. To better demonstrate, localize and evaluate suspicious lesions, apical-lordotic and oblique views are useful, and conventional tomography is of particular value. When only 100 mm radiographs taken with a mobile x-ray machine were available Fourie et al.[8] found that 21 out of 59 patients with culture positive sputa showed no radiographic evidence suggestive of tuberculosis;

- the film reader must be experienced in chest radiography, must have a thorough knowledge of the radiographic features of pulmonary tuberculosis, must be critical and meticulous, and must have a high degree of suspicion;

- all previous radiographs must be available for review and comparison to help with the detection of early radiographic abnormalities and to evaluate abnormalities;

- the radiographic features must never be interpreted in isolation but must always be integrated with the clinical findings, results of special investigations, response to treatment and the clinical problem;

- a diagnosis of pulmonary tuberculosis may be suggested on the radiographic features, but ideally a definitive diagnosis of pulmonary tuberculosis should only be made by demonstrating tubercle bacilli in sputum or gastric washings. This is not always possible, especially in primary pulmonary tuberculosis and in the early stages of post-primary pulmonary tuberculosis, and rarely even in advanced post-primary pulmonary tuberculosis, so that bronchoscopy with bronchial brushings, transbronchial biopsy or even open lung biopsy may be required. It is, however, not always justifiable to go to such extremes to obtain absolute diagnostic certainty and under certain circumstances a diagnosis of pulmonary tuberculosis can be made with a high degree of confidence if the radiographic features are correlated with all available data.

The radiographic features of pulmonary tuberculosis are infinitely variable and stretch over an endless spectrum from an apparently normal radiograph in an asymptomatic patient to a completely destroyed lung with pulmonary arterial hypertension and cor pulmonale in a dying patient. To make sense of such an endless spectrum it is necessary to classify the radiographic changes into manageable groups.

CLASSIFICATION

From a radiographic point of view a meaningful, workable classification of pulmonary tuberculosis is best achieved by grouping together cases with similar pathogenesis, morbid anatomical changes and radiographic features.

The following classification system is suggested:

- *primary pulmonary tuberculosis.* This refers to the primary focus in the lungs (Ghon focus) together with the reaction in the draining lymph nodes and the complications which occur as a direct result of the infection;
- *post-primary pulmonary tuberculosis.* This refers to pulmonary tuberculosis which develops at variable intervals after a patient has had a primary tuberculous infection which has either become quiescent or has apparently healed;
- *transitional pulmonary tuberculosis.* This refers to that minority of cases where primary pulmonary tuberculosis gradually and uninterruptedly, over a period of months or a year or so, progresses to the clinical and radiographic picture of post-primary pulmonary tuberculosis;
- *congenital or neonatal pulmonary tuberculosis.* Congenital pulmonary tuberculosis, where the infection is acquired in utero or during birth, is grouped together with neonatal pulmonary tuberculosis, where massive infection occurs within a few days of birth, because it is difficult and sometimes impossible in practice to differentiate between them.

Primary and post-primary pulmonary tuberculosis can usually be differentiated on clinical, epidemiological, morbid-anatomical, prognostic and radiographic grounds. Certain individual identical pathological and radiographic features, such as pleural effusion, miliary tuberculosis and pericardial effusion are, however, found in primary and post-primary pulmonary tuberculosis. These features cannot by themselves aid the differentiation between primary and post-primary tuberculosis, and therefore primary and post-primary tuberculosis can sometimes not be differentiated on radiographic grounds alone. The differentiation can then only be made if it is known when tuberculin skin test conversion occurred.

The time interval between primary tuberculosis and the development of post-primary tuberculosis varies widely, from a few months to many years. In a minority of cases primary pulmonary tuberculosis may progress to the clinical and radiographic picture of post-primary pulmonary tuberculosis without a latent intervening period of apparent quiescence or healing. These cases are usually referred to as cases of progressive primary pulmonary tuberculosis but are here classified as being cases of transitional pulmonary tuberculosis.

Primary pulmonary tuberculosis

Where the prevalence of tuberculosis in a community is high, primary pulmonary tuberculosis is usually seen in children, but as the prevalence of tuberculosis decreases, primary tuberculosis is seen in progressively older age groups, even into old age. In South Africa most cases of primary tuberculosis are still seen in children but it is not uncommon to find primary tuberculosis in middle-aged or elderly people. Radiographic features of primary pulmonary tuberculosis, as seen in children, teenagers, adults and the elderly are essentially the same although there are differences in the incidence of certain features in different age groups. For example, miliary tuberculosis and hilar adenopathy are more common in children than in older age groups. However, these differences are not of practical importance.

The radiographic features of primary pulmonary tuberculosis can be classified by grouping together cases with similar features.

A chest radiograph with no detectable abnormality

Patients in this group usually fall in grade 2 of the American Thoracic Society classification of tuberculosis, that is, 'tuberculous infection, no disease. Significant reaction to tuberculin skin test, negative bacteriological studies, no clinical and/or roentgenographic manifestations of tuberculosis'. However, ailing children with a normal chest radiograph in whom tubercle bacilli were cultured from gastric washings have been seen by the author.

The complete primary complex

The primary focus (Ghon focus) in the lung and the enlarged draining lymph nodes, i.e. the complete primary complex, are radiographically detectable. The Ghon focus can be seen anywhere in the lung without any marked predilection for any lung, lobe or segment. It usually presents as a non-specific, ill-defined area of veiling 1 to 2 cm in diameter. The accompanying lymph node enlargement may involve hilar and/or mediastinal nodes. In the vast majority of cases the Ghon focus and the lymph nodes heal completely over a period of months and no radiographic abnormality remains. However, occasionally a small fibrotic or calcified nodule remains in the lungs, and calcification in the nodes is not rare. Radiographically the complete primary complex is seldom seen.

Enlarged hilar and/or mediastinal lymph nodes only

Enlargement of any group of lymph nodes draining the lung without a visible parenchymal focus commonly occurs in primary pulmonary tuberculosis.

Unilateral hilar node enlargement is common; bilateral hilar node enlargement is sometimes seen.

Mediastinal node enlargement usually involves the right paratracheal nodes but occasionally the right and left paratracheal nodes may be involved. Paratracheal node enlargement is usually found together with hilar node enlargement but may rarely be found without the accompanying enlargement of the hilar nodes.

The enlarged nodes may be so small that they are difficult to detect radiographically, or they may present as big masses. They may be sharply or poorly defined and on occasion may seem to fade away into the adjacent lung. They may be smoothly rounded or lobulated.

The infection in the nodes may spread by contiguity to involve adjacent structures and so give rise to tuberculous pleural effusion, tuberculous pericardial effusion, traction diverticulum of the oesophagus or (rarely) phrenic nerve palsy. Because of the anatomical distribution of the lymph nodes, the most commonly involved structure is part of the tracheo-bronchial tree.

Over a period of months or years the nodes heal and may no longer be radiographically detectable, but remaining calcification may persist.

Lympho-bronchial lesions

This refers to a spectrum of lesions which are usually referred to as endobronchial tuberculosis, or segmental lesions. In the past they were called epituberculosis.

The lesions develop when a tuberculous infected lymph node involves a bronchus.

The classical radiographic picture is that of a homogeneously opaque lobe of more or less normal size, together with enlargement of the accompanying lymph nodes and narrowing of the lobar bronchus.

Around this classical picture there is a wide spectrum of variations which depends on the degree of bronchial obstruction, whether the node has eroded into the bronchus, whether caseous material has been extruded into the bronchus, the physical and chemical characteristics of the caseous material, and the number of viable tubercle bacilli in the caseous material.

Instead of one lobe being involved, two lobes or even a whole lung may be involved. Equally, instead of a whole lobe being involved, only a single segment or a number of segments may be involved.

Instead of the lobe or segment being of more or less normal size there may be a moderate or marked loss of volume, but the opposite may also occur so that an abnormally big lobe with a bulging fissure may be found.

Instead of a homogeneously dense opacity a heterogeneous opacity may be found. Sometimes a cavity or cavities may be seen within the opacity, and an air bronchogram may occasionally be seen.

The narrowed or completely obstructed bronchus may sometimes be seen on routine radiographs and can often be successfully demonstrated on high kilovoltage radiographs, and even better on conventional tomographs.

With or without treatment it takes months or even years for an opaque lobe or segment to resolve, and the lobe or segment which has been affected is usually permanently damaged. The degree of residual damage varies from mild to gross destruction. Usually there is some loss of volume, bronchiectasis and fibrosis, and specks of calcification within the lesion and in the offending lymph node are sometimes found.

In rare cases the bronchial obstruction acts as a check valve and instead of an opacity, one then finds a hypertranslucent lobe or lung of increased size.

Because this whole spectrum of appearances depends on involvement of a bronchus by a tuberculous infected lymph node, it is meaningful to refer to the condition as lympho-bronchial tuberculosis rather than to use the usual designations of endo-bronchial tuberculosis or segmental lesions.

Lympho-bronchial tuberculosis is very common and in two published series of primary pulmonary tuberculosis in South Africa these lesions, alone or together with other radiographic abnormalities, were found in 56 per cent[6] and 87 per cent[10] of cases respectively.

Primary cavitating pulmonary tuberculosis

It is uncommon but not rare for tuberculous cavities to develop in the lung during the course of primary pulmonary tuberculosis, but it does occur only in patients with poor resistance. Cavitation can develop by a number of mechanisms, the most common of which, in the author's experience, is lympho-bronchial tuberculosis. Cavitation can also develop as a result of progression of a Ghon focus or as a complication of tuberculous bronchopneumonia. It is highly unlikely that cavitation will develop because of progression and coalescence of miliary tuberculosis lesions, although such an occurrence has been documented.[22]

The radiographic appearance of these cavities depends on their pathogenesis. They may be thin or thick walled; small or large; single or multiple. They may be surrounded by more or less normal lung, or they may occur in a big opacity.

There is nothing characteristic about these tuberculous cavities, and the radiographic feature of cavitation taken in isolation cannot, therefore, differentiate a tuberculous cavity from any other type of cavity.

Tuberculous broncho-pneumonia

Tuberculous broncho-pneumonia presents as ill-defined, confluent opacities, usually widespread throughout both lungs, but not necessarily symmetrically or evenly distributed. The opacities themselves look like broncho-pneumonia of any other aetiology but sometimes there are clues in the form of enlarged lymph nodes, lympho-bronchial lesions or cavitation.

The opacities may be so small, numerous and widespread that they resemble coarse miliary tuberculosis. It may be difficult or impossible to differentiate between tuberculous broncho-pneumonia and miliary tuberculosis on radiological, and sometimes even on pathological grounds.[27]

The origin of the tuberculous broncho-pneumonia may be a detectable cavity which has caused bronchogenic spread, or an enlarged gland which has ruptured into a main bronchus discharging fluid material. Often no source for the tuberculous broncho-pneumonia can be detected.

Miliary (disseminated) tuberculosis

Miliary tuberculosis is but one small part of a very wide spectrum of haematogenous dissemination of tuberculosis. Haematogenous dissemination of tubercle bacilli varies from the occasional blood spread of a few tubercle bacilli without any clinical consequence to overwhelming invasion of the blood stream with innumerable tubercle bacilli that gives rise to a fulminant form of non-reactive tuberculosis which can be looked upon as tuberculous septicaemia. The common and well known miliary tuberculosis picture falls between these two extremes and occurs when a caseous focus ruptures into the blood stream or lymphatic system, permitting a large number of tubercle bacilli to enter the blood stream within a brief period of time.

Conceptually and also for practical reasons it would be better to refer to this whole spectrum of disease states as 'disseminated tuberculosis', but the term 'miliary tuberculosis' has the sanctity of tradition and will therefore be adhered to.

Miliary tuberculosis can occur at any time during the course of tuberculosis and the whole wide spectrum of its radiographic features is the same whether it be a complication of primary or of post-primary tuberculosis. It is being found with increasing frequency in adults, and is particularly a challenging problem in old age.

The radiographic features of miliary tuberculosis vary over a very wide spectrum. The classical picture is that of innumerable, round, same sized, sharply defined opacities of a millimeter or less in diameter widely and evenly distributed throughout both lungs. The opacities may, however, be of pinpoint size or so minute that they are barely detectable, and it may be difficult or impossible to say that the radiograph is abnormal. The chest radiograph, even in retrospect, may show no abnormality but an autopsy done shortly after the radiograph is taken may show miliary tuberculosis throughout both lungs. The opacities may be bigger and less well defined, and may even coalesce to give a picture that is difficult, or impossible, to differentiate from tuberculous broncho-pneumonia on radiographic or even pathological grounds.[27] It has been reported that miliary nodules which have coalesced may rarely break down to give small cavities.[22] The opacities may not be evenly distributed; they may be more prominent in the upper lung zones or they may be more prominent in one lung than in the other. One particularly unusual case has been seen where miliary tubercles were confined to the right upper lobe.

Sometimes the opacities are not all of the same size, and sometimes they are not round but are irregularly shaped.

Miliary tuberculosis is a well known cause of the adult respiratory distress syndrome. A patient with miliary tuberculosis may therefore have diffuse opacification of both lungs, as is characteristically seen in the adult respiratory distress syndrome.

The miliary pattern in the lung may occur without any other radiographic abnormality or there may be other evidence of primary tuberculosis such as enlarged lymph nodes, lympho-bronchial lesions, pleural effusion, etc.

With adequate treatment, and on very rare occasions without treatment, miliary tuberculosis will heal over a period of months leaving a radiographically normal lung. It is questionable if healed miliary tuberculosis ever leaves behind scattered calcifications in the lungs.

It is a tragedy when an eminently treatable but otherwise deadly disease, such as miliary tuberculosis, is diagnosed for the first time at autopsy. However, the chances of this happening can be decreased if the wide radiographic spectrum of changes possible in miliary tuberculosis is kept in mind, if all chest radiographs are critically analysed with a high degree of suspicion, and if all chest radiographs in a series are compared with all previous radiographs, especially the first one of the series. It should always be borne in mind that a patient may die of miliary tuberculosis at a stage when his or her pre-death chest radiograph showed no abnormality.

Tuberculous pleural effusion

The pleural effusions which commonly occur as a complication of primary tuberculosis at any age are characteristically serous effusions with a good prognosis.

A pleural effusion without any other radiographically detectable intra-thoracic abnormality is a common complication of primary pulmonary tuberculosis.

Such an effusion is frequently found in children, adolescents and young adults and is sometimes found in old age but is very rarely found under the age of three years.

The effusion has no distinctive radiographic features and looks like an effusion or empyema due to a variety of causes. It may be small but is often big and may render opaque a whole hemithorax. It is usually unilateral but on rare occasions may be bilateral.

With treatment, and sometimes even without treatment, the effusion usually clears slowly over a period of weeks or months and often leaves a normal pleural cavity. There may be residual pleural thickening which may take many months or years to clear and which may rarely persist indefinitely. Residual limited or extensive pleural calcification seldom occurs.

A pleural effusion occurring at the same time as other radiographic features of primary tuberculosis may be found at any age. Such an effusion is usually small and unilateral but may on rare occasions be bilateral.

Combination patterns

Not uncommonly combinations of two or more of any of the radiographic patterns described above will occur simultaneously. Examples are lympho-bronchial tuberculosis together with a pleural effusion; primary cavitating tuberculosis together with tuberculous broncho-pneumonia; or enlarged lymph nodes together with miliary tuberculosis, tuberculous broncho-pneumonia or pleural effusion.

Unclassifiable patterns

In a minority of cases primary pulmonary tuberculosis presents with bizarre pulmonary opacities in one or both lungs which are not readily identifiable as Ghon foci, lympho-bronchial, broncho-pneumonic, miliary or primary cavitating tuberculous lesions. It is difficult to reconcile these radiographic features with the generally accepted morbid anatomy of pulmonary tuberculosis. These unclassifiable patterns are difficult to explain, difficult to interpret and difficult to recognize as tuberculous in origin.

Other intrathoracic manifestations

During the course of primary pulmonary tuberculosis other intrathoracic manifestations of tuberculosis may be found.

Tuberculous pericarditis with effusion is an uncommon complication. It may occur with or without radiographically detectable pulmonary, pleural or lymph node abnormalities.

Empyema, pneumothorax, hydro-pneumothorax and pyo-pneumothorax are rare complications.

Post-primary pulmonary tuberculosis

The radiographic features of post-primary pulmonary tuberculosis extend over such a wide spectrum, and overlap and intertwine to such an extent that they cannot be arranged in separate groups with similar features as can be done with primary pulmonary tuberculosis.

A useful approach to the radiographic features of post-primary pulmonary tuberculosis is to bear in mind the pathogenesis and basic pathological features of this type of tuberculosis and then to translate these features into their relevant radiographic counterparts.

Commencement in vulnerable segments

In most cases post-primary pulmonary tuberculosis begins in one of the so-called vulnerable segments of the lung, namely the apical or posterior segments of the upper lobes or the apical segment of the lower lobes. The vast majority of cases commence unilaterally, but on rare occasions simultaneous bilateral commencement may occur.

It is very unusual for post-primary pulmonary tuberculosis to begin in the basal segments of the lower lobes, the middle lobe or the lingula of the left upper lobe. When it does so, it is often due to, or associated with, decreased resistance to tuberculosis so that it tends to be associated with diabetes mellitus,[9, 15] old age,[19] blacks,[9] pregnant women,[9] and decreased cell mediated immunity as in AIDS.[20, 23]

At the site of commencement the lesion increases in size, and spread then occurs directly so that surrounding satellite nodular or streaky lesions develop in the immediate vicinity. Bronchogenic spread often occurs so that distant lesions develop in the same lobe or lung, and frequently in the opposite lung. Occasionally there is haematogenous spread which leads to widespread lesions throughout the body. Post-primary pulmonary tuberculosis develops in more than 90 per cent of cases as a result of reactivation of a dormant lesion dating back to the time of primary infection. It very rarely develops as a result of reinfection by inhalation of tubercle bacilli. Even when previous radiographs are available it is most unusual to be able to identify the focus from which reactivation started.

Tuberculous inflammation

The tuberculous inflammatory reaction starts as a protein- and cellular-rich exudate which fills the terminal air spaces and involves the alveolar walls and interlobular and intersegmental septa. At its very earliest stage this presents radiographically as a small ill-defined area of veiling which is often difficult to recognize, especially when there is an overlying rib or clavicle. Should there be any suspicion of a lesion an apical-lordotic view, reversed apical view, and conventional tomography should be done. This area of slight veiling gradually (over weeks or months) increases in size and density, becoming a more obvious alveolar opacity. A tuberculous caseating granulo-matous process develops together with the exudative reaction. The lesion now becomes more sharply defined, increases in size more slowly, and is heterogeneous in density. Nodular and streaky opacities of varying sizes tend to develop around the initial alveolar density.

In the older radiological literature the pathological process of inflammatory exuda-tion was sometimes referred to as an 'exuda-tive lesion' and the pathological process of caseating granuloma formation as a 'produc-tive lesion'. Radiographically it is impossible to differentiate between the two pathologi-cal processes, which in any case always occur together in varying degrees, so that the radiological terms 'exudative lesion' and 'productive lesion' should be discarded.

These tuberculous inflammatory opaci-ties are usually ill-defined but may at times be well-defined; they are usually heteroge-neous but may sometimes be homoge-neously dense; it is rare, but not unknown, to see an air bronchogram within them; they are usually non-segmental, but they may be segmental and may even involve a whole lobe. On their radiographic appear-ance alone it is not possible to differentiate these tuberculous lesions from inflamma-tory processes of any other aetiology, and often not even from malignant processes.

Caseation

Pathologically caseation is a hallmark of tuberculosis, but there is no way in which caseation can be detected radiographically.

Calcification

Caseous material tends to calcify and radio-graphically detectable areas of calcification varying in size from a pin head to a centi-meter or more in diameter scattered throughout pulmonary lesions are not un-common in post-primary pulmonary tuber-culosis. However, it is said that calcification in post-primary pulmonary tuberculosis is less common than in primary pulmonary tuberculosis.[27] Conventional tomography is a useful method for demonstrating ques-tionable calcification.

Cavitation

There is a very strong tendency for caseous material to erupt into a bronchus and to be expectorated, resulting in a cavity in the lung. Radiographically cavitation is a very important feature of post-primary pul-monary tuberculosis. These cavities are often a few centimeters in diameter and are usually quite easily identified.

Sometimes it is difficult or impossible to be sure whether a small area of apparent increased translucency is an optical illusion due to overlapping shadows, a true cavity arising from any of a number of possible causes, a bulla, a bleb, or a dilated bron-chus due to bronchiectasis. In such cases conventional tomography is of great value in differential diagnosis.

Tuberculous cavities vary in size from less than 1 cm to 10 cm or more in diameter.

The wall of a tuberculous cavity is usu-ally a few millimeters thick, but this thick-ness may vary markedly: not uncommonly it is pencil-line thin (less than 1 mm) and not infrequently it fades away into a sur-rounding opacity so that the thickness of the wall cannot be determined. The inside of the wall is usually smooth, but some-times it is irregular and undulating.

The cavities are usually empty and do not contain fluid, but it is not at all uncom-mon for a cavity to contain fluid and show a fluid level.

Sometimes a tuberculous cavity contains a homogeneously opaque, smoothly round or lobulated mass which is usually freely mobile but may on rare occasions be fixed to the wall. Such a mass is usually a myce-toma, most commonly due to *Aspergillus fumigatus*, but occasionally due to a blood clot. Should haemorrhage occur, inhalation of blood may give widespread alveolar opacities which may be indistinguishable from broncho-pneumonic spread, except that they fade quickly.

Just as with the earliest manifestations of post-primary pulmonary tuberculosis, tuberculous cavities are most commonly found in the so-called vulnerable segments of the lungs but they may be found anywhere in the lungs.

Cavitation often involves one upper lung zone, where one or more cavities may be found, but it may also involve both upper lung zones with one or more cavities in each zone. Sometimes cavitation in upper lung zones is accompanied by cavitation in lower lung zones (upper and lower lung zones being defined as above and below the level of the hila). Rarely, tuberculous cavitation is found in a lower lung zone without cavitation or any other radiographic abnormality in an upper lung zone.

The lung immediately surrounding and in the vicinity of a tuberculous cavity usually shows some degree of streaky or nodular opacification which may be ill- or well-defined. There is often evidence of fibrosis. Sometimes the cavity is surrounded by a homogeneously dense opacity which may involve a considerable part of a lobe, and on rare occasions even a whole lobe.

Together with cavitation there is often evidence of bronchogenic spread to the rest of the same lobe or lung, and frequently to the opposite lung, especially to the lower half.

A tuberculous cavity itself, considered in isolation, has no radiographic features that can reliably differentiate between tuberculous, pyogenic, fungal or malignant cavities. However, when the characteristics of the cavity are considered together with the position, changes in the surrounding lung, evidence of bronchogenic spread and other radiographic features commonly found in post-primary pulmonary tuberculosis, a suggestion of tuberculosis can often be made with a considerable degree of confidence.

Fibrosis

Fibrosis is an integral part of the pathology of tuberculosis and when extensive tuberculosis heals, there may be widespread, gross, permanent fibrosis.

Fibrosis is characterized radiographically by dense, sharply defined, fine or coarse linear, curvi-linear or nodular opacities. There is usually accompanying loss of volume of a segment, lobe or lung. The loss of volume results in displacement of blood vessels, especially the main pulmonary arteries, fissures and trachea. Radiographically there is nothing to differentiate tuberculous from non-tuberculous fibrosis except that in and around an area of tuberculous fibrosis there may be specks or small nodules of calcification, and thickening of the adjacent pleura is a common finding.

Bronchogenic spread

Bronchogenic spread is a very common finding in post-primary pulmonary tuberculosis. It usually occurs when there is cavitation but may occur without radiographically demonstrable cavitation.

Bronchogenic spread manifests itself as areas of veiling or frank opacification which are usually poorly defined and tend to coalesce but which may be well defined and discrete. These opacities may be found scattered throughout one lobe, the whole of one lung, or both lungs. The lesions are often more obvious in the lower than the upper lung zones. A common presentation is a cavity in one upper lung zone with bronchogenic spread to the lower lung zone of the opposite lung.

Endobronchial tuberculosis

As part of bronchogenic spread tuberculous ulcers may form in any part of the tracheo-bronchial tree giving the post-primary form of endobronchial tuberculosis, which is different from the so-called endobronchial tuberculosis of primary pulmonary tuberculosis.

With healing, broncho-stenosis tends to develop and, when this involves a lobar or segmental bronchus, lobar or segmental collapse tends to occur. The degree of collapse due to broncho-stenosis may be much more severe than that caused by fibrosis, and it may occur with or without obvious radiographic abnormalities in the collapsed lobe. It is necessary to do bronchoscopy to rule out other causes of collapse, especially carcinoma of the bronchus.

Miliary tuberculosis

Haematogenous spread and consequent miliary tuberculosis is much less common in post-primary pulmonary tuberculosis than in primary pulmonary tuberculosis, but is not rare. The pathogenesis is the same as in primary tuberculosis but it occurs more frequently from an extra-thoracic focus. It may occur with or without other evidence of pulmonary tuberculosis. The whole wide spectrum of radiographic features of miliary tuberculosis is the same, irrespective of whether it is a complication of primary or of post-primary tuberculosis. Therefore, the description of miliary tuberculosis as given in the section on primary pulmonary tuberculosis will not be repeated here.

Miliary tuberculosis is traditionally so closely associated with primary pulmonary tuberculosis that there is a real danger that miliary tuberculosis as a complication of post-primary pulmonary tuberculosis may be overlooked in middle-aged or elderly people, especially when it presents with the less commonly found radiographic features.

No appreciable degree of lymphadenopathy

At postmortem a slight degree of hilar and/or mediastinal lymphadenopathy may be found in post-primary pulmonary tuberculosis but more often than not the lymph nodes are completely normal in size.[27] It is however a dictum which should be adhered to that radiographically detectable hilar and/or mediastinal lymphadenopathy is not found in post-primary pulmonary tuberculosis. From this it follows that if a patient, especially an adult or aged person, has pulmonary tuberculosis as well as hilar and/or mediastinal lymphadenopathy, then he or she is suffering from primary pulmonary tuberculosis, or from post-primary pulmonary tuberculosis *together* with another cause for the lymphadenopathy.

Chronicity

In post-primary pulmonary tuberculosis there is characteristically a continuous, long drawn-out battle between host and organism. This battle extends over years, with alternating periods of progression and of healing, and may result in a lobe or even a whole lung being severely damaged or completely destroyed.

Progression is characterized by the extension of parenchymal opacities, appearance of new opacities, an increase in size of existing cavities, formation of new cavities and the development of complications such as pneumothorax, pyopneumothorax, empyema, pleural effusion and haemorrhage.

Healing is characterized by the clearing of parenchymal opacities, the diminution in size and obliteration of cavities, and increasing fibrosis.

Sometimes there may be healing in one area of a lung while there is progression in another.

Characteristically the disease is chronic and the shifting in the line of battle occurs over a period of years. At times the course may be subacute, but with a considerable degree of progression or healing occurring within a month or two. Rarely the course may be acute, and fulminating with very marked progression within a few weeks from an inconspicuous opacity to opacification with cavitation involving half a lung. It is most unusual for there to be a marked degree of improvement within a few weeks.

This continuous interplay of progression and healing extending over months and years results in combinations of radiographic pictures which span an endless spectrum.

Bronchiectasis

Parenchymal destruction, fibrosis and damage to bronchi with or without bronchostenosis leads to bronchiectasis, which is a common complication of long-standing, quiescent or healed post-primary pulmonary tuberculosis.

A definitive diagnosis of bronchiectasis should not be made on conventional radiographs.

It should also be borne in mind that the radiographic features of bronchiectasis may simulate small cavities and that bronchiectasis may cause haemoptysis.

Pneumothorax, hydropneumothorax and pyopneumothorax

Pneumothorax is not an uncommon complication of post-primary pulmonary tuberculosis and usually occurs when there is extensive tuberculous pulmonary parenchymal damage. Rarely a so-called 'spontaneous' or 'simple' pneumothorax is found without any radiographically detectable pulmonary abnormality, but tuberculosis is diagnosed from histology of biopsy material at thoracotomy.[14] It is arguable whether such cases are examples of primary or post-primary pulmonary tuberculosis.

A tuberculous hydro-pneumothorax or tuberculous pyo-pneumothorax may develop as a complication of a tuberculous pneumothorax.

Pleural effusion and empyema

A protein-rich exudative pleural effusion with scanty inflammatory cells, such as is commonly found during the course of primary pulmonary tuberculosis, is a rare complication of post-primary pulmonary tuberculosis. When it is a complication of post-primary tuberculosis there are accompanying parenchymal pulmonary abnormalities. When a serous tuberculous pleural effusion occurs without parenchymal pulmonary abnormalities it should be regarded as a manifestation of primary tuberculosis.

A frank tuberculous empyema, such a rare complication of primary pulmonary tuberculosis, is a not uncommon complication of post-primary pulmonary tuberculosis. It usually occurs together with advanced parenchymal pulmonary abnormalities but may occur without them. A tuberculous empyema may occur with or without an accompanying broncho-pleural fistula and accompanying pneumothorax.

A tuberculous pleural effusion or empyema is usually unilateral but, very rarely, may be bilateral.

A late complication of a pleural effusion or empyema is localized or extensive pleural calcification.

Taken by themselves and in isolation there are no radiographic criteria which can differentiate tuberculous pneumothorax, hydro-pneumothorax, pleural effusion or empyema from their non-tuberculous counterparts.

Tuberculous pericarditis

Tuberculous pericarditis can occur as a complication of post-primary tuberculosis, and localized or extensive pericardial calcification with or without constrictive pericarditis may be found as a late residue.

Transitional pulmonary tuberculosis

In a minority of cases primary pulmonary tuberculosis progresses slowly and uninterruptedly over a period of months to reach a chronic destructive stage in which cavitation is a prominent feature. These cavities may develop in any segment of either lung. When a patient is seen for the first time in this stage without previous radiographs and when there is no knowledge of when tuberculin conversion occurred, it is often impossible to decide whether it is a case of primary or post-primary pulmonary tuberculosis. These cases are usually referred to as cases of 'progressive primary pulmonary tuberculosis' but, because of the uncertainty as to whether or not they are truly cases of primary pulmonary tuberculosis, they are perhaps better called cases of 'transitional pulmonary tuberculosis'.

The radiographic features of these cases are a combination and intermingling of the features of primary and post-primary pulmonary tuberculosis as already described.

Congenital and neonatal pulmonary tuberculosis

There are varying criteria, mainly pathological and environmental, for putting congenital and neonatal pulmonary tuberculosis in different categories but because they cannot be differentiated radiographically, they are grouped together in this chapter.

In congenital tuberculosis the infection is acquired in utero or during passage through the birth canal. Tubercle bacilli may gain access to the foetus by aspiration of infected liquor amnii or infected genital secretions, in which case tuberculous bronchopneumonic foci, usually together with hilar adenopathy, will result. Infection may also occur via the umbilical vein from the placenta, in which case primary foci develop in the liver with adenopathy in the porta hepatis and these cases may or may not show haematogenous spread to the lungs. Infection may also be acquired by ingestion of infected liquor amnii or infected genital secretions, in which case primary foci will be in the gastrointestinal tract with enlarged mesenteric glands which may or may not show haematogenous spread to the lungs. The mother, at the time of delivery, may have pulmonary, genital or disseminated tuberculosis but on rare occasions she may be symptom-free and without any clinical evidence of tuberculosis. Even examination of the placenta may fail to reveal evidence of tuberculosis.

In neonatal tuberculosis the infection is acquired immediately or shortly post-partum, usually from a heavily infective mother or member of the family but the duration of exposure may be as short as a few hours.

Congenital and neonatal pulmonary tuberculosis may present radiographically with multiple or innumerable confluent opacities giving a broncho-pneumonic pattern. It may also present with a miliary pattern, numerous nodular densities or large confluent densities. Rarely an opacity in one lobe may increase in size and spread to other lobes or to both lungs.[2] The radiographic patterns overlap and are non-specific, and may resemble pulmonary opacities from any other cause. Hilar and/or mediastinal lymphadenopathy is difficult to recognize in the neonate and in practice does not contribute significantly to the diagnosis.

Cases of congenital and neonatal pulmonary tuberculosis are rare but three such cases aged eight days, 14 days and 18 days respectively have been seen at Bellville's Tygerberg Hospital. In two cases tubercle bacilli were obtained from gastric washings and from tracheal aspiration in the third. In two of these patients the pulmonary opacities were best described as being bronchopneumonic in type and in one they were miliary in type. Enlarged hilar and/or mediastinal glands could not be detected.

The diagnosis of congenital or neonatal pulmonary tuberculosis is rarely made during life. An awareness of the condition and a diligent search for tubercle bacilli in any newborn who shows widespread pulmonary opacities, especially if the mother has tuberculosis or the baby is born in a tuberculous environment, will result in cases being diagnosed and treated.

PULMONARY TUBERCULOSIS IN HIGH RISK GROUPS

Resistance to tuberculosis may be lowered by many conditions which depress cell-mediated immunity. This results in the individual being at higher risk of developing tuberculosis, and it also alters the immune response to the tubercle bacillus and so changes the usual pathologic and radiographic features of the disease. All segments of the lungs now become more vulnerable, and post-primary pulmonary tuberculosis may commence in any pulmonary segment. The progression of tuberculosis is also altered and the disease process may be much more aggressive, acute and rapidly spreading. These high risk patients frequently show patterns of post-primary pulmonary tuberculosis which are infrequent in the general population.

As the incidence of tuberculosis in a community decreases, these high risk groups become of increasing importance.

The most important conditions which singly or in combination put people at high risk of developing post-primary pulmonary tuberculosis are silicosis, diabetes mellitus, alcoholism, old age, and AIDS.

The radiographic appearances of pulmonary tuberculosis in these conditions only will be considered, and it must be remembered that many other conditions such as poor living conditions, malnutrition, gastrectomy, intercurrent debilitating disease (especially malignant disease) and immunosuppressive and corticosteroid therapy make people more susceptible to pulmonary tuberculosis than the general population. For many reasons inmates of jails, especially alcoholics, are at very high risk.

Silicosis

There is increased susceptibility to tuberculosis in miners, especially those with silicosis. At the turn of the century tuberculosis was a scourge in South African gold miners and even today tuberculosis is still an important and common complication of silicosis.

The usual presentation of pulmonary tuberculosis in people with silicosis, as seen in South Africa, does not differ from that which is seen in non-silicotic subjects.[5, 25] Radiographically it may be difficult to differentiate between tuberculous and silicotic lesions. It is particularly difficult to differentiate between nodular or miliary tuberculosis and silicotic nodulation. According to Thomas[26] the greatest difficulty is with silicosis category 2/2 q/q. He states that if silicotic nodulation extends right up to the lung apices, one should always be suspicious of coexistent tuberculosis, or of nodular tuberculosis without silicosis.

It may also be difficult to differentiate between tuberculosis and progressive massive fibrosis, particularly if it is a unilateral lesion, 1 to 5 cm in diameter, in an upper lung zone.[26] According to Thomas[26] progressive massive fibrosis lesions in South African silicosis almost never break down, and such a cavitating lesion should be regarded as highly suspicious of tuberculosis or some other cavitating disease.

The radiographic features which should arouse suspicion of tuberculosis in a person exposed to silica with or without silicosis are: nodulation extending right up to one or both lung apices; a unilateral upper lung zone opacity; marked asymmetry of pulmonary lesions; and especially a cavitating lesion. The principle that should be adhered to is that in a silica-exposed person any pulmonary opacity which does not fit in well with the usual radiographic features of silicosis should make one highly suspicious of tuberculosis 'and even cases of apparently classic uncomplicated silicosis should have the sputum examined for tubercle bacilli at intervals'.[25]

It is also disturbing that active tuberculous lesions are occasionally found at autopsy in silicotic subjects who have shown no radiographic features suggestive of tuberculosis in life.[25]

Diabetes mellitus

Before the discovery of insulin and effective anti-tuberculous drugs, tuberculosis was a scourge of diabetics, and even today it is a rather frequent complication of diabetes.

The radiographic features of post-primary pulmonary tuberculosis in diabetics may be the same as that commonly seen in the general population, but certain features commonly seen in diabetics are less frequently or rarely seen in non-diabetics.

In diabetics cavitating tuberculosis confined to the lower lung fields is not uncommon.

Le Roux[15] states that cavitating pulmonary tuberculosis is common in diabetics and that the cavities can occur anywhere in the lungs (for example, the posterior basal segments of lower lobes, middle lobe or lingula) and that this 'perverse distribution of cavitating pulmonary tuberculosis' is common in Indian and black diabetics.

Marais from Bloemfontein[17] reported on seven black or coloured diabetics with tuberculosis. Two had involvement with cavitation in the lower lung fields only, while five had extensive involvement of all lung fields.

Further afield Weaver in Atlanta, Georgia[28] reported that four out of 20 adult patients with pulmonary tuberculosis and diabetes had involvement of the lower lobes only. In an additional patient, only the right middle lobe was involved. Only one of 182 non-diabetic patients with pulmonary tuberculosis had involvement only of the lower lobes. She advises that 'in adult patients found to have lower lobe tuberculosis, diabetes should be strongly suspected'.

Alcoholism

Post-primary pulmonary tuberculosis is common in chronic alcoholics. In this population group there are many factors that favour the development and progression of tuberculosis and mitigate against effective treatment, such as poor nutrition, overcrowding, intercurrent illness, neglect of symptoms, non-compliance with treatment and probably many more. The effect of alcohol itself cannot therefore be unravelled and no features peculiar to tuberculosis in alcoholics can be identified, except that by the time the diagnosis is made, the pulmonary involvement is usually at a sadly advanced stage, that there is poor response to treatment, and that relapse and progression are common.

Old age

In South Africa pulmonary tuberculosis in children and adolescents is still distressingly common, but at the same time post-primary pulmonary tuberculosis and, to a lesser extent, primary pulmonary tuberculosis are becoming increasingly frequent in older age groups. In 1988 Morris and Nell[19] reported the prevalence of pulmonary tuberculosis in residents of old-age homes in East London. An alarmingly high incidence of 798 per 100 000 for whites and 10 344 per 100 000 for coloureds was found against a nationwide incidence of 16 per 100 000 for whites. Elderly people, especially men, living in old age homes face a particularly high risk of developing tuberculosis.[19]

In South Africa the vast majority of cases of pulmonary tuberculosis in the aged are of post-primary tuberculosis due to reactivation of a primary infection of decades ago or are due to flare up of a post-primary infection which has been quiescent.

In some rare instances, cases of primary pulmonary tuberculosis occur even in the seventh and eighth decades.

Primary pulmonary tuberculosis at this age is most likely a true primary infection, but there is a possibility that some may be cases where the immune system has lost its memory of the primary infection of decades ago and that re-introduction of tubercle bacilli then results in a second primary infection.

'Unusual' or 'atypical' radiographic features of pulmonary tuberculosis in adults and the aged have been described.[11, 12, 18, 19, 22, 30] Many of the described cases are of primary tuberculosis occurring in old age and the radiographic features are quite usual for primary pulmonary tuberculosis and can only be regarded as 'unusual' or 'atypical' if measured by the standards applicable to post-primary pulmonary tuberculosis. Because primary tuberculosis in the aged is

rare and the radiographic features are similar to those in younger age groups, the rest of this section will be devoted to post-primary tuberculosis.

In the aged the clinical and the radiographic spectrum of post-primary pulmonary tuberculosis is even wider than in younger age groups. The traditional teaching that a common source of tuberculosis in an extended family is a grandfather with 'chronic bronchitis' who is not obviously ill and whose chest radiograph shows no obvious abnormality is still true.

The radiographic changes of post-primary pulmonary tuberculosis in the aged may be the same as those frequently found at any other age. However, many of the changes that are frequently seen in the aged are rarely seen in younger people and are often not suggestive of active pulmonary tuberculosis. The following radiographic features in the aged should suggest a serious possibility of active pulmonary tuberculosis:

- linear, nodular or irregular opacities, suggestive of fibrotic changes, anywhere in the lung fields;
- streaky densities with or without tubular or round areas of increased translucency in the lower lung fields suggestive of bronchiectasis;
- ill-defined, patchy densities in one or both lower lung fields or widespread throughout one or both lungs suggestive of bronchopneumonia;
- an irregular ill-defined or sharply defined opacity anywhere in the lung field, but especially in an upper lung zone, suggestive of carcinoma of the bronchus;
- miliary or nodular opacities evenly or unevenly distributed throughout the lung fields, or even a suspicion of miliary shadowing.

Haematogenous spread of tuberculosis in the elderly is not uncommon and such patients may have normal chest radiographs and the diagnosis may first be made at autopsy.

Rarely no radiographic abnormality can be detected in spite of the fact that sputum is smear and culture positive for tubercle bacilli.

Morris and Nell[19] have reported on 12 tuberculotic inmates of geriatric homes: one had a normal chest radiograph; one had apical confluent densities with cavitation typical of post-primary pulmonary tuberculosis; while 'in ten there were basal inflammatory infiltrates or patchy fibrotic changes (in one a small pleural effusion was present)'.

Pulmonary tuberculosis in the aged often lurks unsuspected and may be found together with other diseases. Any unexplained radiographic abnormality in the lungs of old people, however bizarre and in whatever pulmonary segment, should lead to a diligent search for previous chest radiographs which may hold a clue as to the diagnosis, to repeated sputum examinations and to serial radiography.

AIDS

Because of their depressed cellular, and to a lesser extent humoral, immunity, patients with AIDS are at high risk of developing infections by opportunistic organisms as well as by ordinary pathogens and of developing pulmonary neoplasms. Pulmonary infections, due to whatever organism, and neoplasms, of whatever nature, may occur concurrently and their individual radiographic features can usually not be unravelled.

Patients with AIDS are at high risk of developing mycobacterial infections. In the United States it has been stated[20] that about 10 per cent will develop infection with *Mycobacterium tuberculosis* and about 20 per cent with mycobacteria other than tuberculosis (MOTT) especially *Mycobacterium avium-intracellularae*. Such infection may occur before, at the time of, or after the diagnosis of AIDS has been made.

The presentation, clinical course and radiographic findings of mycobacterial infections in patients with AIDS are different from those commonly found in patients without AIDS.

Radiographic features of pulmonary mycobacterial infections in AIDS patients in South Africa have not been well documented. The findings to be described in this section have been obtained from the literature, especially that of the United States.[7, 16,] [20, 23] These findings will probably hold good for South Africa, but as experience is gained they may have to be changed.

Because of the depressed cell-mediated immunity, reactivation of a long dormant infection or the occurrence of a true second reinfection gives the picture of primary pulmonary tuberculosis rather than of post-primary pulmonary tuberculosis.

In the general population the radiographic features of infection with MOTT are indistinguishable from those seen in post-primary pulmonary tuberculosis, but there is no pattern comparable to that seen in primary pulmonary tuberculosis. In patients with AIDS, infection with MOTT can give hilar and/or mediastinal lymphadenopathy with or without opacities localized to mid- and lower lung fields reminiscent of primary pulmonary tuberculosis. The radiographic features of all stages of pulmonary infection with *Mycobacterium tuberculosis* and MOTT in patients with AIDS are indistinguishable and are here considered together.

Hilar and/or mediastinal lymphadenopathy, sometimes of marked degree, is common and may occur with or without pulmonary parenchymal opacities. Bilateral hilar adenopathy is not uncommon.

The pulmonary parenchymal opacities may be small and diffusely distributed or may be large and localized and may involve a whole lobe or lobes. These opacities are often localized to the mid and lower lung fields. Opacities localized to upper lung zones are extremely rare. It is very rare for these opacities to undergo cavitation. When these opacities clear up, as they often do on treatment, there is no residual fibrosis.

A miliary pulmonary pattern may be seen but sometimes miliary spread is found at autopsy without pre-mortem evidence of it on a chest radiograph.

Pleural effusions are not frequent and tend to be small. A pericardial effusion may develop. Disseminated infection with extra-pulmonary involvement is common (especially so with MOTT) and may occur without radiologically detectable pulmonary abnormalities. Patients may have positive sputum cultures for mycobacteria even though their chest radiographs show no detectable abnormalities.

The pulmonary radiographic features of mycobacterial infections in AIDS patients are non-specific and non-suggestive and may even be absent. Because infection with *Mycobacterium tuberculosis* responds well to treatment, every effort should be made to diagnose or exclude tuberculosis in patients with AIDS.

As more experience is gained with mycobacterial infections in HIV positive patients with varying degrees of suppression of immunity, a rational picture will probably emerge. The author would postulate a scenario similar to that which follows.

There will be a wide spectrum of radiographic appearances which will overlap and intertwine, and which will correlate roughly with the degree of suppression of immunity.

At one end of the spectrum there will be patients with a mild degree of immune suppression, and they will show increased susceptibility to infection with *Mycobacterium tuberculosis*. Their radiographic features will be similar to those seen in the general population.

At the other end of the spectrum will be patients with the most severe degree of suppression of immunity. They will show an increased susceptibility to infection with all species of mycobacteria, and especially non-tuberculous mycobacteria. Those infected with *M. tuberculosis*, whether they have a primary infection, reactivation of a previous infection or a true re-infection, will show the radiographic features of primary tuberculosis with particularly prominent intrathoracic lymphadenopathy and an increased incidence of disseminated tuberculosis. Those infected with non-tuberculous mycobacteria will show intrathoracic lymphadenopathy with or without any opacities in the mid- and lower- lungfields, reminiscent of primary tuberculosis.

Those with intermediate degrees of immunity suppression will show an increased incidence of infection with *M. tuberculosis* and non-tuberculous mycobacteria. They will show features similar to post-primary tuberculosis in the general population. The pulmonary opacities will, however, tend not to cavitate, will be more widespread and may be confined to the mid- and lower- lungfields; there will be less tendency to fibrosis and an increased tendency towards extra-thoracic spread.

With the increasing prevalence of HIV positive patients it may become prudent to test all patients with mycobacterial infection for HIV infection.

PULMONARY TUBERCULOMA

This refers to a chronic tuberculous focus containing a variable amount of caseous material, with or without calcification, surrounded by a fibrous capsule. It may arise during the course of primary or post-primary pulmonary tuberculosis.

Such a tuberculoma is usually an incidental finding on a chest radiograph, and may be detected at any age from childhood to old age but is rare in children. It can occur in any pulmonary segment but is more frequent in the upper lung zones.

A tuberculoma is usually a solitary mass lesion but two or three and on rare occasions more may be found, in which case they are commonly grouped in close proximity. It is usually a smoothly round or oval or slightly lobulated sharply circumscribed mass 0,5 to 4 cm or even more in diameter. It may be poorly defined and a case has been seen with a spiculated outline most suggestive of carcinoma.

Areas of calcification within or in the vicinity of the lesion are often found.

Small discrete nodules or irregularly shaped shadows (so-called 'satellite' lesions) in the immediate vicinity of the lesion are found in up to 80 per cent of cases.[9] Fibrotic strands near the lesion or in the upper lung are commonly found.

A tuberculoma may remain unchanged for many years, may become smaller and more densely calcified over a period of years, or may break down, spread and cavitate.

The differential diagnosis is that of any mass lesion, and in this respect comparison with previous radiographs is of paramount importance. Although a combination of clinical and radiographic data may suggest the diagnosis of tuberculoma a definitive diagnosis can only be made by obtaining material for histological and bacteriological examination.

PULMONARY TUBERCULOSIS AND CARCINOMA OF THE BRONCHUS

The co-existence of pulmonary tuberculosis, active or quiescent, and carcinoma of the bronchus is not uncommon. Both conditions are common in South Africa and in most cases the association is probably purely coincidental, but there may well be a cause and effect relationship.

A so-called 'scar' carcinoma may develop in an old fibrotic tuberculous lesion in a patient with or without current active pulmonary tuberculosis. This concept is currently losing ground because the scar in many so called 'scar carcinomas' may be the result rather than the cause of the carcinoma.[27]

Carcinoma of the bronchus developing independently, or as scar carcinoma, may invade quiescent tuberculous foci and reactivate them, giving rise to active pulmonary tuberculosis. Carcinoma of the bronchus may also cause debilitation and decreased resistance so that reactivation of tuberculosis may occur.

The finding of tubercle bacilli does not rule out a co-existent carcinoma of the bronchus.

Because of the wide spectrum of radiographic abnormalities that may be found in both post-primary pulmonary tuberculosis and in carcinoma of the bronchus, it is often difficult on radiographic grounds alone to differentiate one from the other. Where both occur together the diagnostic difficulty is compounded.

It is important always to bear in mind that pulmonary tuberculosis, either quiescent or active, may co-exist with carcinoma of the bronchus. The progression of radiographic shadows, or the appearance of new shadows in a person known to have or to have had pulmonary tuberculosis, may be due to carcinoma of the bronchus and not to flare up of old tuberculosis or non-response to anti-tuberculous drugs. The following clues to the possibility that the two conditions might exist together, should be diligently sought:

- the appearance of a new radiographic shadow in a patient who is under treatment for pulmonary tuberculosis, and where the previously known tuberculous lesions are responding satisfactorily to treatment should seriously raise the possibility of carcinoma of the bronchus. This becomes even more likely if the new shadow is very dense and occurs in an anterior or basal segment or in the middle lobe or lingula;
- the appearance of lobar collapse in a patient with pulmonary tuberculosis should lead to bronchoscopy;
- the appearance of a hilar mass or hilar and/or mediastinal lymphadenopathy during the course of post-primary pulmonary tuberculosis should seriously raise suspicion of a carcinoma of the bronchus;
- in a patient with tuberculosis, whether quiescent or active, a sharply circumscribed opacity or a shadow that is homogeneously dense may be a tuberculoma but should suggest carcinoma of the bronchus;
- a thick walled cavity with a rugged interior surface may be a tuberculous cavity but is more likely to be carcinoma of the bronchus and should be further investigated with this provisional diagnosis in mind;
- the development of a pleural effusion during treatment for pulmonary tuberculosis should point to carcinoma of the bronchus rather than to non-response to treatment;
- paralysis of a diaphragm or destruction of a rib should indicate carcinoma of the bronchus rather than tuberculosis;
- clinically, in a patient with tuberculosis, the development of finger clubbing, chest pain and a persistent rhonchus should raise the suspicion of carcinoma of the bronchus.

PULMONARY TUBERCULOSIS AS AN UNEXPECTED DIAGNOSIS ('UNUSUAL' OR 'ATYPICAL' FEATURES OF PULMONARY TUBERCULOSIS)

The radiographic features of pulmonary tuberculosis stretch over an endless spectrum. The pattern of the disease depends on the interplay between organism and host and may be modified by dose of organisms, age, nutritional status, race, living conditions, alcoholism, immunological status, diabetes, silicosis and probably a host of other factors. The frequency with which the numerous different radiographic patterns of pulmonary tuberculosis is seen depends largely on patient selection and the frequency varies between patients seen in general practice, a general hospital, a teaching hospital, a tuberculosis clinic, a tuberculosis sanatorium, a creche, an old age home, and so on. Features which may be common in one setting may well be uncommon in another. What may be regarded as 'unusual', 'uncommon' or 'atypical' features of pulmonary tuberculosis is usually due to patient selection, lack of experience of the clinician or radiologist or preconceived ideas, rather than a deviation from the wide spectrum of radiographic presentation of pulmonary tuberculosis.

Even amongst clinicians with wide experience of pulmonary tuberculosis, the finding of tubercle bacilli may come unexpectedly under the following conditions:

- a chest radiograph on which no radiographic abnormality can be detected;
- pulmonary parenchymal opacities which appear, progress or clear rapidly in weeks rather than months;
- radiographic changes suggestive of carcinoma of the bronchus and where carcinoma has been proved by bronchoscopy and biopsy;
- a spontaneous pneumothorax with no radiographically detectable abnormality in the lung;
- insignificant, non-specific, streaky opacities in one or both lower lobes;
- a big, dense opacity in which there is a fluid-containing cavity with an irregular wall and no abnormality in the rest of the lungs;
- bizarre pulmonary parenchymal abnormalities which are difficult to correlate with the generally accepted pathological changes of pulmonary tuberculosis;
- one or more well- or poorly-circumscribed homogeneously dense opacities which do not contain any calcification in otherwise normal lungs;
- widespread diffuse alveolar opacities throughout both lungs, resembling shock lung;
- widespread extensive destruction of one whole lung with a combination of cavities, bronchiectasis and fibrosis, but with the other lung radiographically normal.

PULMONARY NON-TUBERCULOUS MYCOBACTERIAL DISEASES

Non-tuberculous mycobacteria (mycobacteria other than tuberculosis, MOTT), of which *M. kansassii*, *M. avium-intracellularae*, *M. scrofulaceum* and *M. xenopi* are the most common, occur widely in nature, in soil and on fodder.

As saprophytes they may colonize the oro-pharyngo-tracheo-bronchial system of normal asymptomatic people or of people with pre-existing pulmonary diseases, such as chronic bronchitis, emphysema, bronchiectasis, pneumoconiosis or pulmonary fibrosis. They may be cultured from the secretions of the respiratory tract of people without any evidence of tissue invasion. Kleeberg[13] reported that 'from the 8 850 sputum samples collected randomly, mostly from healthy African adults, 604 strains of MOTT were cultured, a fact indicating a prevalence of seven per cent' and that '10 per cent of African children react specifically to avium PPD tuberculin'.

These usually saprophytic organisms may become pathogens and invade tissue, usually when there is reduced local resistance as a result of structural lung damage or when there is reduced general resistance due to depressed cell-mediated immunity. On rare occasions they invade apparently healthy individuals. Culture of MOTT from tracheo-bronchial secretions does not mean that the patient is suffering from disease produced by these bacteria. Strict criteria, on which there is unfortunately not universal agreement, are necessary to differentiate between saprophytic colonization and pathologic invasion by these organisms.

The transmission and pathogenesis of MOTT infection is not clear. These organisms may cause a disease state similar to post-primary pulmonary tuberculosis but they do not cause a disease state comparable to primary pulmonary tuberculosis.

While MOTT abound in South Africa, disease produced by these organisms is very rare. Nel *et al.*[21] reported five cases in South African miners. Kleeberg[13] stated that 'a conservative estimate is that 0,004 per cent of lung tuberculosis [in South Africa] is caused by non-tuberculous mycobacteria'. He also stated that 'at the Tuberculosis Research Institute, Pretoria, cases of true mycobacteriosis were proved only 19 times in the past 15 years'. As recently as September 1988 Plit, Woolf and Miller[24] stated that 'reports of non-tuberculous mycobacterial disease of the lung [in South Africa] are sparse', and they could find only three confirmed and seven possible cases among patients with pulmonary tuberculosis referred for treatment to the Rietfontein Hospital over a five year period.

The incidence of infection by *Mycobacterium tuberculosis* in South Africa as a whole is decreasing and it may well be that, as the incidence decreases, the incidence of infection by MOTT will rise as is currently happening in developed countries.[3]

In South Africa there should be an increased awareness of the possibility of pulmonary infection by MOTT and the 1980 statement by Fourie *et al.*[8] that 'there is no evidence that non-tuberculous mycobacterial infections present any health threat to the Xhosa of Transkei despite appreciable exposure' needs to be reassessed.

Although disease produced by MOTT is indistinguishable from post-primary pulmonary tuberculosis on clinical, histological and radiographic grounds, there are differences in the incidence of certain radiographic features. The following radiographic features are more commonly found in infection with MOTT than in infection with *M. tuberculosis*:[1, 3, 4, 29]

- a small thin-walled cavity or multiple thin-walled cavities with little or no surrounding reaction;
- cavities in lower lung fields;
- a solitary opacity in a lower lobe, middle lobe or lingula;
- multiple patchy nodular opacities in upper and lower lung fields without upper lobe preponderance.

Mycobacterial infections other than tuberculosis are often resistant to treatment, and under treatment the pulmonary abnormalities may remain unchanged or may even spread.

Pre-existing pulmonary disease, especially emphysema, chronic bronchitis and pneumoconiosis is said to be more common in MOTT infection than in tuberculosis.

The following radiographic findings are more common in post-primary pulmonary tuberculosis than in MOTT infections: cavities larger than 5 cm in diameter; thick walled cavities; pleural effusions; empyema; and haematogenous spread.

Statistically these differences are valid but in any individual patient it is impossible to differentiate between post-primary pulmonary tuberculosis and infection due to MOTT on radiographic, clinical or pathological grounds.

ASSESSMENT OF ACTIVITY

As a general rule activity should not be assessed radiographically — certainly not on a single radiograph — and not even on a series of radiographs stretching over years. However, at the extremes of the spectrum of activity a radiographic assessment of activity may be made with some confidence.

A cavity in an area of opacification or with surrounding alveolar opacities can usually be regarded with confidence as a sign of activity. Very rarely a cavity may become sterilized, acquire an epithelial lining and persist, so that even a cavity by itself does not invariably indicate activity.

Dense, sharply defined linear strand-like opacities with displacement of vessels, bronchi and fissures indicating a long standing fibrotic change, with or without scattered calcified foci usually indicate chronic fibro-calcific non-active tuberculosis. Tubercle bacilli may rarely be cultured from such a lesion which may flare up at any time, so that even these radiographic findings do not always indicate inactivity.

If activity cannot be accurately judged radiographically even at the extremes of the spectrum, so much the less can it be judged between the extremes.

In the routine follow-up of patients under treatment for tuberculosis, or in patients with quiescent tuberculosis, radiographs should be taken at long intervals of time. Each new radiograph should be compared with all previous radiographs and especially with the first radiograph of the series. It is then usually possible to determine whether the situation is improving or regressing. Rarely it may be found that while improvement can be seen in one area, regression is occurring in another. Sometimes no apparent radiographic change may take place for many months, even though the patient shows satisfactory clinical improvement.

The determination of activity of pulmonary tuberculosis is a bacteriological, laboratory and clinical exercise rather than a radiographic exercise.

Radiographically it cannot be determined whether a lesion has healed, and it should not be reported as such for any lesion may flare up at any time. Categoric statements that a lesion is active, inactive, quiescent or healed should not be made. Statements such as 'old, chronic fibro-calcific tuberculosis' should be used with caution as they may be taken to imply a healed, inactive lesion.

It is suggested that radiographic opinions on activity be limited to one of the following statements:

- 'must be regarded as active';
- 'probably active';
- 'radiographically stable or unchanged';
- 'activity indeterminate';
- 'probably inactive'.

'Inactive' or 'healed' should never be reported.

SPECIAL IMAGING TECHNIQUES
Apical-lordotic, reversed apical and oblique views

These simple techniques are of considerable value in the better demonstration and localization of questionable lesions, especially in upper lung zones.

High kilovoltage radiography

This is very useful for showing bronchi narrowed by enlarged lymph nodes, especially in children.

Conventional tomography

This is a very useful technique for demonstrating suspicious lesions and for better defining and evaluating opacities, cavities, calcifications, bronchi and questionable mycetomas.

Bronchography

In the context of tuberculosis, bronchography is limited to the demonstration of compression or occlusion of bronchi by glands, the demonstration of broncho-stenosis or bronchiectasis, and occasionally to outline an intracavitary mycetoma. It is becoming outdated and should rarely be used.

Fluoroscopy

Fluoroscopy is very seldom necessary in the work-up of a patient with tuberculosis and should be reserved for the demonstration of the mobility of thoracic and intra-thoracic structures, and as an aid during a variety of diagnostic techniques such as bronchoscopy, bronchography and needle biopsy of pleura or lung.

Computerized tomography

Computerized tomography is rarely called for in the work up of a patient with tuberculosis, but it is very useful for demonstrating enlarged lymph nodes, evaluating a questionable mycetoma, localizing encapsulated pleural effusions, and evaluating suspected bronchiectasis.

Ultrasonography

The use of ultrasonography in tuberculosis is limited to the demonstration of pleural and pericardial effusions.

Magnetic resonance imaging

Currently magnetic resonance imaging plays no role in the work-up of a patient with tuberculosis.

CONCLUSIONS

Radiographically pulmonary tuberculosis may simulate almost any pulmonary disease and it may occur concurrently with any other disease. The diagnosis of pulmonary tuberculosis is usually suggested by changes found on a radiograph of the chest. Under ideal conditions a definitive diagnosis of pulmonary tuberculosis should only be made by the isolation of *Mycobacterium tuberculosis.* In practice this is not always possible, especially in primary pulmonary tuberculosis and in the early stages of post-primary pulmonary tuberculosis. A diagnosis must then be made, and acted upon, by correlating the radiographic findings with the clinical picture, risk of infection in the environment, presence of high risk factors, skin tests, histological examination of biopsy material and response to treatment. Conventional radiography remains of great value in the diagnosis and management of pulmonary tuberculosis.

The radiographic features of pulmonary tuberculosis are so many that a workable classification has been given to help in the interpretation of the innumerable radiographic patterns. Some of these patterns or combinations of patterns are so suggestive of pulmonary tuberculosis that the diagnosis may be suggested with a considerable degree of confidence. However, some of the patterns are so non-suggestive that an eventual diagnosis of tuberculosis comes as a surprise. Those who only diagnose pulmonary tuberculosis when the radiographic features are suggestive will under-diagnose. Those who regard all radiographic abnormalities, however bizarre, as indicative of pulmonary tuberculosis, will over-diagnose. It is debatable what does more harm to the patient and the community: over-diagnosis with consequent unnecessary treatment and delay in making the right diagnosis, or under-diagnosis with delay in instituting effective treatment and allowing the disease to spread in the patient and in the community. The art lies in striking a healthy balance between over-and under-diagnosis.

With its infinite variety of clinical, radiographic and pathological features and with the problems associated with demonstrating the tubercle bacillus, pulmonary tuberculosis keeps the clinician, pathologist, microbiologist and especially the radiologist humble.

REFERENCES

1 Albelda S M *et al.*, 1985. Expanding spectrum of pulmonary disease caused by nontuberculous Mycobacteria. *Radiology.* 157, 289–96.

2 Amick F E *et al.*, 1950. Congenital tuberculosis. *Pediatrics.* 6, 384–90.

3 Anderson D H *et al.*, 1975. Pulmonary lesions due to opportunist mycobacteria. *Clinical Radiology.* 26, 461–9.

4 Christensen E E *et al.*, 1981. Initial roentgenographic manifestations of pulmonary Mycobacterium tuberculosis. *M. kansasii* and *M. intracellularis* infections. *Chest.* 80, 132–6.

5 Cowie R L, 1989. Ernest Oppenheimer Hospital, Welkom. Personal communication.

6 Donald P R, Ball J B & Burger P J, 1985. Bacteriologically confirmed pulmonary tuberculosis in childhood. *South African Medical Journal.* 67, 588–90.

7 Federle M P, 1988. A radiologist looks at AIDS: imaging evaluation based on symptom complexes. *Radiology.* 166, 553–62.

8 Fourie P B *et al.*, 1980. Follow-up tuberculosis prevalence survey of Transkei. *Tubercle* 61, 71–9

9 Fraser R G & Paré J A P, 1978. *Diagnosis of Diseases of the Chest.* London: W B Saunders.

10 Freiman I, Geefhuysen J & Solomon A, 1975. The radiological presentation of pulmonary tuberculosis in children. *South African Medical Journal.* 49, 1703–6.

11 Hadlock F P *et al.*, 1980. Unusual radiographic findings in adult pulmonary tuberculosis. *American Journal of Roentgenology.* 134, 1015–8.

12 Khan M A *et al.*, 1977. Clinical and roentgenographic spectrum of pulmonary tuberculosis in the adult. *American Journal of Medicine.* 62, 31–8.

13 Kleeberg H H, 1981. Epidemiology of mycobacteria other than tubercle bacilli in South Africa. *Review of Infectious Diseases.* 3, 1008–12.

14 Le Roux B T, 1982. Pulmonary tuberculosis as a present-day thoracic surgical problem. *South African Medical Journal.* Spec. ed. 17 Nov. 1982, 24–5.

15 Le Roux B T, 1989. University of Natal, Durban. Personal communication.

16 Louie E L, Rice L B & Holzman R S, 1986. Tuberculosis in non-Haitian patients with acquired immunodeficiency syndrome. *Chest.* 90, 542–5.

17 Marais R M, 1980. Diabetes mellitus in black and coloured tuberculosis patients. *South African Medical Journal.* 57, 483–4.
18 Miller W T & MacGregor R R, 1978. Tuberculosis: frequency of unusual radiographic findings. *American Journal of Roentgenology.* 130, 867–75.
19 Morris C D W & Nell H, 1988. Epidemic of pulmonary tuberculosis in geriatric homes. *South African Medical Journal.* 74, 117–20.
20 Naidich D P *et al.,* 1987. Radiographic manifestations of pulmonary disease in the acquired immunodeficiency syndrom (AIDS). *Seminars in Roentgenology.* 22, 14–30.
21 Nel E E *et al.,* 1977. Pulmonary disease associated with Mycobacteria other than tubercle bacilli in miners. *South African Medical Journal.* 51, 779–83.
22 Palmer, P E S, 1979. Pulmonary tuberculosis — usual and unusual radiographic presentations. *Seminars in Roentgenology.* 14, 204–43.
23 Pitchenik A E & Robinson H A, 1985. The radiographic appearance of tuberculosis in patients with the acquired immune deficiency syndrome (AIDS) and pre-AIDS. *American Review of Respiratory Diseases.* 131, 393–6.
24 Plit M L, Woolf M, Miller G B, 1988. Pulmonary non-tuberculous mycobacterial disease. *South African Medical Journal.* 74, 217–9.
25 Solomon A & Kreel L, 1989. *Radiology of Occupational Chest Disease.* Springer-Verlag.
26 Thomas R G, 1989. The Rand Mutual Hospital, Johannesburg. Personal communication.
27 Van der Walt, J J, 1989. Tygerberg Hospital and University of Stellenbosch. Personal communication.
28 Weaver R A, 1974. Unusual radiographic presentation of pulmonary tuberculosis in diabetic patients. *American Review of Respiratory Diseases.* 109, 162–3.
29 Wiot J F & Spitz H B, 1973. Atypical pulmonary tuberculosis. *Radiological Clinics of North America.* 11, 191–6.
30 Woodring J H, 1986. Update: the radiographic features of pulmonary tuberculosis. *American Journal of Roentgenology.* 146; 497–506.

CHAPTER 14

Immunological aspects of the host response to *Mycobacterium tuberculosis* infection

G M Ainslie and E D Bateman

INTRODUCTION

Mycobacteria, like other intracellular organisms, survive and thrive in host tissues by subverting mechanisms that are designed to kill them. This may be viewed as a form of parasitism, albeit failed, because untreated a significant proportion of infected hosts will die.

Mycobacterium tuberculosis is a master of disguise, having a complex cell wall with molecules in different layers that are capable of inducing a variety of tissue responses. As will be described, some of these provoke the production of antibodies that are ineffective in the elimination of the organism, others are directly toxic to host cells or initiate mechanisms which suppress the immune response, while a third group establishes cell-mediated tissue-destructive delayed hypersensitivity. Finally, the most significant group of antigens are those that induce host protective or anti-mycobacterial responses.

It is reasonable to question the relevance of studying the immunology of tuberculosis when the pressing need is to implement control and treatment programmes. Several benefits may be cited, and these are listed in Table 14.1. They show that an improved understanding of immunological mechanisms potentially impacts upon many aspects of patient care.

In this chapter, we focus upon the recruitment of host defences after infection with mycobacteria, and their link with the observed pathology. Then we summarize current views of the role of individual cell types in tuberculous immunity (monocyte/macrophages, T and B lymphocytes, natural killer cells and neutrophils), and the role of heat shock protein, tumour necrosis factor and vitamin D. Also discussed is the current understanding of the relationship between cell-mediated protection and delayed hypersensitivity, of anergy and suppressor mechanisms, and of important immune regulatory or modifying factors. These issues provide a backdrop for understanding new approaches to the diagnosis and treatment of this disease.

THE LINK BETWEEN NATURAL HISTORY OF INFECTION AND IMMUNITY

Primary infection and 'innate' immunity (Figure 14.1)

Primary infection occurs when a previously unexposed host inhales respirable particles called droplet nuclei in which mycobacteria are suspended.[10] The first cells that the organisms encounter are resident phagocytic cells of the lower respiratory tract — neutrophils and naive non-activated alveolar macrophages. After phagocytosis organisms remain viable intracellularly, and replicate.[32] Whether or not this encounter progresses to the so-called primary infection depends on the dose and virulence of the organism,[15] and the efficiency with which the phagocytes deal with them. The latter is termed 'innate resistance' or immunity and is influenced by genetics, age and sex.

Table 14.1
Practical value of understanding the immunology of tuberculosis

GOAL	PHENOMENON	COMMENT
Diagnosis	Tuberculin reaction	Improved interpretation of reactions and anergy.
	Serum antibodies to mycobacterial antigens.	A large number of mycobacterial antigens are being tested (e.g. ELISA technique) and are nearing clinical usefulness for diagnosing infection and/or disease.
	Detection of mycobacterial antigens in blood, body fluids and tissues.	Promising progress is being made, particularly for body fluids e.g. CSF. Detection of DNA by molecular biologic methods, e.g. polymerase chain reaction, is most sensitive and potentially useful.
Prophylaxis	Recognition of risk of infection	Targeted prophylaxis may be practised with the understanding of genetic factors and the nature of risk in AIDS, protein malnutrition and drug-induced immunosuppression.
Treatment	Fulminating disease, adult respiratory distress syndrome and worsening after initiation of treatment.	Treatment should be aimed at reduction of tissue-destructive effects of excessive delayed hypersensitivity and release of tumour necrosis factor (TNF).
	Need for adjuncts to treatment	The basis for the value of vitamin D, iron, magnesium and an adequate protein intake is being understood.
	Enhancing elimination of mycobacteria.	Specific immunomodulation of the 'protective' antimycobacterial mechanisms is becoming a possibility.

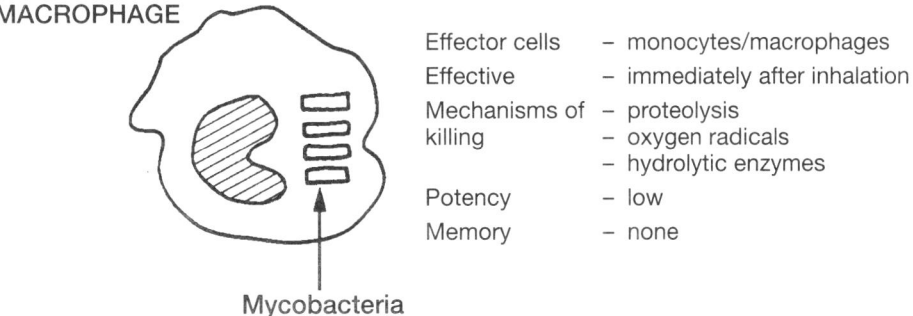

MACROPHAGE

Effector cells — monocytes/macrophages
Effective — immediately after inhalation
Mechanisms of — proteolysis
killing — oxygen radicals
— hydrolytic enzymes
Potency — low
Memory — none

Mycobacteria

Figure 14.1. Innate immunity.

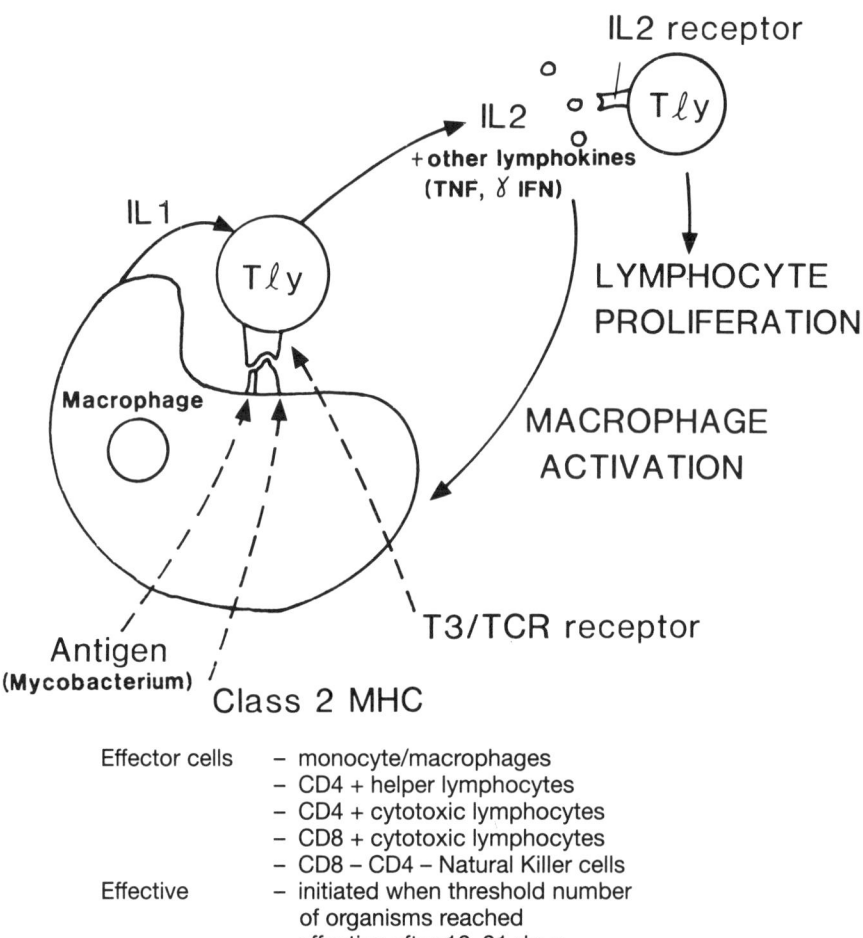

Effector cells	– monocyte/macrophages
	– CD4 + helper lymphocytes
	– CD4 + cytotoxic lymphocytes
	– CD8 + cytotoxic lymphocytes
	– CD8 – CD4 – Natural Killer cells
Effective	– initiated when threshold number of organisms reached
	– effective after 10–21 days
Mechanisms of killing	– proteolysis
	– oxygen radicals
	– cytolysis
Potency	– great
Memory	– long-lived CD4 + memory cells

Figure 14.2. Specific acquired immunity. Legend:

T ly	= T lymphocytes;		γIFN	=	Gamma interferon
IL1	= Interleukin 1;		T3	=	CD3
IL2	= Interleukin 2;		TCR	=	T cell receptor
TNF	= Tumour necrosis factor;		MHC	=	Major histocompatibility complex

Primary disease and 'specific acquired' immunity

An effective 'specific acquired immune response' is only mounted when organisms proliferate and reach a critical 'threshold' number at the primary site — 10^4 colony forming units (CFUs) in guinea pigs and 10^7 in murine lungs.[11] From this primary site, organisms are transported within phagocytes, via lymphatics, to regional lymph nodes. During a silent bacteraemia organisms seed to other parts of the lungs and all over the body. Specific acquired immunity develops over the next few weeks in all these areas, including the regional lymph nodes. This determines whether tuberculous 'disease' will develop. In 85 to 95 per cent of persons the organisms in all locations are contained or killed,[14] the risk of progression to disease being highest early in the first year after infection. The risk decreases over years, but as many of the organisms are not killed but remain dormant in old foci (especially lung upper zones), a risk (less than five per cent) of reactivation and progression remains. This occurs when the host immunity becomes depressed by malnutrition, other disease and drugs.[10]

Several steps are involved in the development of specific acquired cell-mediated immunity (see Figure 14.2). Tubercle bacilli in regional lymph nodes and elsewhere are engulfed by macrophages, partially degraded, and their antigens 'processed'. These latter are 'presented' to T lymphocytes, of which antigen-specific clones proliferate by a complex series of mechanisms (described in detail later). Monocytes are attracted to the site of infection and become activated, enabling them to more efficiently kill or contain mycobacteria [14, 15] and allow the development of 'local acquired immunity'. This is non-specific (i.e. macrophages activated by mycobacteria also have increased ability to kill other organisms).

The accumulation of these proliferating T cells and macrophages in small foci, a dynamic process occurring over 10 to 21 days, is called 'accelerated tubercle formation'.[11] These granulomas are clusters of tightly packed cells, which allow the transmission and reception of complex stimulatory and inhibitory signals.[10] Activated macrophages may differentiate and acquire certain specific external characteristics — they may become epithelioid cells, or fuse together to form multinucleated Langerhans-type giant cells characteristic of the tuberculous granuloma. Granulomas form in infections where insoluble antigen persists, as in tuberculosis.[10]

Generalized or 'systemic immunity' develops as these important components of cellular immunity spill over from the local sites of infection into the circulation. Of these components, specific T lymphocytes are the most important.[14, 15] At least two populations are recognizable in the draining lymph nodes and spleen: (a) short-lived T cells which circulate in the blood and migrate to the inflamed areas; and (b) long-lived memory T cells which circulate via the lymphatics and do not enter the disease sites,[35] the latter being responsible for the accelerated summoning of T lymphocytes and other cells during future encounters with the organism.

A second component of acquired-specific immunity is the development of 'delayed hypersensitivity'. Whereas the first component protects the host, the second is tissue-damaging and is characterized by caseous necrosis, liquefaction and exudation.[14, 15] As can be expected in hypersensitivity reactions, the tissue effect is proportional to the load of organisms: small bacterial loads cause a compact proliferative response with granuloma formation; while larger loads cause increasing caseation and liquefaction. Caseous lesions are avascular, acidic and contain few macrophages; but fortunately mycobacteria replicate poorly within them. The caseous material in small foci can be cleared by macrophages, but larger ones are removed by enzyme digestion or they become encapsulated by fibrous tissue.[14] Liquefaction results from hydrolysis of protein, lipid and nucleic acid components of caseous tissue by cellular products, such as tumour necrosis factor (TNF), and the hydrolytic enzymes and toxic oxygen radicals of macrophages and neutrophils.[15]

Post-primary disease and dissemination

Progression of the primary disease within weeks or months is termed post-primary disease, and may be either local or distant. Local spread is due to spillage of caseous or liquefied material. In contrast to areas of caseation, liquefied tissue permits extracellular multiplication of organisms. These may reach very large numbers[14] and when the lesion ruptures into bronchi or blood vessels may result in local or miliary spread.[10] The outcome in secondarily seeded areas depends upon the local levels of acquired specific protective immunity — the accumulation of activated macrophages at these sites. Some heal while others progress.[15]

Healing is associated with infiltration of fibroblasts and the laying down of collagen and calcium.[10] Dormant tubercle bacilli are often walled off in these lesions, but are prone to later reactivation should conditions become favourable. In time, organisms are destroyed, either spontaneously or as a result of therapy, and the protective cell-mediated immunity wanes. This is accompanied by decreasing numbers of sensitized T lymphocytes in the tissues, lymph nodes and blood.[15] However, a level of continuing specific immunity is ensured because, in addition to dormant viable or effete bacteria in walled-off disease foci, the processes of follicular dendritic cells of draining lymph nodes and spleen contain persistent mycobacterial antigen.[40]

Death in untreated disease is not due to the toxic effects of mycobacteria *per se* (large numbers of heat-killed organisms can be injected intravenously into mice with no ill effect[11]). In T cell-depleted hosts death results from extensive inflammatory consolidation of the lungs and elsewhere with large aberrant foamy macrophages filled with viable acid fast bacilli. This process can be reversed by the transfusion of immune or non-immune T cells. In normal non-T cell-depleted hosts death occurs as a result of the harmful effects of uncontrolled delayed hypersensitivity. Tissue destruction, adult respiratory distress syndrome, shock and cachexia are prominent.[10, 15, 60, 72]

Secondary or adult-type pulmonary tuberculosis

Infection in a previously BCG-vaccinated, or reactivation in an exposed host takes the following course. Organisms initially proliferate relatively unchecked until a threshold number of bacilli (10^3 CFUs in guinea pigs) is reached (usually by two weeks), when an effective immune response is triggered.[70] The rate of growth of the virulent organisms is then slowed. Although the components of the immune response are the same as in the primary infection, they are more rapid, vigorous and effective in localizing disease. Dissemination in the lungs and elsewhere is markedly decreased,[11, 60, 70] and, because the delayed hypersensitivity component is also better developed, local tissue destruction with cavitation is more rapid and common than in primary infection.

CELLULAR IMMUNE MECHANISMS

The above description provides a background for the study in greater detail of the major players (cells and molecules) and rules of play (mechanisms) of immune responses to *M. tuberculosis*.

Macrophages

Macrophages are capable of acquiring widely differing functions (e.g. phagocytosis, killing, secretion of enzymes and cytokines, processing and presentation of antigens) under the influence of local modifying factors, which, in tuberculosis, include mycobacterial antigens, T cells and soluble mediators such as interferon [38] and vitamin D.[60]

Phagocytosis

Phagocytosis by macrophages requires the triggering of a cell surface molecule or 'adherence receptor' similar to the Fc receptor required for antibodies. There are several types belonging to the 'integrin' superfamily.[55]

After engaging the organism, the latter is ingested by a process of internalization of the macrophage membrane, and so forms a phagosome.

Processing of organism/antigens

Phagosomes fuse with lysosomes containing proteolytic enzymes and toxic oxygen radicals. Some bacilli die, and their complex cell walls are disrupted while individual protein and lipopolysaccharide components or antigens undergo a variable degree of change.[55]

Some of these products are transported back to the macrophage cell membrane and linked to surface molecules or antigens called DR or Class 2 HLA, part of the major histocompatibility complex (MHC).

Antigen presentation

Once linked in this way, the antigens are ready to be 'presented' to lymphocytes (see Figure 14.2). Such presentation is MHC-restricted, which means that it will only occur when the Class 2 HLA of the macrophage matches that of the T cells. In addition to this a second signal is required from the macrophage to activate the T cell: release of interleukin 1 (IL1).[42] Once activated, the T cells begin to proliferate, secrete other soluble mediators (lymphokines), and express new cell surface molecules. The lymphokines include interleukin 2 (IL2), gamma-interferon (IFN), monocyte chemotactic factor (MCF), macrophage migration inhibitory factor (MMIF), and tumour necrosis factor (TNF). The cell surface molecules include IL2 receptor, both IL2 and its receptor being required for ongoing T cell proliferation to a stimulus or antigen (i.e. clonal expansion), while the other lymphokines attract and activate macrophages.[10, 15]

Mycobacterial killing

A crucial question concerning the role of the macrophages in the immune response to tuberculosis is whether or not they are able to *kill* mycobacteria.[35] Activated mouse peritoneal and bone marrow macrophages have been shown to inhibit mycobacterial growth. Activation may be stimulated by crude lymphokines, tuberculin-responsive T cell lines from lymph nodes of immunized mice, or gamma-interferon.[60] The observed inhibition of growth may involve the slowing of replication (bacterial stasis), or actual killing of organisms. Studies using human cells have been less impressive.[60] Non-activated monocytes from blood show a variable but weak effect on mycobacterial

replication which can be enhanced by crude lymphokines, gamma-interferon and vitamin D, and depressed by corticosteroids. Human bronchoalveolar lavage macrophages have a similar weak action. The reasons for this poor activity of the cells most likely to first make contact with viable mycobacteria is puzzling, and may simply be technical (perhaps because of incorrect proportions of organism, macrophages or T cells, or failure to use the correct lymphokines). Alternatively, macrophages may not be the main players in the process. Recent research suggests that cytotoxic T lymphocytes may play a leading role in mycobacterial killing by lysing macrophages that contain viable organisms.[32]

The mechanism by which macrophages inhibit mycobacterial intracellular growth is unclear. An important role is probably played by oxygen compounds, such as hydrogen peroxide, resistance to which has been described in more virulent tubercle bacilli.[6]

Lymphocytes

T Lymphocytes

T lymphocytes involved in tuberculous immunity should not be viewed as a single cell type, but as a variety of cells with widely divergent and even opposing functions. Before considering the varieties recognized in tuberculous infections, it is important to understand the features by which these subsets are recognized and the overlapping functions of each.

Subsets of T lymphocytes are distinguished according to their glycoprotein cell surface markers (receptors), called clusters of differentiation (CD).[55] All T cells have CD3 which exists as part of the antigen binding complex (TCR), but other CD surface molecules differ in the various subpopulations (e.g. CD4 and CD8). These are often referred to as 'helper/inducer' and 'suppressor/cytotoxic' subsets respectively. The 'helper' CD4+ subset is further subdivided into those that induce help and those that induce suppression. However, it is now appreciated that these markers do not provide a rigid definition of the function of cells (for example, some CD4+ cells are cytotoxic[55]). Other surface markers only appear on T cells after various stages of activation, such as CD25 (also known as Tac and the receptor for interleukin 2) and HLA - DR (also known as Class 2 HLA).

Unlike B cells, T cells do not recognize antigen unless it has been processed and presented together with MHC (HLA in humans) on the surface of other cells.[55] Most cells express Class 1 HLA and can therefore present antigens to CD8+ T cells. However only a few cells (called 'antigen-presenting cells') express Class 2 HLA which is needed to present antigens to CD4+ T cells.

Some of the CD glycoproteins are 'cell adhesive molecules', which enhance the interaction of antigen-presenting cells and lymphocytes.[55] This is the role of CD4 and CD8, which are the receptors respectively for the ligands MHC Class 2 and Class 1. Positive and negative feedback of these receptors probably occurs as an immune regulating mechanism.

Both CD4+ and CD8+ T cells have been shown to play a role in protection from tuberculosis.[33, 49] CD4+ lymphocytes are probably the most important in that mice depleted of CD4+ cells fare as badly as those depleted of both subsets.[33] Also, in Mantoux-positive normal humans, 72 per cent of the peripheral blood T cells reactive to PPD (purified protein derivative) and BCG are CD4+, while only eight per cent are CD8+.[4]

CD4+ T cells

Several different varieties of CD4+ cells have been recognized in tuberculous infections. These include lymphocytes in draining lymph nodes where protective T cells are generated,[61] and those in tuberculous pleural effusions.[66] Similarly, although the majority of T cells in peripheral blood and bronchoalveolar lavage of patients with disseminated TB are CD8+ at diagnosis, there is during recovery an impressive switch to CD4+ cells.[2] Moreover, the dominant protective T cell after intravenous challenge with mycobacteria in mice is L3T4+ Lyt2– (the equivalent of CD4+). There is reasonable evidence that the long term memory cells are also CD4+.[49] *In vitro*, CD4+ T cell lines and clones responsive to *M. tuberculosis*

and its antigens have been generated in mice[33] and humans.[39] These cells secrete lymphokines (e.g. gamma-interferon and interleukin 2) that activate macrophages to inhibit mycobacterial growth. CD4+ mycobacterial-reactive human T cell clones are also generated by the 65 kDa heat shock protein of mycobacteria.[39]

Finally, most lymphocytes in tuberculosis with cytotoxic capability are CD4+.[28, 52] This cytotoxicity, which is class 2-MHC restricted, involves lysis of target cells through direct contact between them and the lymphocytes. Death of mycobacteria after cytolysis of the macrophages containing them may be achieved by exposing the organisms to proteolytic enzymes or superoxide radicals,[32] effective phagocytosis and killing by other more activated macrophages [20], and direct kill by membrane attack.[24]

CD8+ T cells

There is considerable evidence of increased CD8+ T cells in the peripheral blood of patients with severe tuberculosis,[68, 71] and of even higher numbers of these cells in the lungs of patients with tuberculosis.[2]

Mice immunized with mycobacteria produce CD8+ in addition to CD4+ clones.[33] Some activate bone marrow macrophages to inhibit mycobacteria by releasing gamma-interferon, while others use a lymphokine-independent mechanism. Most cause antigen-specific Class 1 MHC-restricted target cell lysis. However, there is as yet no evidence for CD8+ cytotoxic T cells in humans,[32, 57] but failure to demonstrate such cells might be technical.

Natural killer cells (NK cells)

Natural killer T cells have a gamma-delta instead of an alpha-beta TCR, seldom express CD4 or CD8, and do not need antigen to be presented in association with either Class 1 or 2 MHC molecules.[30] Their function is to recognize cell surface changes (usually bound antigen), and to eliminate the cells concerned. They may also produce lymphokines, e.g. IL2, IL4 and gamma-interferon. The latter in turn can stimulate NK differentiation.[46]

Evidence concerning the numbers of NK cells in tuberculosis is conflicting.[18, 46] BCG immunization elevates NK cells [46] and there is evidence for direct killing of organisms by T cells in humans.[24] There are also CD4–CD8– T lymphocytes in tuberculous effusions.[30] A recent study in mice has shown that mycobacteria-specific CD4– CD8– gamma-delta T cells are generated in the lymph nodes draining footpads immunized with *M. tuberculosis*.[30] They were shown to respond to the 65 kDa heat shock protein component of mycobacteria. They were 10 times more active than alpha-beta T cells in the primary response against tuberculous infection, but were not present in the secondary response. Since they are generated early and do not require antigen presentation via MHC products, they probably play an important role in the early response to tuberculosis.

B Lymphocytes

Antibodies against mycobacteria are found consistently in tuberculosis provided sensitive methods are employed. However, their specificity is poor, as they are also found in normal subjects and patients with other diseases, because of shared antigens with environmental mycobacteria and other organisms.[26] It is thought that they play little role in protective immunity.[11, 26] Circulating immune complexes containing IgM, G and A may be found.[18, 26] Antibody and immune complex levels are highest in patients with advanced, severe disease and anergy.[18, 26]

Although the main function of B cells is to produce immunoglobulins, they may also present soluble (e.g. PPD) and particulate antigens (such as whole mycobacteria).[39] It is unlikely that B cell processing and presentation of antigen is important.

Neutrophils

The role of neutrophils in tuberculosis is unclear. They appear early in disease foci, often before macrophages arrive,[18] and, like macrophages, release chemotactic factors which summon both neutrophils and monocytes to the site of infection. They might collaborate in other ways. For example, macrophages are able to take up neutrophil peroxidase found in cellular debris, and might utilize this to kill mycobacteria.[18]

Soluble products

Tumour necrosis factor

Tissue necrosis, both within microgranulomas and in organs is a characteristic feature of the pathology of tuberculosis, especially in cases with a high bacterial load. *Mycobacterium tuberculosis* does not possess powerful tissue toxins [62] and it is likely that the principal cause of necrosis is TNF released from lymphocytes [15] and activated macrophages.[62] The release of TNF from the latter is triggered by various stimuli such as lipopolysaccharide, toxins, fungal and other antigens. However, macrophages must first have been 'primed' by gamma-interferon or vitamin D.[62]

TNF is considered to be the major mediator in the adult respiratory distress syndrome, fever, weight loss and septic shock.[60, 72] Prostaglandins, which inhibit TNF release, may act as regulators of tissue necrosis *in vivo*.[62]

Heat shock protein

Heat shock proteins (HSPs) are a group of proteins released by cells after exposure to a variety of stressful stimuli, such as high temperature, hypoxia, pH change, inadequate nutrition, toxic oxygen radicals and viral and bacterial infections.[56] They are constitutively present in all normal cells and help protect them from these stressful phenomena by acting as molecular chaperones for proteins, preventing unfolding and degradation, and by influencing transport and assembly. A possible role in antigen presentation has also been suggested.

There is a striking similarity between the HSP of widely differing living organisms. For example, the HSP of *M. tuberculosis*, a 65 kDa molecule, shares 50 per cent of the amino acid sequence of human HSP.[76] Not surprisingly, they show immunological crossreactivity. Since both the host and *M. tuberculosis* release HSP during infection, there is potential for the induction of autoimmunity and self-directed cytotoxicity.

HSP is specifically recognized by the gamma-delta subset of T lymphocytes, which are important in the early response to infection as they are not HLA-restricted.[30] In this way HSP may act as a primer for cytotoxic T lymphocytes[52] and NK cells.[1]

Vitamin D

Vitamin D has recently been shown to be an important immune modulator with the ability to affect the function of both macrophages and lymphocytes. It enhances the ability of monocytes to inhibit mycobacterial growth,[60] and stimulates macrophage differentiation, giant cell formation and hydrogen peroxide production.[5] Studies of its effect on lymphocyte function have yielded conflicting results — some showing decreased antigen-stimulated lymphocyte transformation, and others the reverse.[5] Depression of sensitized T-lymphocyte activity at sites of disease activity may serve to limit damage from delayed hypersensitivity.

Clinical evidence of benefit from Vitamin D therapy is scanty. It improves the healing of tuberculous skin disease, but there is a vigorous early febrile response with raised ESR and local inflammation.[60] These early effects may be due to TNF, as Vitamin D, like gamma-interferon, primes macrophages for TNF release.

The question of Vitamin D replacement is further confused by the changes in its metabolism that are found in tuberculosis. As in other granulomatous diseases (such as sarcoidosis), macrophages under the influence of gamma-interferon synthesize the enzyme 1–alpha hydroxylase, thereby enabling them to convert the inactive circulating 25–hydroxy vitamin D_3 (cholecalciferol) to the active metabolite 1, 25 dihydroxy vitamin D_3 (calcitriol).[60] Furthermore, there is loss of the feedback control that normally limits over-production of active calcitriol. This explains the occasional cases of hypercalcaemia found in tuberculosis.[60] Elevated calcitriol has been demonstrated in tuberculous, but not other exudative pleural effusions.[5]

PROTECTION VERSUS DELAYED HYPERSENSITIVITY

Protection against tuberculosis requires the development of cell-mediated immunity (acquired cellular resistance), both this and delayed hypersensitivity being mediated by antigen-specific T lymphocytes.[11, 39] Both usually develop simultaneously and involve the release of lymphokines which activate macrophages.[11] Protection results from the increased intracellular bacteriostatic/cidal activity of macrophages, while delayed hypersensitivity is more associated with inflammation and tissue damage via macrophage release of TNF, proteolytic enzymes, oxygen radicals and coagulation factors.[14, 15, 60]

Some investigators [11, 49] believe that both are inextricably linked in that they appear to be mediated by a single lymphocyte population. If this is so, the relative predominance of protection or delayed hypersensitivity might be related to the antigenic load alone — high local concentration of antigen causes predominantly delayed hypersensitivity and tissue destruction, while a low concentration causes more cellular protection.[14, 15]

There is, however, strong evidence against a single population of T lymphocytes mediating both phenomena.

- Different species of animals have differing levels of delayed hypersensitivity (DH) and resistance to *M. tuberculosis*. Rats develop little DH but marked resistance, whereas guinea pigs are the opposite. Humans display both marked DH and resistance.[14]
- In several different experimental models, one has been induced, transferred or attenuated without the other.[11, 74]
- Systemic resistance persists in spite of waning skin reactivity to tuberculin.[35, 64]
- In several animal studies different subpopulations of T cells have been shown to confer protection, DH and immunological memory.[49, 51]
- Finally, DH and protection appear to be induced by different antigenic components of mycobacteria (see Figure 14.3): PPD components induce DH but no protection, while immunity without DH results from RNA-ribosomal protein extracts of the organism.[54, 64, 74]

Protective immunity and delayed hypersensitivity are thus best considered as separate processes that occur in response to different antigens. They develop in parallel but on occasions one may dominate. The strength of each reaction may be influenced

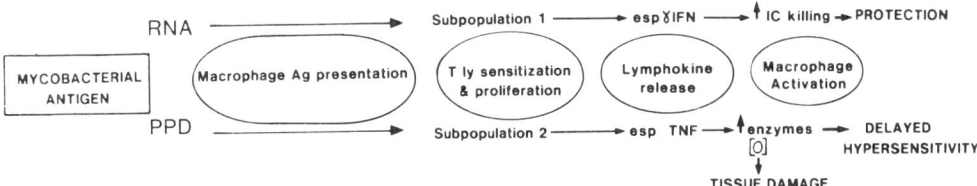

Figure 14.3. Comparison of components and stages of development of protective immunity and delayed hypersensitivity. Legend:

RNA	= Ribonucleic acid	Ag	= Antigen
PPD	= Purified protein derivative	T Ly	= T lymphocyte
γIFN	= Gamma interferon	TNF	= Tumour necrosis factor
IC	= Intracellular	[O]	= Oxygen radicals

by genetic differences, antigenic load, route of infection and modifying drugs or other disease.

CLINICAL AND IMMUNO-LOGICAL SIGNIFICANCE OF THE TUBERCULIN REACTION

The tuberculin skin test is considered to be a useful clinical indicator of delayed hypersensitivity to *M. tuberculosis*. A positive test has a strong correlation with transformation of peripheral blood lymphocytes to PPD *in vitro*. The ease with which it is performed, its reproducibility, and its low cost will continue to ensure that it remains the chief means of evaluating the immunological status of exposed or at risk persons, both for clinical and epidemiological purposes. In addition, the information about the host-organism relationship that its widespread use has provided over many decades has been of great value. A positive test is considered diagnostic of tuberculous infection either past or present, but not of tuberculous disease. The incubation period between infection and the appearance of skin sensitivity to tuberculin protein varies from four to eight weeks.[58]

Failure to develop the delayed hypersensitivity skin reaction in the face of obvious infection and/or disease is termed 'anergy'. The incidence of anergy in newly-diagnosed cases of tuberculosis varies in different studies from nil to 30 per cent,[10, 14] this variation being due to differences in the

populations tested, the technique, dose of PPD and criteria for positivity. In most studies a high frequency of anergy (e.g. 50 per cent) is found in patients with advanced, disseminated disease.[13, 39] Other factors which increase the incidence of anergy are malnutrition, uraemia, viral disease, diabetes mellitus, sarcoidosis, increased age, malignancy (e.g. lymphoma), AIDS and immunosuppressive drugs, such as steroids and cyclophosphomide.[3, 11, 25, 64] Anergy is usually non-specific and also applies to other common antigens, such as candida and mumps.[13] The presence of anergy in a patient with known tuberculous disease is considered by some to imply a poor prognosis.[11] While this may be true of disseminated (miliary) disease, and possibly of extensive pulmonary disease, it is not true in milder localized forms of pulmonary involvement and patients with tuberculous pleural effusions, a third of whom may show anergy at the time of diagnosis.[13]

Anergy is associated with enhanced antibody production but decreased T cell proliferation to PPD and other mycobacterial antigens, and decreased T cell secretion of interleukin 2 and gamma-interferon.[10, 13]

Anergy typically occurs early in the disease process and both the positive skin test and T cell proliferative responses return after successful therapy, beginning as early as two weeks.[13] Occasionally anergy may persist, and may be attributed to a larger load of organisms in the lungs or elsewhere.[11] As has already been mentioned, anergy or the lack of delayed hypersensitivity is not synonymous with poor protective immunity to tuberculosis.[11, 35, 64]

SUPPRESSOR MECHANISMS

The presence of anergy and depressed T cell proliferative responses in patients and experimental animals with tuberculosis suggest that there is a component of immunosuppression. This may be mediated by a number of different mechanisms involving combinations of T cells; B cells; adherent macrophages/monocytes; soluble components, mycobacterial or antibodies/immune complexes; and sequestration of cells into some body compartments away from other areas of need. The evidence that each of these might be relevant is briefly reviewed.

Suppressor T cells

Suppressor T cell induction in mice requires a threshold number of viable mycobacteria in the spleen[73] and can be prevented, even in heavily infected animals, by anti-tuberculous drugs given prior to the development of delayed hypersensitivity.[11] This is associated with skin anergy and decreased lymphocyte transformation to both PPD and mitogens. A study has shown that mice infected with excess mycobacteria switch to the production of predominantly suppressor T cells.[59] It would appear that suppressor T cells are a feature of early and overwhelming infection.

Humans with tuberculosis, especially those with severe and disseminated disease, have decreased numbers of circulating T cells with low CD4+ and increased CD8+ subsets.[2, 68] CD8+ lymphocytes are also elevated in the lungs of patients with both localized and disseminated pulmonary tuberculosis.[2] Functionally suppressive T cells have been demonstrated in the peripheral blood in several studies.[13, 31, 67] T cells are the main cause of suppression in 80 per cent of tuberculous patients with a poor proliferative response to PPD.[22] Circulating CD8+ suppressor T cells appear to act by releasing soluble suppressor factors or lymphokines, which inhibit lymphocyte proliferation and NK cell induction by interfering with the lymphokine cascade at several levels, including the depressed release of IL1, IL2 and gamma-interferon, and downgraded IL2 receptor expression.[22, 39]

Suppressor B cells

B cells have been shown to suppress the T cell response to mycobacterial antigens.[10]

Suppressor adherent macrophages/monocytes

The property of adherence is characteristic of macrophages and monocytes. In mice, adherent cells with a suppressor function are found in the spleens of animals inoculated with mycobacteria.[73]

Circulating adherent suppressor cells are also a feature in human disease where anergy is present, and these cells are considered to contribute to the poor lymphocyte proliferation to PPD.[20] They have decreased expression of DR and function poorly as antigen-processing cells,[18, 22, 75] possibly because they are immature and poorly differentiated.[22, 75] Interleukin 1 might also be involved, as its secretion by monocytes is enhanced in tuberculosis and it has been shown to depress T cell proliferation to PPD in a dose-dependent manner.[22] Adherent cells are also implicated in the diminished IL2 production and receptor expression by T cells in tuberculosis.[22]

Suppressor function may be mediated by a particular sub-population of macrophage (e.g. immature or permanently programmed cells), and/or by specific suppressive mycobacterial antigens ingested by the macrophages and then released into surrounding tissues.[75] The immune response genes may also play an important role.[36]

It is worth noting that the functions of adherent cells might themselves be altered by the organisms. Viable mycobacteria are able to inhibit fusion of phagosomes and lysosomes within macrophages,[6] and they also impair macrophage chemotaxis,[18] and inhibit lymphokine secretion and bacteriostasis.[33]

Soluble components

Suppressive soluble serum components may either be anti-idiotypic antibodies (antibodies directed against one or more of the patients' own antibodies),[39] mycobacterial antigens or immune complexes of both.[21] Suppressive mycobacterial antigens include the major carbohydrate lipopolysaccharide cell wall components, such as arabinomannan, arabinogalactan,[13] phosphatidyl choline and phosphatidyl ethanolamine.[77] As opposed to the cellular mechanisms of suppression, antigen- or immune complex-mediated suppression is antigen-non-specific and prostaglandin-mediated.[21]

Sequestration

In certain conditions, for example in sarcoidosis, cells in the peripheral blood and skin appear to be hyporesponsive, as antigen-reactive cells are sequestered in the lungs and other sites of inflammation. This sort of compartmentalization is not found in tuberculosis and does not account for the

suppression seen. In tuberculous pleural effusions, large numbers of highly active CD4+ T cells accumulate in pleural fluid as a result of local proliferation,[21, 23] and the same is probably true of the increased CD8+ cells in the lungs versus blood and pleural fluid in miliary disease.[2] Normal numbers of reactive cells are present in areas where suppression has been demonstrated (such as blood), and their responsiveness returns once suppressor cells have been removed.[13, 22]

Interaction of suppressor mechanisms in tuberculosis

It should be clear from the above discussion that the potential exists for many complex interactions between the various suppressor mechanisms. Such actions may occur in

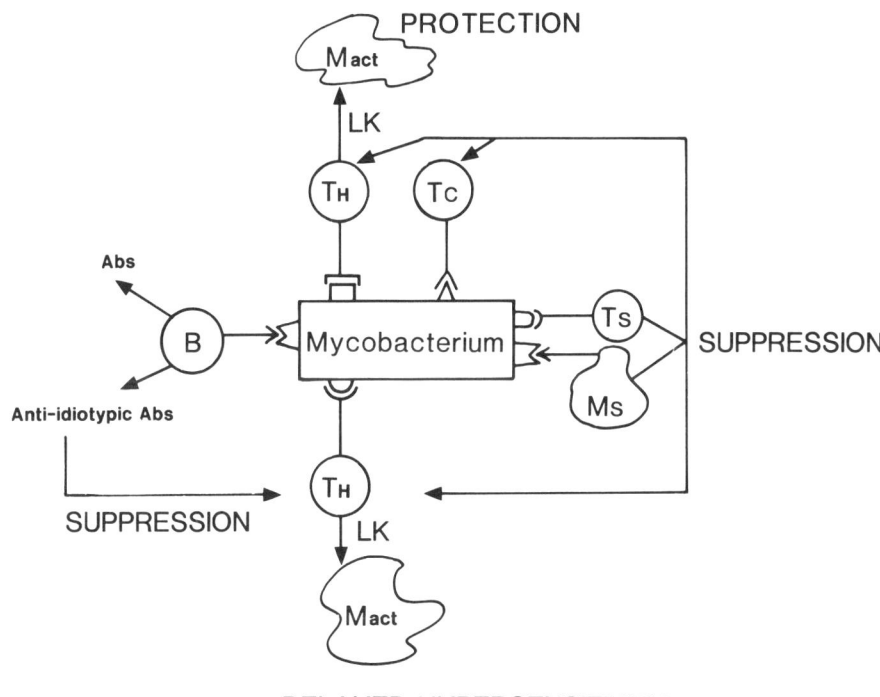

Figure 14.4. Role of suppression in the balance between protection and delayed hypersensitivity/tissue damage. Legend:

Mact	= Activated macrophage	Ts	= Suppressor T lymphocyte
Ms	= Suppressor macrophage	B	= B lymphocyte
Th	= Helper T lymphocyte	Abs	= Antibodies
Tc	= Cytotoxic T lymphocyte	LK	= Lymphokines

parallel (concurrently), or in series (one leading to another). For example, adherent cells might release mycobacterial products which lead to the induction of suppressor T cells. Different mechanisms might be involved in different patients, depending upon the immune response genes, the dose of mycobacteria and the route of inoculation. Some of the possible relationships between protective and delayed hypersensitivity mechanisms and the ways in which these components of the immune response might be suppressed are depicted in Figure 14.4.

Suppression rather than helper mechanisms may be mediated by specific mycobacterial antigens or even different spatially-separated epitopes on the same molecule.[39, 53] As enhanced antibody levels are associated with depressed cellular immunity and delayed hypersensitivity in tuberculosis,[22] this may suggest that epitopes recognized by antibodies are immunosuppressive. Suppression appears to be dominant under certain disease conditions, such as advanced disease with high bacterial load.[10, 59] These are also the conditions which favour the induction of delayed

hypersensitivity with its marked tissue-destructive effects. In this setting, the presence of suppression would serve as an important protective mechanism against host-induced tissue damage. The price paid for this reduction of injury might be the slower development of T helper cell-induced protection against the organism and its subsequent killing. Similar reduction of the harmful effects of DH, with the risk of delayed antimycobacterial effect, is achieved by the early use of corticosteroids in certain forms of fulminant disseminated disease.

MODIFYING FACTORS

Factors that influence the host response to tuberculosis are listed in Table 14.2. The most important ones will be discussed.

Genetic effects

Several studies have shown ethnic differences in susceptibility to tuberculosis,[10, 29] but there are many confounding variables such as socio-economic status, overcrowding, malnutrition, alcohol and other disease. Studies in the United States have shown that blacks have a two to three times higher incidence of positive Mantoux skin reactions

Table 14.2
Factors modifying the host response to tuberculosis

ORGANISM

1. Viability (dead organisms have antigens but produce different responses)
2. Virulence (ability of the organism to replicate and escape host defence mechanisms)
3. Dose
4. Route of inoculation

HOST

A) Intrinsic
1. Genetic
    (i)   innate ability of macrophages
    (ii) HLA-linked macrophage and lymphocyte function and interaction
2. Hormonal, e.g. oestrogens and glucocorticoids (these affect the maturation and function of cells, especially macrophages)
3. Age
B) Extrinsic
1. Nutrition
2. Other disease
3. Drugs
4. Vaccination

than whites, even when controlled for age, sex and socio-economic status.[58] Such differences might also be explained by the phasic shift of the epidemic wave — the developing world is currently experiencing the peak of infection while the infected cohort has already died off in the first world.[6, 15] This hypothesis does not explain co-segregation of known chromosomal markers with tuberculosis in families and outbred populations and evidence of similar disease susceptibility in twin studies.[47, 69]

There is also much evidence for genetic influence amongst animals. Increased or decreased immunity to tuberculosis is seen in different strains of rabbits and mice.[11, 14] Back-crossing experiments suggest that genetic factors that determine resistance to tuberculosis are multiple, additive and are more dominant than those governing susceptibility.[14, 69]

Resistance to tuberculosis has two different regulatory mechanisms, affecting both MHC-independent innate and MHC-linked acquired immunity (involving co-operation between macrophages and lymphocytes as described above).[33]

Multiple 'immune response' genes are involved, the most important of which are those coding for the MHC.[16, 69] Associations between HLA markers and tuberculosis incidence, pattern and severity have been shown, but these vary in different populations.[14, 16]

Class 2 genes determine which mycobacterial antigens are engaged, the efficacy of antigen-presenting cells, which T cell subsets are activated and the intensity of mediator production.

From the above, it is apparent that the balance between suppression and help, and consequently the course and expression of tuberculous disease, may be governed by allelic differences in Class 2 molecules.[16, 18]

It is likely that there are other important regulatory genes that determine susceptibility to tuberculosis. For instance, in mice, susceptibility to mycobacterial infection has been found to depend on a single autosomal dominant gene — the BCG gene[69] — and there is evidence for a similar gene in humans. The mouse BCG gene also controls early host response to other intra-

cellular pathogens, such as *Leishmania*. It determines the innate ability of macrophages to inhibit mycobacterial growth. Macrophage activation involves a series of events whereby cells in varying degrees of differentiation become receptive to primary and activating signals.[41] The resistant BCG allele endows macrophages with a more advanced level of activation than does the susceptible allele which requires lymphokine priming from sensitized T cells. In addition, this gene might also play a role in the specific T cell-dependent acquired immune response.[69]

Age

Tuberculosis is more common in the young and the elderly,[15] but some believe that this effect is related to the time phase of the epidemic wave mentioned above.[6] However, there is also evidence of a defective immune response in the elderly. The incidence of tuberculin skin anergy in the aged is high,[3, 58] circulating suppressor T cell numbers are increased,[9] and studies in mice show diminished T cell function against tuberculosis.[50] It is possible that poor nutrition in the elderly also plays a role.[8]

Nutrition

Poor nutrition is associated with an increased incidence of tuberculosis.[15, 29] Epidemiological studies have shown no difference in the infection rate but increased incidence of disease in the tall and thin.[19] Animal studies suggest that malnutrition must be extreme before susceptibility to tuberculosis increases.[6] More important is the presence of protein deprivation which causes skin anergy, decreased lymphoid tissue and T lymphocyte numbers and function, decreased CD4+ helper cells, decreased NK activity and depressed phagocytosis.[8, 11, 17] B cell numbers are normal but there is polyclonal hypergammaglobulinaemia and increased circulating immune complexes.[17]

Other significant deficiency states which have a bearing upon susceptibility to tuberculosis are those involving iron (associated with depressed phagocytosis[17]), vitamins C and D (depressed macrophage function [5, 35, 60]) and zinc (reduced lymphocyte function[17]).

Other disease

Tuberculosis is more common in certain conditions such as malignancy (especially Hodgkin's Disease),[15] diabetes mellitus,[6, 15] silicosis[6] and AIDS.[25] These conditions are also associated with increased frequency of anergy,[3, 10, 25] suggesting a defect in cell-mediated immunity. The ingestion of silica by macrophages has been shown to depress their antimycobacterial function.[27]

Human immunodeficiency virus infection

The human immunodeficiency virus (HIV) preferentially infects T lymphocytes via the CD4 receptor and then progressively destroys these cells.[7, 25] It can cause almost any type of immunological abnormality, especially cell-mediated, rendering the lung in particular very prone to infection.[7] The most important abnormality, which correlates with the incidence of opportunistic lung infections, is the decreased number of circulating lymphocytes, especially the CD4+ helper subset,[78] which is also the dominant cell in anti-tuberculosis protection.[4, 33] There is also skin anergy,[25] abnormal lymphocyte proliferation,[78] and decreased secretion of lymphokines.[44] In the bronchoalveolar fluid of AIDS patients the total number of lymphocytes may be normal or increased, but CD4+ lymphocytes are decreased, and the CD8+ lymphocytes are relatively increased.[78] Of interest is that increased susceptibility to tuberculosis occurs long before these abnormalities are established, i.e. in early HIV infection.[44] This might be due to the direct inhibitory effect of HIV infection on alveolar macrophages.[63]

Most TB in HIV-positive hosts is due to endogenous reactivation of previously controlled infection, rather than to newly acquired disease.[7, 44] However, there is also a high incidence of progression to active disease from newly encountered organisms. It has been calculated that there is a 30 per cent rather than the usual five per cent early progression from infection to disease.[43]

Drugs

Immunosuppressive drugs

Patients taking immunosuppressive drugs, such as corticosteroids and cyclo-phosphamide, are at increased risk of developing tuberculosis.[6, 15] However, at least one study of asthmatics taking steroids failed to show an increased incidence of tuberculosis in spite of a fall in tuberculin skin reactivity.[65] Corticosteroids have many effects on the immune system, and cause anergy,[3, 11, 65] which occurs within three weeks with doses greater than 15 mg of prednisone per day, but is less likely to occur with alternate day therapy.[65] Data on the effect of corticosteroids on macrophage inhibition of mycobacterial growth is conflicting.[60, 64] Cyclophosphamide has been shown to induce suppressor T lymphocytes which can adoptively inhibit delayed hypersensitivity.[45]

Anti-tuberculous drugs

Successful anti-tuberculous chemotherapy reverses the skin anergy (and diminished *in vitro* lymphocyte transformation to both PPD and mitogens) found in some patients with tuberculosis, especially those with severe disease.[11, 34] In animal studies the earlier the therapy is begun, the better the restoration of blastogenic responses in spleen T cells.[12] Indeed, therapy with rifampicin or INH begun immediately at the time of infection prevents the development of delayed hypersensitivity and the induction of suppressor T cells.[12] Successful treatment also increases previously low circulating T lymphocytes to normal, and reverses the low CD4:8 ratio.[6, 31, 68] This occurs to an even greater extent in the lungs of patients with miliary tuberculosis responding to treatment.[2] On the other hand, rifampicin is occasionally associated with sudden death in therapy, especially in the malnourished and alcoholic.[48] This could possibly be due to the drug causing increased kill of organisms with massive TNF release on a background of a damaged liver, which predisposes to TNF damage.[37]

CONCLUSION

The study of tuberculosis poses a great challenge to immunologists, as each new discovery exposes deeper and more complex issues of this host-parasite relationship. The host response may be viewed as a delicate balance between the positive effects of cell-mediated protective immunity and the potentially harmful effects of delayed hypersensitivity. Suppressor mechanisms become involved, both from the organism's endeavour to escape destruction, and the host's need to regulate uncontrolled tissue damage. These considerations can be expected to heavily influence current and future modifications to treatment and control programmes.

REFERENCES

1 Ab B K, Kiessling R, Van Embden J D, Thole J E, Kumararatne D S, Pisa P, Wondimu A & Ottenhof T H, 1990. Induction of antigen-specific CD4+ HLA-DR- restricted cytotoxic T lymphocytes as well as non-specific non-restricted killer cells by the recombinant mycobacterial 65–kDa heat-shock protein. *European Journal of Immunology*. 20, 369–77.

2 Ainslie G M, Bateman E D & Solomon J A, 1986. Variation in T lymphocyte numbers and subsets in different forms and stages of pulmonary tuberculosis. *American Review of Respiratory Disease*. 133, 39.

3 American Thoracic Society, 1981. The tuberculin skin test. *American Review of Respiratory Disease*. 124, 356–63.

4 Bach M A, Pennec J M, Flageul B, Wallach D & Cottenot F, 1985. Specificity study of PPD-reactive human T cell line and clones. *Immunology Letters*. 9, 81–5.

5 Barnes P F, Modlin R L, Bikle D D & Adams J S, 1989. Transpleural gradient of 1,25–dihydroxy vitamin D in tuberculous pleuritis. *Journal of Clinical Investigation*. 83, 1527–32.

6 Bates J H, 1982. Tuberculosis: Susceptibility and resistance. *American Review of Respiratory Disease*. 125, 20–4.

7 Chaisson R E, Schecter G F, Theuer C P, Rutherford G W, Echenberg D F & Hopewell P C, 1987. Tuberculosis in patients with the acquired immunodeficiency syndrome: clinical features, response to therapy and survival. *American Review of Respiratory Disease*. 136, 570–4.

8 Chandra R K, 1983. Nutrition, immunity, and infection: present knowledge and future directions. *Lancet*. (i), 688–91.

9 Chandra R K, Joshi I, Au B, Woodford G & Chandra S, 1982. Nutrition and immunocompetence of the elderly. Effect of short term nutritional supplementation on cell-mediated immunity and lymphocyte subsets. *Nutrition Research*. 2, 223–32.

10 Chaparas S D, 1982. Immunity in tuberculosis. *Bulletin of the World Health Organization*. 60, 447–62.

11 Collins F M, 1982. The immunology of tuberculosis. *American Review of Respiratory Disease*. 125, 42–9.

12 Collins F M & Watson S R, 1980. Effect of chemotherapy on suppressor T-cells in BCG-infected mice. *Immunology*. 40, 529–37.

13 Daniel T M, 1980. The immunology of tuberculosis. *Clinics in Chest Medicine*. 1, 189–201.

14 Dannenberg A M Jr, 1982. Pathogenesis of pulmonary tuberculosis. *American Review of Respiratory Disease*. 125, 25–9.

15 Dannenberg A M Jr, 1989. Immune mechanisms in the pathogenesis of pulmonary tuberculosis. *Reviews of Infectious Diseases*. 11, S369–78.

16 De Vries R R P, 1989. Regulation of T cell responsiveness against mycobacterial antigens by HLA Class 2 immune response genes. *Reviews of Infectious Diseases*. 11, S400–3.

17 Dowd P S & Heatley R V, 1984. The influence of undernutrition on immunity. *Clinical Science*. 66, 241–8.

18 Edwards D & Kirkpatrick C H, 1986. The immunology of mycobacterial diseases. *American Review of Respiratory Disease*. 134, 1062–71.

19 Edwards L B, Livesay V T, Acquaviva F A & Palmer C E, 1971. Height, weight, tuberculosis infection and tuberculous disease. *Archives of Environmental Health*. 22, 106–12.

20 Ellner J J, 1978. Suppressor adherent cells in human tuberculosis. *Journal of Immunology*. 121, 2573–9.

21 Ellner J J, 1986. Immune dysregulation in human tuberculosis. *Journal of Laboratory and Clinical Medicine*. 108, 142–9.

22 Ellner J J & Wallis R S, 1989. Immunologic aspects of mycobacterial infections. *Reviews of Infectious Diseases*. 11, S455–9.

23 Fujiwara H, Okuda Y, Fukukawa T & Tsukuguchi I, 1982. *In vitro* tuberculin reactivity of lymphocytes from patients with tuberculous pleurisy. *Infection and Immunity.* 35, 402–9.

24 Garcia-Penarrubia P, Koster F T, Kelly R O, McDowell T & Bankhurst A D, 1989. Antibacterial activity of human natural killer cells. *Journal of Experimental Medicine.* 169, 99–113.

25 Glatt A E, Chirgwin K & Landesman S H, 1988. Current concepts. Treatment of infections associated with human immunodeficiency virus. *New England Journal of Medicine.* 318, 1439–48.

26 Grange J M, 1984. The humoral immune response in tuberculosis: its nature, biological role and diagnostic usefulness. *Advances in Tuberculosis Research.* 21, 1–78.

27 Gros P, Skamene E & Forget A, 1983. Cellular mechanisms of genetically controlled host resistance to *Mycobacterium bovis* (BCG). *Journal of Immunology.* 131, 1966–72.

28 Hank J A & Sondel P M, 1982. Soluble bacterial antigen induces specific helper and cytotoxic responses by human lymphocytes *in vitro. Journal of Immunology.* 128, 2734–8.

29 Hopewell P C, 1988. Mycobacterial diseases. *In*: Murray J F & Nadel J A, eds. *Textbook of Respiratory Medicine.* Philadelphia: W.B. Saunders.

30 Janis E M, Kaufmann S H E, Schwartz R H & Pardoll D M, 1989. Activation of gamma-delta T cells in the primary immune response to *Mycobacterium tuberculosis. Science.* 244, 713–6.

31 Katz P, Goldstein R A & Fauci A S, 1979. Immunoregulation in infection caused by *Mycobacterium tuberculosis*: the presence of suppressor monocytes and alteration of subpopulations of T lymphocytes. *Journal of Infectious Diseases.* 140, 12–21.

32 Kaufmann S H E, 1988. CD8+ T lymphocytes in intracellular microbial infections. *Immunology Today.* 9, 168–74.

33 Kaufmann S H E, 1989. *In vitro* analysis of the cellular mechanisms involved in immunity to tuberculosis. *Reviews of Infectious Diseases.* 11, S448–54.

34 Khomenko A G, Averbach M M, Litvinov V I, Gergert B J & Chukanov V I, 1984. Effects of chemotherapy on the immunological characteristics of patients with primary destructive pulmonary tuberculosis. *Bulletin of the World Health Organization.* 62, 763–71.

35 Lagrange P H, 1981. Tuberculosis: Immunological and clinical aspects. *In*: Humber D P, ed. *Immunological Aspects of Leprosy, Tuberculosis and Leishmaniasis.* Amsterdam: Exerpta Medica, International Congress Series 574.

36 Lamb J R, Lathigra R, Rothbard J B, Sweetser D, Young R A, Ivanyi J & Young D B, 1989. Identification of mycobacterial antigens recognised by T lymphocytes. *Reviews of Infectious Diseases.* 11, S 443–7.

37 Lehmann V, Freudenberg M A & Galanos C, 1987. Lethal toxicity of lipopolysaccharide and tumor necrosis factor in normal and D-galactosamine-treated mice. *Journal of Experimental Medicine.* 165, 657–63.

38 Lipscomb M F, Lyons C R, Nunes G, Ball E J, Stastny P, Vial W, Lem V, Weissler J, Miller L M & Toews G B, 1986. Human alveolar macrophages: HLA-DR-positive macrophages that are poor stimulators of a primary mixed leucocyte reaction. *Journal of Immunology.* 136, 497–504.

39 Lombardi G, Del Gallo F, Vismara D, Piccolella E & Colizzi V, 1987. Immunology of tuberculosis: New directions in research. *La Ricerca in Clinico e in Laboratorio.* 17, 1–15.

40 Mandel T E, Phipps R P, Abbot A & Tew J G, 1980. The follicular dendritic cell: long term antigen retention during immunity. *Immunological Review.* 53, 29–59.

41 Meltzer M S & Nacy C A, 1985. Macrophage cytotoxicity against tumor cell and microbial targets: genetic control of the activation network. *Progress in Leukocyte Biology.* 3, 595–604.

42 Mizel S B, 1982. Interleukin 1 and T cell activation. *Immunological Review.* 63, 51.

43 Murray J F, 1989. The white plague: down and out or up and coming? *American Review of Respiratory Disease.* 140, 1788–95.

44 Murray J F & Mills J, 1990. Pulmonary infectious complications of human immunodeficiency virus infection. Part 1. *American Review of Respiratory Disease.* 143, 1356–72.

45 Nakamura R M & Tokunaga T, 1980. Induction of suppressor T-cells in delayed-type hypersensitivity to *Mycobacterium bovis* BCG in low responder mice. *Infection and Immunity.* 28, 331–5.

46 Onwubalili J K & Scott G M, 1985. Natural killer cell activity in tuberculosis. *British Journal of Diseases of the Chest.* 79, 67–76.

47 Onwubalili J K, Scott G M & Robinson J A, 1985. Deficient immune interferon production in tuberculosis. *Clinical and Experimental Immunology.* 59, 405–13.

48 Onwubalili J K, Scott G M & Smith H, 1986. Acute respiratory distress related to chemotherapy of advanced pulmonary tuberculosis: A study of two cases and review of the literature. *Quarterly Journal of Medicine.* 230, 599–610.

49 Orme I M, 1987. The kinetics of emergence and loss of mediator T lymphocytes acquired in the

response to infection with *Mycobacterium tuberculosis. Journal of Immunology.* 138, 293–8.

50 Orme I M, 1987. Aging and immunity to tuberculosis: increased susceptibility of old mice reflects a decreased capacity to generate mediator T lymphocytes. *Journal of Immunology.* 138, 4414–8.

51 Orme I M & Collins F M, 1984. Adoptive protection of the *Mycobacterium tuberculosis*-infected lung. *Cellular Immunology.* 84, 113–20.

52 Ottenhoff T H M, Ab B K, Van Embden J D A, Thole J E R & Kiessling R, 1988. The recombinant 65–kD heat shock protein of *Mycobacterium bovis* Bacillus Calmette-Guérin/*M. tuberculosis* is a target molecule for CD4+ cytotoxic T lymphocytes that lyse human monocytes. *Journal of Experimental Medicine.* 168, 1947–52.

53 Ottenhoff T H M, Converse P J, Gebre N, Wondimu A, Ehrenberg J P & Kiessling R, 1989. T cell responses to fractionated *Mycobacterium leprae* antigens in leprosy. The lepromatous nonresponder defect can be overcome *in vitro* by stimulation with fractionated *M. leprae* components. *European Journal of Immunology.* 19, 707–13.

54 Pancholi P, Vinayak V K & Khuller G K, 1989. Immunogenicity of ribonucleic acid-protein fraction of *Mycobacterium tuberculosis* encapsulated in liposomes. *Medical Microbiology.* 29, 131–8.

55 Piessens W F, 1989. Introduction to the immunology of tuberculosis. *Reviews of Infectious Diseases.* 11, S436–42.

56 Polla B S, 1988. A role for heat shock proteins in inflammation? *Immunology Today.* 9, 134–7.

57 Rees A, Scoging A, Mehlert A, Young D B & Ivanyi J, 1988. Specificity of proliferative response of human CD8 clones to mycobacterial antigens. *European Journal of Immunology.* 18, 1881–7.

58 Reichman L B, 1979. Tuberculin skin testing: the state of the art. *Chest* 76, 764–70.

59 Rook G A W, 1975. The immunological consequences of antigen overload in experimental mycobacterial-infections in mice. *Clinical and Experimental Immunology.* 19, 167–78.

60 Rook G A W, 1988. Role of activated macrophages in the immunopathology of tuberculosis. *British Medical Bulletin.* 44, 611–23.

61 Rook G A W, Carswell J W & Stanford J L, 1976. Preliminary evidence for the trapping of antigen-specific lymphocytes in the lymphoid tissue of 'anergic' tuberculosis patients. *Clinical and Experimental Immunology.* 26, 129–32.

62 Rook G A W, Taverne J, Leveton C & Steele J, 1987. The role of gamma-interferon, vitamin D₃ metabolites and tumour necrosis factor in the pathogenesis of tuberculosis. *Immunology.* 62, 229–34.

63 Salahuddin S Z, Rose R M, Groopman J E, Markham P D & Gallo R C, 1986. Human T lymphotropic virus type III infection of human alveolar macrophages. *Blood.* 68, 281–4.

64 Sbarbaro J A, 1979. Tuberculosis. *In*: Simmons D, ed. *Current Pulmonology.* Vol. 1. Boston: Houghton-Mifflin.

65 Schatz M, Patterson R, Kloner R, *et al*, 1976. The prevalence of tuberculin tests in a steroid-treated asthmatic population. *Annals of Internal Medicine.* 84, 261–5.

66 Shimokata K, Kishimoto H, Takagi E & Tsunekawa H, 1986. Determination of the T-cell subset producing gamma-interferon in tuberculous pleural effusion. *Microbiological Immunology.* 30, 353–61.

67 Shiratsuchi H & Tsuyaguchi I, 1984. Analysis of T cell subsets by monoclonal antibodies in patients with tuberculosis after *in vitro* stimulation with purified protein derivative of tuberculin. *Clinical and Experimental Immunology.* 57, 271–8.

68 Singhal M, Banavalikar J N, Sharma S & Saha K, 1989. Peripheral blood T lymphocyte subpopulations in patients with tuberculosis and the effect of chemotherapy. *Tubercle.* 70, 171–8.

69 Skamene E, 1989. Genetic control of susceptibility to mycobacterial infections. *Reviews of Infectious Diseases.* 11, S394–9.

70 Smith D W & Wiegeshaus E H, 1989. What animal models can teach us about the pathogenesis of tuberculosis in humans. *Reviews of Infectious Diseases.* 11, S385–93.

71 Swanson Beck J, Potts R C, Kardjito T & Grange J M, 1985. T4 lymphopaenia in patients with active pulmonary tuberculosis. *Clinical and Experimental Immunology.* 60, 49–54.

72 Tracey K J, Cerami A & Lowry S F, 1988. Tumour necrosis factor and septic shock and adult respiratory distress syndrome (editorial). *American Review of Respiratory Disease.* 138, 1377–8.

73 Turcotte R, 1981. Evidence for two distinct populations of suppressor cells in the spleens of *Mycobacterium bovis* BCG-sensitized mice. *Infection and Immunity.* 34, 315–22.

74 Turk J L, 1983. Dissociation between allergy and immunity in mycobacterial infections. *Leprosy Review.* 54, 1–8.

75 Tweardy D J, Schacter B Z & Ellner J J, 1984. Association of altered dynamics of monocyte surface expression of human leucocyte antigen DR with immunosuppression in tuberculosis. *Journal of Infectious Diseases.* 149, 31–7.

76 Van Eden W, Hogervorst E J M, Van der Zee R, Van Embden J D A, Hensen E J & Cohen I R, 1989. The mycobacterial 65 kD heat-shock protein and auto-immune arthritis. *Rheumatology International.* 9, 187–91.

77 Wadee A A, Sher R & Rabson A R, 1980. Production of a suppressor factor by human adherent cells treated with mycobacteria. *Journal of Immunology.* 125, 1380–6.

78 Wallace J M, Barbers R G, Oishi J S & Prince H, 1984. Cellular and T-lymphocyte subpopulation profiles in bronchoalveolar lavage fluid from patients with acquired immunodeficiency syndrome and pneumonitis. *American Review of Respiratory Disease.* 130, 786–90.

CHAPTER 15

Diagnostic considerations in management and epidemiology

P R Donald

INTRODUCTION

Diagnosis has been variously defined as 'the art of distinguishing one disease from another' and 'the determination of the nature of a case of disease'.[34] The approach to the diagnosis of tuberculosis does not differ from that required for other diseases, resting firmly as it does upon the established procedures of history taking, clinical examination, side-room investigations and special investigations. However, the diagnosis of tuberculosis in an adult should be accepted with reluctance in the absence of bacteriological confirmation, especially as the approach to the diagnosis of tuberculosis is also somewhat complicated by the availability of the tuberculin test which makes it possible to distinguish those persons who are infected with *Mycobacterium tuberculosis* and are thus potentially, if not actually, diseased.

The South African Department of National Health and Population Development suggests the following definition for *a case of tuberculosis:*

> *... a person in whom the disease has been proven bacteriologically, radiologically, histologically and/or cytologically or in whom a pleural effusion responded to antituberculous therapy where other efforts at diagnosis failed.*

A *suspect case* is:

> *... a person with symptoms suggestive of tuberculosis, namely productive cough plus two of weight loss, loss of appetite, shortness of breath, chest pain, lassitude or night sweats or a radiological picture suggestive of tuberculosis.*

In the case of children those with a strongly positive tuberculin test (Mantoux ≥15mm induration) 'and other suggestive signs or symptoms or investigations are also regarded as cases'.[17]

HISTORY

Close contact with an adult suffering from cavitating smear positive disease

It has been estimated that each infectious tuberculosis patient may infect between 10 and 20 other persons, and that about 70 per cent of close contacts (i.e. bedroom or home contacts) will be infected by the time of diagnosis.[86] Of those infected, at least 10 to 15 per cent are likely to become diseased within two years of infection.

A history of contact is of particular importance in young children under two years of age because of their susceptibility to the development of disseminated tuberculous disease. Five per cent of infected children under two years of age will develop miliary tuberculosis or tuberculous meningitis.[6, 12]

Conversely, the finding of a strongly positive tuberculin test in a young child should lead to a search for a source of infection. The child's home should be the principal focus for the search.

Persistent cough of more than three weeks duration

Cough is an all too common symptom of respiratory tract disease in both adults and children. Persistent cough of more than three weeks duration must, however, lead to tuberculosis being considered as a possible cause. It is an important public health message that every *persistent* cough should be evaluated by a doctor. Non-productive initially, the cough may later become productive and ultimately bloodstained. Alternative diagnoses include chronic bronchitis, pulmonary neoplasmas and bronchiectasis, especially in adults. In children other infections such as pertussis and atypical pneumonias caused by *Mycoplasma pneumoniae, Chlamydia trachomatis* and a variety of viruses may present with persistent cough lasting for several months. Occasionally pertussis may give rise to hilar adenopathy, causing further confusion.

In children persistent or recurrent coughing (particularly nocturnal) with or without wheezing is often a manifestation of asthma. However, primary tuberculosis may also cause bouts of coughing and wheezing as the result of hilar adenopathy and airway narrowing. In one series of pulmonary

tuberculosis proven bacteriologically 17 per cent of children presented with wheezing.[29]

Loss of weight or, in children, failure to gain adequately in weight

There is a long established association between tuberculosis and loss of weight, which is well illustrated by the vernacular name 'consumption'. Clinical descriptions of tuberculosis frequently refer to the malnourished condition of the patient. Although loss of weight is not invariably present in adults with tuberculosis it may be an early symptom of tuberculosis, and regular weighing has been suggested as a simple method of surveillance to detect the development of disease. In the later stages of the disease the patient will frequently become emaciated.

In one South African study recent weight loss as a 'peripheral feature' was present in more than half of a group of 50 newly

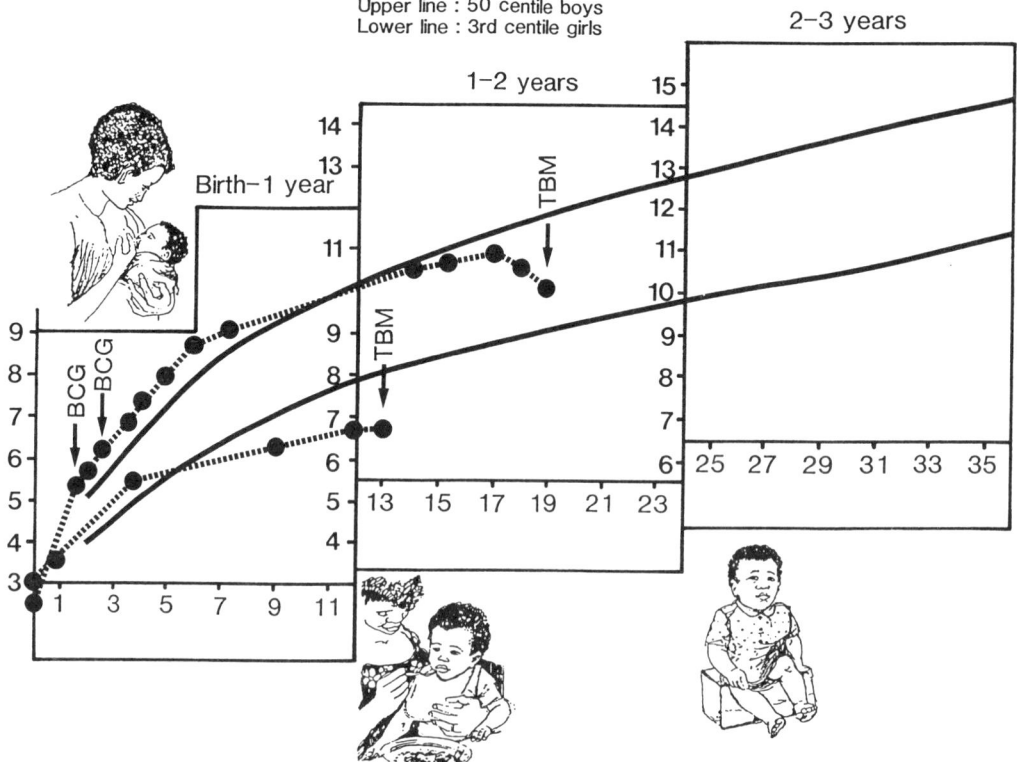

Figure 15.1. Road to Health Chart of two children, revealing inadequate weight gain for some time prior to diagnosis of TBM.

diagnosed pulmonary tuberculosis patients.[65] In another study, however, only one case of tuberculosis was diagnosed out of 300 patients investigated after routine weighing had shown weight loss.[19] Although little precise data is available from developing communities, studies of adults presenting with involuntary weight loss in developed communities have not shown tuberculosis to be a prominent cause (only two per cent of cases in one series).[64]

In children in developing communities, failure to gain adequately in weight or loss of weight can often reflect a multiplicity of socio-economic problems interwoven with infection by agents other than *Mycobacterium tuberculosis*. It is, however, the firm opinion of paediatricians practising in areas with a high incidence of tuberculosis that children who fail to gain weight or who lose weight must be investigated for possible tuberculous disease.[67, 70] This is demonstrated by the fact that in one study two-thirds of 50 children with probable pulmonary tuberculosis presenting to a clinic in an area with a very high incidence of tuberculosis (greater than 700/100 000) were failing to gain in weight or had experienced recent weight loss.[47]

A majority of children presenting with tuberculous meningitis has been shown to have been failing to gain adequately in weight for some time prior to diagnosis.[33] The course of events in two such children is illustrated in Figure 15.1. Timely investigation of these children might have prevented the progression of their disease.

Kwashiorkor with its concomitant weight loss is also frequently associated with tuberculosis and 10 per cent or more of kwashiorkor-affected children will have underlying or complicating tuberculosis.[57, 80] Undiagnosed tuberculosis may be a reason why children with kwashiorkor fail to respond to dietary therapy.

Finally, it must be emphasized that adequate weight gain in a child, or absence of loss of weight in an adult, by no means excludes the diagnosis of tuberculosis.

Immunosuppression

Any defect in cell-mediated immunity will aid the activation of latent tuberculosis.

When considering the diagnosis of tuberculosis, enquiry should be made as to the use of cortico-steroids or other immunosuppressant drugs. Diabetes mellitus, previous gastrectomy or the recent experience of mentally or physically stressful situations may have a similar deleterious effect upon resistance to tuberculosis.

Protein-energy malnutrition, particularly in the form of kwashiorkor, leads to suppression of cellular immunity[90] and tuberculosis should be actively sought in patients suffering from these conditions.

It is the conviction of paediatricians practising in developing communities that both measles and whooping cough (pertussis) predispose to the activation of latent tuberculosis.[37] In the case of measles, tuberculin hypersensitivity is depressed,[103] and there is a considerable drain upon the child's energy resources, leading in turn to loss of weight.[35, 36] Widespread inflammatory damage to the lungs may be sustained as a result of the measles itself and of secondary bacterial and viral infection.[26, 53] Individual cases and some epidemiological evidence support the contention that this damage leads to an increased susceptibility to tuberculosis.[4, 15] However, close analysis of the published data supporting this association has led some to question whether measles really does predispose specifically to tuberculosis.[39]

In the case of pertussis, destructive changes throughout the lungs, together with a prolonged course frequently accompanied by loss of weight, is sufficient reason to expect the activation of tuberculosis,[69] but once again this association has been questioned.[16]

Infection with the human immunodeficiency virus (HIV) and the development of the acquired immunodeficiency syndrome (AIDS) undoubtedly leads to an increased risk of developing tuberculosis,[92, 107] an association which is of diagnostic significance for both tuberculosis and AIDS.

Amongst AIDS patients, tuberculosis is one of the most frequent opportunistic infections. In North America this has often been caused by the *Mycobacterium avium-intracellulare* complex but where there is a high prevalence of *Mycobacterium tuberculosis* infections. In most developing countries this will be found to be the responsible organism in most instances.

The manifestations of tuberculosis in AIDS patients often differ from those usually associated with 'adult' type tuberculosis. An increased incidence of extra-pulmonary manifestations is to be expected, and sputum smears are reported to be less frequently positive, while there is a tendency to lower or midzone infiltrates on chest radiography.[92]

For its part tuberculosis may serve as a sentinel infection for the detection of AIDS. Studies from Africa and the Caribbean have found between 20 and 60 per cent of tuberculosis patients to be HIV positive, and tuberculosis will frequently be the first clinical manifestation of AIDS.[107] Confirmation of the diagnosis of tuberculosis in AIDS patients may require the examination of a wide range of specimens including sputum, bronchial washings, lung biopsy, bone marrow aspirate, blood, urine, stool, cerebrospinal fluid or brain biopsy. False negative tuberculin testing results may be encountered.

Other symptoms

Other symptoms frequently associated with tuberculosis which should be inquired after include night-sweats, lethargy, pain in the chest (which may be pleuritic in nature) and amenorrhoea.

CLINICAL EXAMINATION

Clinical examination may not reveal any abnormalities in early pulmonary tuberculosis, but with progression signs of lobar consolidation or a pleural effusion may appear. However, these are in no way specific for tuberculosis. Phlyctenular conjunctivitis and erythema nodosum are somewhat more specific but may also result from infection with other agents. In more advanced complicated disease, clubbing may be found in association with signs of bronchiectasis or cor pulmonale.

SIDE-ROOM INVESTIGATIONS

These will usually contribute little to the specific diagnosis of tuberculosis, but

should not be neglected. In a patient with few other clinical signs a raised erythrocyte sedimentation rate (ESR) may draw attention to the necessity for further investigation. However, a normal ESR does not exclude the diagnosis of tuberculosis and in one South African series more than 25 per cent of newly diagnosed pulmonary tuberculosis patients had an ESR of less than 20 m/hour.[19]

SPECIAL INVESTIGATIONS
Bacteriology

Culture of *Mycobacterium tuberculosis* from sputum or other body secretions or tissues is the gold standard for the diagnosis of tuberculosis. Every effort should be made to obtain such evidence in any patient where tuberculosis is suspected. Traditionally three sputum specimens are submitted for culture and microscopy for the presence of acid-fast bacilli, and where it is financially feasible this practice should be continued as the number of confirmed cases may be increased by 25–30 per cent when three specimens rather than one are submitted.[56]

Sputum microscopy for acid-fast bacilli has the virtue of speed, but will detect only those cases where large numbers of bacilli are being excreted. Depending upon circumstances these may represent only half of the cases ultimately confirmed by culture,[40] but they are nonetheless important as they are responsible for the survival of the disease in the community. In developing countries with severe financial restraints it has been suggested that reliance should be placed solely upon sputum microscopy for the diagnosis of tuberculosis; the argument being that the identification of these cases will remove from the community those patients who are responsible for the infection of others.[96] This takes little account of the fact that those cases confirmed by culture, but negative on direct microscopy, will almost inevitably progress to a more advanced stage within a relatively short space of time and will then themselves become a source of infection.

Great emphasis is placed upon sputum culture in the South African Tuberculosis Control Programme, both for the diagnosis of the individual patient and in prevalence surveys.[40]

In children *Mycobacterium tuberculosis* will be cultured or identified on microscopy in only a minority of cases. Despite this, confirmation of the disease should be vigorously sought. As young children do not readily produce sputum, recourse must be had to the collection of three consecutive early morning gastric aspirates for culture and direct microscopy. The lesions of primary tuberculosis do not, in the absence of cavitation, contain large numbers of organisms and *Mycobacterium tuberculosis* can therefore only be cultured from a minority of children with undoubted primary tuberculosis, and can be identified on microscopy in an even smaller number. The results obtained will vary according to the 'intensity and quality' of the examination.[95] Following a thorough bacteriological examination of a group of children with suspected pulmonary tuberculosis aged 0–14 years in Saskatchewan, *Mycobacterium tuberculosis* was cultured from 32 per cent of children but visualized on microscopy in only two per cent.[3] A similar degree of success in culturing *Mycobacterium tuberculosis* from children with undoubted primary tuberculosis has been reported by others.[72]

The use of laryngeal swabs is claimed to increase the number of positive cultures obtained in children, but their application by unskilled workers could be dangerous to the patient.[61]

Chest radiography

While chest radiography is by no means essential to the diagnosis of pulmonary tuberculosis, it does serve to provide corroborative evidence which may be substantiated by later sputum microscopy and culture. It is also important to note that chest radiography is the only way the early stages of pulmonary tuberculosis can be detected at a time when the patient is asymptomatic, before any severe degree of lung damage has taken place, and before the patient has become a source of infection to others.[20] It must, however, again be emphasized that no matter how typical of tuberculosis the chest radiography may be, bacteriological confirmation of the diagnosis by culture of sputum must be sought. The 'overdiagnosis' of tuberculosis solely on radiological grounds is an all too common problem.[28, 43]

Mass miniature chest radiography was frequently used in the past as a means of case finding, but this has now been shown not to be cost effective, except in certain high risk situations such as old age homes.[71] Far more use is now being made of sputum culture for mass screening purposes.

In childhood, chest radiography is, together with the tuberculin test, the most important means of diagnosing tuberculosis, but problems are not infrequently encountered in the interpretation of films due to rotation, poor inspiration, or under- or over-penetration. Attention to these technical details makes the life of the clinician much easier.

Tuberculin testing

Implications of a positive tuberculin test

Cell-mediated delayed hypersensitivity to tuberculo-protein develops shortly after infection with *Mycobacterium tuberculosis*, and this can be demonstrated by the tuberculin test. However, it must be pointed out that a tuberculin test, no matter how strongly positive it might be, constitutes evidence of tuberculous infection only and not of disease. Although tuberculin testing is of relatively little diagnostic value in the adult, it does form an essential part of the evaluation of the young child with suspected tuberculosis.

Risk of disease following infection

It is well established that the first two years after infection with *Mycobacterium tuberculosis* hold the greatest risk for progression of the infection to disease. The risk that disease will develop is particularly high in children under two years of age, and disease at this age is particularly likely to take the form of miliary tuberculosis or tuberculous meningitis.[12, 100]

The increased risk of serious disease to which infected young children are exposed is reflected by mortality data gathered before the advent of antituberculous chemotherapy. Arnold Rich in the United States reported an annual mortality of 49,2 per thousand infected children under one year of age as against 1,2 for those between one and four years of age and less than 1,0 thereafter.[84] Bentley and collaborators found in an in-depth study of tuberculosis in London during the decade 1940–50 that there was a mortality of 59,6 per thousand for those under one year of age, 7,7 for those aged between one and four years and less than 1,0 for older children.[6] A similar trend of susceptibility can been seen in South African data for the period 1970–80. The annual case fatality ratio (percentage) for children under one year of age varied from five to 10 per cent and from two to four per cent for those aged between one and four years and was less than two per cent for older children.[58]

In an Indian study of tuberculosis in family contacts of sputum positive patients in the five year period after diagnosis, an attack rate of 20 per cent was found in contacts under five years of age compared to eight per cent or less in older contacts.[27]

Cammock and Miller in an evaluation of tuberculosis in young children in Newcastle, England between 1945 and 1949 found infected children aged under two years to have a risk of approximately one in 20 of developing miliary tuberculosis or tuberculous meningitis.[12]

As a strongly positive tuberculin test in a child under five years of age indicates infection with *Mycobacterium tuberculosis*, such children, because of the risks involved, deserve to be treated as if suffering from tuberculous disease irrespective of other findings.

False negative reactions

False negative tuberculin reactions may result from the use of an incorrect technique when administering the test or from any depression of cell-mediated immunity such as that associated with the use of cortico-steroids, malnutrition, viral infections such as measles, or immunization with live virus vaccines (measles and rubella for example); anergy may also be encountered during overwhelming tuberculous infection. Further, a small percentage of otherwise normal individuals appear to be unable to respond to tuberculin. It should therefore be clear that a negative tuberculin test does not mean that the patient is not infected by *Mycobacterium tuberculosis.*

The booster effect

Repeated tuberculin testing of individuals uninfected with *Mycobacterium tuberculosis* will not lead to the development of a positive tuberculin test. However, tuberculin hypersensitivity may wane over a period of time, appear negative on retesting, but on further retesting give a positive result or a greater induration than the previous test.[98] This 'booster' effect is most common in older individuals and may be seen as soon as one week after the previous tuberculin test. Where it becomes important to distinguish a boosted response, the procedure of two-stage testing may be adopted: a second tuberculin test being performed within a week of the first. If the two tests give the same result, then an increased induration at later testing is not due to boosting but to infection by a mycobacterial agent.

Different forms of tuberculin testing

Three forms of tuberculin testing are in widespread use in South Africa at present — the Mantoux test, the Tine test and the Heaf test.

The Mantoux test

This is the most accurate form of tuberculin testing and enables the investigator to inject a precise amount of tuberculo-protein intradermally. In South Africa at present, use will most often be made of 5 units Tween 80 stabilized PPD.

After cleaning the skin with acetone or ether, a tuberculin syringe with a short 25 G needle is used to inject 0,1 mls of PPD into the anterior surface of the forearm at the junction of the mid and upper thirds. If correctly given, the injection should raise a wheal 5 mm or more in diameter which will disappear within two hours.

The test should be read 48–72 hours after administration. The diameter (not the erythema) is measured transverse to the length of the forearm and the result recorded in millimeters together with the strength of PPD used.

Interpretation of the Mantoux test. Tuberculin hypersensitivity may result from infection with *Mycobacterium tuberculosis* or a variety of other non-tuberculous mycobacteria, such as *Mycobacterium avium-intracellulare* or from BCG vaccination. The interpretation of induration resulting from a tuberculin test will therefore be influenced by the occurrence within a particular region of other 'environmental' mycobacteria and by the widespread use of BCG vaccine.

When tuberculous patients from a number of different countries are Mantoux tested with five units PPD a normal distribution will be obtained around a mean with a range from approximately 10 to 25 mm.[104] In some geographical areas (and particularly coastal tropical areas) a number of positive reactions with induration varying from 6 to 12 mm are encountered; these are thought to result from infections by non-tuberculous mycobacteria.[38, 104]

BCG is known to induce tuberculin hypersensitivity and one of the objections to its use is that this hypersensitivity may negate the value of the tuberculin test. The degree and duration of hypersensitivity induced by BCG will vary according to the potency of the vaccine, the manner of its administration and possibly genetic factors in its recipients.[44, 91] Furthermore, repeated tuberculin testing, further BCG vaccination or infection with *Mycobacterium tuberculosis* or other mycobacteria may boost the resulting tuberculin hypersensitivity.[44, 45, 89] Despite these complicating factors it is probable that, where BCG-induced hypersensitivity is present (and BCG is possibly the most successfully administered vaccine in South Africa), it is usually represented by Mantoux reactions of between 6 and 14 mm.[41, 93]

It is thus suggested that, where BCG has been widely administered (as in South Africa) and where non-tuberculous mycobacteria are common, Mantoux reactions of more than 15 mm should be accepted as resulting from *Mycobacterium tuberculosis* infection.[41, 93] Similarly, Heaf test results of grade III or IV should be regarded as resulting from *Mycobacterium tuberculosis* infection.[13] However, despite the widespread use of BCG and the occurrence of non-tuberculous mycobacteria the tuberculin test remains a valuable diagnostic and epidemiological tool provided that possible 'cross reactions' at lower levels of induration are kept in mind.[60]

The Tine test

The Tine test, because of its relative simplicity, has its greatest value as a screening test, as for example, in a paediatric outpatient department where a large number of children must be tuberculin tested. It is a commercially available disposable multiple puncture tuberculin testing apparatus. Four sterile steel prongs or 'tines' are coated with tuberculin (in the past old tuberculin was used to coat the tines but in recent years PPD has been used) and these deliver the tuberculin into the skin when the apparatus is evenly pressed onto it for two seconds. Upon removing the apparatus four puncture marks and a circular depression caused by the base-plate of the apparatus should be visible. The Tine test is also read after 48 to 72 hours.

Interpretation of the Tine test. It is recommended by the manufacturers that any induration of ≥2 mm around a tine puncture should be regarded as 'positive'. A coalescent ring of induration involving all four tine punctures and giving rise to a solid dome-shaped swelling is probably equivalent to an induration of ≥15 mm following Mantoux testing; and it is desirable that this should be confirmed by Mantoux testing.

The Heaf test

The multiple puncture Heaf test was described in 1951 by Frederick Heaf and has been a valuable screening test in the past. However, with the advent of AIDS it is likely that the test will fall into disuse. The Heaf gun is a multiple-puncture spring-loaded device which causes six needles to pierce the skin and carry an amount of tuberculin more or less equal to 10 units PPD into the skin.

The test is also read after 48 to 72 hours and its grading is well established.

Grade I
Induration is palpable around at least four puncture sites.

Grade II

A ring of induration has been formed.

Grade III

A solid dome-shaped swelling is formed.

Grade IV

Vesiculation or even ulceration is present in addition to induration.

In the presence of BCG immunization a grade III or IV reaction is accepted as indicating *Mycobacterium tuberculosis* infection.

Immunological techniques

Immunological techniques have been used in attempts to diagnose tuberculosis almost since the discovery of *Mycobacterium tuberculosis* by Robert Koch in 1882. In 1898 Arloing and Courmant described an agglutination technique for the detection of anti-tuberculous antibodies using whole *Mycobacterium tuberculosis* organisms, but they encountered a false positivity rate of 30 per cent.[1] Since then increasingly sophisticated methods, such as haemagglutination,[66] gel diffusion,[77] bentonite flocculation,[99] fluorescent antibody techniques,[74] radioimmunoassay,[75] and ELISA[76] have been applied to the problem. However, until recently the problems of false positivity or false negativity have negated the large scale clinical usefulness of the procedures.

The identification and purification of specific highly purified mycobacterial antigens[23, 24] and the development of monoclonal antibodies[48] again raised hopes of increased diagnostic accuracy. Using an ELISA with antibody to *Mycobacterium tuberculosis*, antigen 5 for the identification of antibodies in certain groups of subjects with pulmonary tuberculosis, a sensitivity of nearly 90 per cent was found. It was, however, thought that the specificity of the test would fall to close to 80 per cent in areas of high tuberculosis prevalence.[5] Following another study of the serodiagnosis of tuberculosis by radioimmunoassay the opinion was expressed that it was 'unlikely that antibody assays alone would prove useful in the diagnosis of this disease'.[106]

As a result of the problems encountered in developing simple reliable methods for the detection of antibodies against mycobacterial antigens, attempts have also been made to identify specific immune complexes as a better indication of tuberculous activity. Such immune complexes can indeed be identified in pulmonary tuberculosis patients and have been found to be significantly higher in patients than in healthy controls, but the precise value of such assays in the clinical world remains to be determined.[7]

An alternative to the detection of antibody to mycobacterial antigens is the detection of the antigens themselves, and a number of investigators have now evaluated a variety of diagnostic methods for this purpose. In 1982 Kadival *et al.* described a radioimmunoassay using a commercially available anti-BCG immunoglobulin fraction (Dakopatts A/S Copenhagen) and a cell sonicate antigen of *Mycobacterium tuberculosis* strain H37RV.[52] Used in sputum the assay had sufficient sensitivity to detect 1×10^3 organisms/ml, or 1 ng/ml of sonicate antigen when used in cerebrospinal fluid in tuberculous meningitis, but the assay was unsuccessful. More recently these same workers have developed a biotin-avidin radioimmunoassay with a sensitivity to less than 20 ng/ml tuberculous antigen, which enabled them to detect antigen in 15 of 19 cerebrospinal fluid samples from TBM patients evaluated (79 per cent). Only two of 56 control samples (four per cent) contained detectable antigen.[51]

An ELISA which also uses commercially available anti-BCG immunoglobulin and BCG for the detection of mycobacterial antigens in the cerebrospinal fluid of TBM patients was described by Mexican workers in 1983. In a relatively small number of cases this had a sensitivity of 81 per cent and a specificity of 95 per cent.[87] A year later a latex particle agglutination test using monoclonal antibody for the detection of a specific mycobacterial plasma membrane antigen in cerebrospinal fluid was described, and this also had very satisfactory sensitivity and specificity.[55] Despite their promise, neither of the above tests has become as yet commercially available or found large scale clinical application. A competition ELISA for the detection of mycobacterial antigen has also been recently described. This showed no false negative results and only one false positive when evaluated in a variety of tuberculous exudates.[82]

Given the antigenic complexity of *Mycobacterium tuberculosis* and other mycobacteria – more than 60 immunologically active antigens which could give rise to antibody formation have now been identified[25] – it is not surprising that considerable difficulty has been experienced in developing totally satisfactory repeatable immunological methods for the diagnosis of tuberculosis. It is also apparent that tuberculosis – like leprosy – is characterized by a spectrum of immune responses.[59] On the one hand this may be mainly cell-mediated with minimal antibody production ('tuberculoid'), while on the other hand a poor cell-mediated response may be associated with an enormous production of antibody ('lepromatous'). Furthermore, it is also possible that the nature of the response and the tuberculous antigens to which the body will respond may be determined by an initial 'priming' of the immune system – environmental mycobacteria may play a role in this.[85, 94] However, it is also known that mycobacteria share antigens with some other micro-organisms and that these antigens may be responsible for certain of the false positive results encountered in immunologic antigen detection systems.[68]

With the ever increasing knowledge of immune functions and a deepening of our knowledge of the structure of mycobacteria it would appear to be only a question of time before sensitive and specific immunologic tests become freely available for the diagnosis of the various forms of tuberculosis.

Adenosine deaminase activity

Adenosine deaminase (ADA) is an enzyme found in most mammalian tissues and is thought to have a prominent role in cell growth and division, and in lymphocyte proliferation in particular.[49] Increased serum and plasma ADA activity has been found in patients and experimental animals with cancer,[88] and particularly high levels have been reported in patients with infectious mononucleosis and miliary tuberculosis.[54, 73]

It has been known for some time that cerebrospinal fluid ADA activity is often increased in TBM, but infrequently in virus or aseptic meningitis.[46, 78] However, while some have reported values within normal limits (less than 6 u/l) in bacterial meningitis,[8, 83] others have found raised levels in bacterial meningitis cerebrospinal fluid evaluated prior to the initiation of therapy.[18, 31, 49, 62] A relationship to cerebrospinal fluid protein concentration has also been shown,[31, 54, 62] and sequential sampling of cerebrospinal fluid during direct ventricular drainage has indicated a tendency for cerebrospinal fluid protein concentration and ADA activity to move in parallel.[30]

It therefore seems probable that the increased cerebrospinal fluid ADA activity found in TBM represents an 'increase of the protein permeability through the vascular barrier between blood and fluid (cerebrospinal fluid)'.[46] Cerebrospinal fluid ADA activity greater than 6 u/l is not found in normal cerebrospinal fluid and is very unusual in aseptic or viral meningitis, although values above this level may be found in TBM or bacterial meningitis or in the presence of some other malignant or infectious involvement of the meninges. Values of less than 6 u/l do not, however, exclude TBM, and cerebrospinal fluid ADA activity values should, as with other cerebrospinal fluid investigations, be interpreted in the light of the patient's clinical condition.

ADA activity is also increased in tuberculous pleural effusions[78] and is of diagnostic value in that it aids their differentiation from effusions resulting from secondary malignant tumours of the pleura, from mesothelioma and from pulmonary embolisms. ADA activity in tuberculous pleural effusions is not as high as is the level in effusions caused by lymphoproliferative disorders and it does not differ from that found in para-infective effusions.[63] ADA activity is higher than 40 u/l in 90 per cent of tuberculous or parapneumonic effusions, but in only 10 per cent of those effusions that result from a malignancy. When an effusion is found to be mainly lymphocytic on microscopy, an ADA activity greater than 60 u/l is very suggestive of a tuberculous origin.

The bromide partition test

Differential permeability of the blood-brain barrier for bromide in a variety of diseases

Table 15.1
Suggested hierarchical classification of childhood tuberculosis

1. SUSPECTED TUBERCULOSIS
   Any child with a suspicious chest radiograph where doubt exists as to the radiological findings or quality of the plate.

2. PROBABLE TUBERCULOSIS
   Any child with a suspicious chest radiograph together with weight loss or failure to gain adequately, or a history of contact with an adult case of tuberculosis or with a strongly positive tuberculin test (Mantoux ≥15 mm);
   or any child with a good quality chest radiograph showing changes undoubtedly due to tuberculosis, such as hilar or paratracheal adenopathy or a miliary picture;
   or with histological evidence of tuberculosis on biopsy.

3. CONFIRMED TUBERCULOSIS
   Those children with a positive culture of *Mycobacterium tuberculosis*.

was first investigated in 1929, and increased permeability was found in tuberculous meningitis and neurosyphilis.[101] These findings were confirmed by later workers,[50] and the use of the bromide partition ratio as a diagnostic aid was assessed by Taylor *et al.* in 1954. They considered the test 'helpful' in differentiating TBM from other non-purulent meningitides.[97] In 33 patients values lower than 1,6 were found in all but three instances, and similar results have been reported by other investigators.[14] The test has been refined by the use of a bromide radioisotope 82[BR],[18, 21, 105] and overall sensitivity and specificity have exceeded 90 per cent. False positives may occur in pyogenic meningitis and occasionally in mumps meningitis.[18, 102] The test is particularly valuable in that positive results may be found in TBM for up to five months after the start of treatment.[18]

Other diagnostic techniques

Other diagnostic techniques described in the literature include electron capture gas chromatography and mass spectrum identification of specific substances in the cerebrospinal fluid for TBM[11] and the detection of tuberculostearic acid, also by gas chromatography and mass spectrometry.[62] Both these techniques are relatively cumbersome and have not found wide application as yet. Recently considerable interest has been

aroused by the possibility of detecting mycobacterial DNA in clinical samples.[110]

The determination of cerebrospinal fluid lactate levels may aid the differentiation of TBM from aseptic meningitis, but normal values may occasionally be encountered in TBM.[32] Lactate dehydrogenase levels are frequently normal in TBM and are of little diagnostic value.[2, 32]

THE DIAGNOSIS OF TUBERCULOSIS IN CHILDHOOD

The diagnosis of tuberculosis in childhood is seldom incontrovertibly proven bacteriologically, and often rests upon accumulated circumstantial evidence.[3, 72, 95] The clinician may also feel it necessary at times to initiate antituberculous therapy in a sick child upon what may appear to be somewhat flimsy grounds. The certainty with which the diagnosis is made and the reliability of the evidence upon which it is based will thus vary from case to case.

The World Health Organization[81] and, more recently, workers in Kenya[22] have suggested the adoption of an hierarchical approach to the diagnosis of tuberculosis in childhood, classifying cases as suspect, probable or confirmed (Table 15.1). The more widespread use of such a system would promote the use of a standard case definition, with advantages for both clinical and epidemiological work.

SUMMARY

Suspicion is the key to the diagnosis of tuberculosis in the individual. This should be aroused by appropriate history or clinical signs and supported by chest radiography, sputum culture and microscopy. For *epidemiological purposes*, as for example in prevalence surveys or the screening of large numbers of patients, reliance should be placed on sputum culture. Mass radiography should be resorted to only for the evaluation of specific limited populations with a high risk of disease. For the evaluation of long term trends, the determination of *the annual risk of infection* is the most valuable procedure and may be supported by the monitoring of a sentinel manifestation such as tuberculous meningitis.

In childhood, the diagnosis of tuberculosis is infrequently confirmed by culture of *Mycobacterium tuberculosis*, while chest radiography supported by tuberculin testing is an important diagnostic tool to detect those young children who are infected and therefore in danger of developing tuberculous disease.

REFERENCES

1 Arloing S & Courmant P, 1898. Sur la recherche et la valeur clinique de l'agglutination du bacille de Koch par le serum sanguim de l'homme. *C R Acad Sci.* 127, 425–8.
2 Aronson S M, 1960. Enzyme determinations in neurologic and neuromuscular disease of infancy and childhood. *Pediatric Clinics of North America.* 7, 527–42.
3 Barnett G D & Styblo K, 1977. Bacteriological and x-ray status of tuberculosis following primary infection acquired during adolescence or later. *Bull IUAT.* 52, 5–15.
4 Bech V, 1962. Measles epidemics in Greenland. *American Journal of Diseases of Childhood.* 103, 252–3.
5 Benjamin R G & Daniel T M, 1982. Serodiagnosis of tuberculosis using the enzyme-linked immunosorbent assay (ELISA) of antibody to *Mycobacterium tuberculosis* antigen 5. *American Review of Respiratory Diseases.* 126, 1013–6.
6 Bentley F J, Grzybowski S & Benjamin B, 1954. Epidemiological considerations. In: *Tuberculosis in Childhood and Adolescence.* London: National Association for the Prevention of Tuberculosis.
7 Bhattacharya A, Ranadive S N, Kale M & Bhattacharya S, 1986. Antibody-based enzyme-linked immunosorbent assay for determination of immune complexes in clinical tuberculosis. *American Review of Respiratory Diseases.* 134, 205–9.
8 Blake J & Berman P, 1982. The use of adenosine deaminase assays in the diagnosis of tuberculosis. *South African Medical Journal.* 62, 19–21.
9 Brailey M, 1940. A study of tuberculous infection and mortality in the children of tuberculous households. *American Journal of Hygiene.* 31, 1–43.
10 Brisson-Noel A, Gicquel B, Lecossier D, Levy-Frebault V, Nassif X & Hance A J, 1989. Rapid diagnosis of tuberculosis by amplification of mycobacterial DNA in clinical samples. *Lancet.* 2, 1069–71.
11 Brooks J B, Choudhary G, Craven R B *et al.*, 1977. Electron capture gas chromatography detection and mass spectrum identification of 3–(2'–ketohexyl) indoline in spinal fluids of patients with tuberculous meningitis. *Journal of Clinical Microbiology.* 5, 625–8.
12 Cammock R M, Miller F J W, 1953. Tuberculosis in young children. *Lancet.* 1, 158–60.
13 Capewell S, Leitch A G, 1986. Tuberculin reactivity in a chest clinic, the effects of age and prior BCG vaccination. *British Journal of Diseases of the Chest.* 80, 37–44.
14 Cheek D , 1956. Further observations on electrolyte changes in tuberculous meningitis. *Pediatrics.* 18, 218–26.
15 Christensen P E, Schmidt H, Jensen O, Bang HO, Andersen V & Jordal B, 1952. An epidemic of measles in southern Greenland. *Acta Medica Scandinavica.* 144, 313–22, 430–49, 450–4.
16 Christie A B, 1987. Whooping cough (pertussis) In: Christie A B (ed.). *Infectious Disease, Epidemiology and Clinical Practice* (4th edn). Edinburgh: Churchill Livingstone.
17 Collie A, 1987. The tuberculosis control programme. *Epidemiological Comments.* 14(8), 2–40.
18 Coovadia Y M, Dawood A. Ellis M E, Coovadia H M & Daniel T M, 1986. Evaluation of adenosine deaminase activity and antibody to *Mycobacterium tuberculosis* antigen 5 in cerebrospinal fluid and the radioactive bromide partition test for the early diagnosis of tuberculosis meningitis. *Archives of Diseases of Childhood.* 61, 428–35.

19 Cowie R L & Escreet B C, 1980. The diagnosis of pulmonary tuberculosis. *South African Medical Journal.* 57, 75–7.

20 Cowie R L, Langton M E & Escreet B C, 1985. Diagnosis of sputum smear- and sputum culture-negative pulmonary tuberculosis. *South African Medical Journal.* 68, 878.

21 Crook A, Duncan H, Gutteridge B & Pallis C, 1960. Use of [82]BR in differential diagnosis of lymphocytic meningitis. *British Medical Journal.* 1, 704–6.

22 Cundall D B, 1986. The diagnosis of pulmonary tuberculosis in malnourished Kenyan children. *Annals of Tropical Paediatrics.* 6, 249–55.

23 Daniel T M & Aderson P A, 1978. The isolation by immuno absorbent affinity chromatography and physiochemical characterization of *Mycobacterium tuberculosis* antigen 5. *American Review of Respiratory Diseases* 117, 533–9.

24 Daniel T M, Ellner J J, Todd L S *et al.*, 1977. Immunobiology and species distribution of *Mycobacterium tuberculosis* antigen 5. *Infectious Immunology.* 24, 72–82.

25 Daniel T M & Janicki B W, 1978. Mycobacterial antigens, A review of their isolation, chemistry and immunological properties. *Microbiology Review.* 42, 84–113.

26 DeBuse P J, Lewis M G &, Mugerwa J W, 1970. Pulmonary complications of measles in Uganda. *Journal of Tropical Pediatrics.* 16, 197–203.

27 Devadatta S, Dawson J J Y, Fox W *et al.*, 1970. Attack rate of tuberculosis in a 5 year period among close family contacts of tuberculous patients under domiciliary treatment with isoniazid plus PAS or isoniazid alone. *Bulletin of the World Health Organization.* 42, 337–51.

28 Dippenaar J, 1986. Overdiagnosis of tuberculosis. *South African Medical Journal.* 70, 839–40.

29 Donald P R, Ball J B & Burger P J, 1985. Bacteriologically confirmed pulmonary tuberculosis in childhood. *South African Medical Journal.* 67, 588–90.

30 Donald P R, Malan C & Schoeman J F, 1987. Adenosine deaminase activity as a diagnostic aid in tuberculous meningitis. *Journal of Infectious Diseases.* 156, 1040–41.

31 Donald P R, Malan C, Van der Walt A & Schoeman J F, 1986. The simultaneous determination of cerebrospinal fluid and plasma adenosine deaminase activity as a diagnostic aid in tuberculous meningitis. *South African Medical Journal.* 69, 505–7.

32 Donald P R & Malan C, 1985. Cerebrospinal fluid lactate and lactate dehydrogenase levels as diagnostic aids in tuberculous meningitis. *South African Medical Journal.* 67, 19–20.

33 Donald P R, Schoeman J F & Van Schalkwyk H J S, 1985. The 'Road to Health' card in tuberculous meningitis. *Journal of Tropical Pediatrics.* 31, 117–20.

34 Dorlands Medical Dictionary, 1988. 7th edn. Philadelphia: W B Saunders Co.

35 Duggan M B, Alwar J & Milner R D G, 1986. The nutritional cost of measles in Africa. *Archives of Diseases of Childhood.* 61, 61–6.

36 Duggan M B & Milner R D G, 1986. Energy cost of measles infection. *Archives of Diseases of Childhood.* 61, 436–39.

37 Ebrahim G J, 1981. *Paediatric Practice in Developing Countries.* Basingstoke:English Language Book Society, Macmillan.

38 Edwards P Q & Edwards L B, 1960. Quantitative aspects of tuberculin sensitivity. *American Review of Respiratory Diseases.* 81 (supplement), 24–32.

39 Flick J A, 1976. Does measles really predispose to tuberculosis? *American Review of Respiratory Diseases.* 114, 257–65.

40 Fourie P B, Gatner E M S, Glatthaar E & Kleeberg H H, 1980. Follow up tuberculosis prevalence survey of Transkei. *Tubercle.* 61, 71–9.

41 Fourie P B, 1983. Patterns of tuberculin hypersensitivity in South Africa. *Tubercle.* 64, 167–79.

42 French G L, Teoh R, Chan C Y, Humphries M J, Cheung S W & O'Mahony G O, 1987. Diagnosis of tuberculous meningitis by detection of tuberculostearic acid in cerebrospinal fluid. *Lancet.* 2, 117–9.

43 Gill G V, Krige L P & Pelly M D E, 1983. Overdiagnosis of tuberculosis. *South African Medical Journal.* 63, 933–5.

44 Grindulis H, Baynham M I D, Scott P H, Thompson R A & Wharton B A, 1984. Tuberculin response two years after BCG vaccination at birth. *Archives of Diseases of Childhood.* 59, 614.

45 Guld J, Waaler H, Sundaresan T K, Kaufmann P C & ten Dam H G, 1968. The duration of BCG-induced tuberculin sensitivity in children and its irrelevance for revaccination. *Bulletin of the World Health Organization.* 39, 829–36.

46 Hankiewicz J & Lesniak M, 1972. Adenosine deaminase in cerebrospinal fluid. *Enzymologia.* 43, 385–95.

47 Hennink M J, Skibbe A & Donald P R, 1988. Failure to gain in weight prior to the diagnosis of pulmonary tuberculosis. *Journal of Tropical Pediatrics.* 34, 108–9.

48 Hewitt J, Coates A R M, Mitchison D A & Ivanyi J, 1982. The use of murine monoclonal antibodies without purification of antigens in the serodiagnosis of tuberculosis. *Journal of Immunological Methodology.* 55, 205–11.

49 Hovi T, Smyth J F, Allison A C & Williams S C, 1976. Role of adenosine deaminase in lymphocyte proliferation. *Clinical and Experimental Immunology.* 23, 395–403.

50 Hunter G, Smith H V & Taylor M, 1954. On the bromide test of permeability of the barrier between blood and cerebrospinal fluid — an assessment. *Biochemistry Journal.* 56, 588–97.

51 Kadival G V, Samuel A M, Telisforo B M S M & Chaparas S D, 1987. Radioimmunoassay for detecting *Mycobacterium tuberculosis* antigen in cerebrospinal fluids of patients with tuberculous meningitis. *Journal of Infectious Diseases.* 155, 608–11.

52 Kadival G V, Samuel A M, Virdi B S *et al.,* 1982. Radioimmunoassay of tuberculous antigen. *Indian Journal of Medical Research.* 75, 765–70.

53 Kipps A & Kaschula R O C, 1976. Virus pneumonia following measles. *South African Medical Journal.* 50, 1083–8.

54 Koehler L H & Benz E J, 1962. Serum adenosine deaminase, methodology and clinical application. *Clinical Chemistry.* 8, 133–40.

55 Krambovitis E, McIllmurray M B, Lock P E, Hendrickse W & Holzel H, 1984. Rapid diagnosis of tuberculous meningitis by latex particle agglutination. *Lancet.* 2, 1229–31.

56 Krasnow I & Wayne L G, 1969. Comparison of methods for tuberculosis bacteriology. *Applied Microbiology.* 18, 915.

57 Krige F K & Donald P R, 1990. Die voortgesette voorkoms van kwashiorkor binne die groter metropolitaanse gebied van Kaapstad. *Geneeskunde.* 32.

58 Kustner H G V, 1981. Tuberculosis in children. *Epidemiological Comments.* 8(10), 2–18.

59 Lenzini L, Rotolli P & Rotolli L, 1977. The spectrum of human tuberculosis. *Clinical and Experimental Immunology.* 27, 230–7.

60 Lifschitz M, 1965. The value of the tuberculin test as a screening test for tuberculosis among BCG vaccinated children. *Pediatrics.* 36, 624–7.

61 Lloyd A V C, 1968. Bacteriological diagnosis of tuberculosis in children. A comparative study of gastric lavage and laryngeal swab methods. *East African Medical Journal.* 45, 140–3.

62 Malan C, Donald P R, Golden M & Taljaard J J F, 1984. Adenosine deaminase levels in cerebrospinal fluid in the diagnosis of tuberculous meningitis. *Journal of Tropical Medicine and Hygiene.* 87, 33–40.

63 Maritz F J, Malan C & Le Roux I, 1982. Adenosine deaminase estimations in the differentiation of pleural effusions. *South African Medical Journal.* 62, 556–8.

64 Marton K I, Sox H C & Krupp J R, 1981. Involuntary weight loss, diagnostic and prognostic significance. *Annals of International Medicine.* 95, 568–74.

65 Mets J T, 1980. The diagnosis of pulmonary tuberculosis. *South African Medical Journal.* 57, 521.

66 Middelbrook G & Dubos R K, 1948. Specific serum agglutination of erythrocytes sensitized with extracts of tubercle bacilli. *Journal of Experimental Medicine.* 88, 521–8.

67 Miller F J W, 1982. The recognition, diagnosis and treatment of tuberculosis in children. In: *Tuberculosis in Children.* Edinburgh: Churchill, Livingstone.

68 Minden P, McClatchy J K & Farr R S, 1972. Shared antigens between heterologous bacterial species. *Infectious Immunology.* 6, 574–82.

69 Morley D, 1973. Whooping cough. In: *Paediatric Priorities in the Developing World.* London: Butterworths.

70 Morley D C, 1959. Childhood tuberculosis in a rural area of West Africa. *West African Medical Journal.* 8, 225–9.

71 Morris C D W & Nell H, 1988. Epidemic of pulmonary tuberculosis in geriatric homes. *South African Medical Journal.* 74, 117–20.

72 Morrison J B, 1973. Natural history of segmental lesions in primary pulmonary tuberculosis. *Archives of Diseases of Childhood.* 48, 90–8.

73 Muller-Beissenhirtz Von W & Keller H, 1966. Die bestimmung der adenosindeaminase im serum. *Deutsche Mediese Wochenschrift.* 91, 159–68.

74 Nassau E & Merrick A J, 1970. The fluorescent antibody test in human tuberculosis, a pilot study. *Tubercle.* 51, 430–6.

75 Nassau E, Parsons E R & Johnson G D, 1975. Detection of antibodies to *Mycobacterium tuberculosis* by solid phase radioimmunoassay. *Journal of Immunological Methodology.* 6, 261–71.

76   Nassau E, Parsons E R & Johnson G D, 1976. The detection of antibodies to Mycobacterium tuberculosis by microplate enzyme-linked immunosorbent assay (ELISA). *Tubercle.* 57, 67–70.

77   Parlett R C & Youmans G P, 1959. An evaluation of the specificity and sensitivity of a gel double-diffusion test for tuberculosis. A double-blind study. *American Review of Respiratory Diseases.* 80, 153–66.

78   Piras M A, Gakis C, Budroni M & Andreoni G, 1978. Adenosine deaminase activity in pleural effusions, an aid to differential diagnosis. *British Medical Journal.* 2, 1751–2.

79   Piras M A & Gakis C, 1973. Cerebrospinal fluid adenosine deaminase activity in tuberculous meningitis. *Enzyme.* 14, 311–7.

80   Pretorius P J, Davel J G A & Coetzee J N, 1956. Some observations on the development of kwashiorkor. *South African Medical Journal.* 30, 396–9.

81   *Provisional Guidelines for the Diagnosis and Classification of the EPI Target Diseases for Primary Health Care Surveillance and Special Studies,* 1983. (EPI/GEN/83/4). Geneva: World Health Organization.

82   Ramkisson A, Coovadia Y M & Coovadia H M, 1988. A competition ELISA for the detection of mycobacterial antigen in tuberculosis exudates. *Tubercle.* 69, 209–12.

83   Ribera E, Martinez-Vazquez J M, Ocana I, Segura R M & Pascual C, 1987. Activity of adenosine deaminase in cerebrospinal fluid for the diagnosis and follow up of tuberculous meningitis in adults. *Journal of Infectious Diseases.* 155, 603–7.

84   Rich A R, 1951. The influence of sex and age. In: *The Pathogenesis of Tuberculosis.* Springfield: Charles C Thomas.

85   Rook G A W, Bahr G M & Stanford J L, 1981. The effect of two distinct forms of cell-mediated response to mycobacteria on the protective efficacy of BCG. *Tubercle.* 62, 63–8.

86   Rouillon A, Perdrizet S & Parrot R, 1976. Transmission of tubercle bacilli, the effects of chemotherapy. *Tubercle,* 57, 275–99.

87   Sada E, Ruiz-Palacios G M, Lopez-Vidal Y & Ponce de Leon S, 1983. Detection of mycobacterial antigens in cerebrospinal fluid of patients with tuberculous meningitis by enzyme-linked immunosorbent assay. *Lancet.* 2, 651–2.

88   Schwartz M K & Bodansky O, 1959. Serum adenosine deaminase activity in cancer. *Proceedings of the Society for Experimental Biology.* 101, 560–2.

89   Sepulveda P L, Burr C, Ferrer X & Sorensen R U, 1988. Booster effect of tuberculin testing in healthy 6–year-old school children vaccinated with *Bacillus Calmette-Guérin* at birth in Santiago, Chile. *Pediatric Infectious Disease Journal.* 7, 578–81.

90   Smythe P M, Schonland M, Brereton-Stiles G G *et al.,* 1971. Thymolymphatic deficiency and depression of cell-mediated immunity in protein- calorie malnutrition. *Lancet.* 2, 939.

91   Snider D E, 1985. Bacille-Calmette-Guérin vaccinations and tuberculin skin tests. *Journal of the American Medical Association.* 253, 3438–9.

92   Snider D E, Hopewell P C, Mills J & Reichman L B, 1987. Mycobacterioses and the acquired immunodeficiency syndrome. *American Review of Respiratory Diseases* 136, 492–6.

93   Snider D E, 1982. The tuberculin skin test. *American Review of Respiratory Diseases.* 125 (supplement), 108–18.

94   Standford J L, Shield M J & Rook G A, 1981. How environmental mycobacteria may predetermine the protective efficacy of BCG. *Tubercle.* 62, 55–62.

95   Styblo K & Sutherland I, 1982. Epidemiology of tuberculosis in children. *Bulletin of the IUAT.* 57, 133–9.

96   Styblo K, 1983. The epidemiological situation of tuberculosis and the impact of control measures. *Bulletin of the IUAT.* 58, 179–86.

97   Taylor M, Smith H V & Hunter G, 1954. The blood-CSF barrier to bromide in diagnosis of tuberculous meningitis. *Lancet.* 1, 700–2.

98   Thompson N J, Glassroth J L, Snider D E & Farer L S, 1979. The booster phenomenon in serial tuberculin testing. *American Review of Respiratory Diseases.* 119, 587–97.

99   Wallace R, Diena B B, Greenberg L & Jassamine A F, 1966. A study of tuberculosis antibodies by bentonite flocculation. *Canadian Medical Association Journal.* 94, 947–50.

100 Wallgren A, 1948. The 'time-table' of tuberculosis. *Tubercle.* 29, 245–51.

101 Walter F K, 1929. Die blut-liquor schranke. Leipzig: G Thieme.

102 Wassermann H P & Van Heerden P R D, 1977. Pampoentjie-meningitis — Broom 82 partisietoets en serebrospinale vog glukose. *South African Medical Journal.* 52, 851–2.

103 Whittle H C, Bradley-Moore A, Fleming A & Greenwood B M, 1973. Effects of measles on the immune response of Nigerian children. *Archives of Diseases of Childhood.* 48, 753–6.

104 WHO Tuberculosis Research Office, 1955. Further studies of geographic variation in naturally acquired tuberculin sensitivity. *Bulletin of the World Health Organization.* 12, 63–83.
105 Wiggelinkhuizen J & Mann M, 1980. The radioactive bromide partition test in the diagnosis of tuberculous meningitis in children. *Journal of Pediatrics.* 97, 843–7.
106 Winters W D & Cox R A, 1981. Serodiagnosis of tuberculosis by radioimmunoassay. *American Review of Respiratory Diseases.* 124, 582–5.
107 World Health Organization, 1989. *Statement on AIDS and Tuberculosis* (WHO/GPA/INF/89). Geneva: World Health Organization.

CHAPTER 16

The evolution of anti-tuberculosis chemotherapy

S R Benatar

The history of anti-tuberculosis chemotherapy begins in the 1940s, when streptomycin was discovered and introduced into clinical medicine at a time when statisticians were beginning to play an important role in the design of clinical trials. The British Medical Research Council led the way with a series of controlled studies that first involved streptomycin and later para-amino-salicylic acid (PAS) and isoniazid (INH). These resulted in the establishment, by the early 1950s, of a combined chemotherapy regimen that used the three drugs to achieve an anticipated 100 per cent cure rate with only rare relapses. By the mid-1950s the characteristics of contemporary management and therapy of pulmonary tuberculosis, as summarized by Fox,[21] were as follows:

- the combined use of PAS, streptomycin and INH for two years or more;
- administration of these drugs in divided doses, two to four times per day;
- many months of in-patient treatment in rural sanatoria with careful attention to diet, rest, and fresh air;
- monthly chest radiographs and frequent tomographic examinations;
- sputum examination — direct smear and culture — on a monthly basis;
- routine sensitivity tests and adjustments made to drug therapy if resistant strains were grown;
- a decline in the use of surgery although many indications for surgery remained. In 1962 the MRC established the optimum duration of therapy for cavitary tuberculosis, thus eliminating the need to resect cavities which remained after adequate chemotherapy. Subsequent to this

the decline in surgery for tuberculosis became more marked; and
- follow up on a regular basis, both clinically and radiographically, after completion of chemotherapy, often for many years.

This treatment programme was expensive and made major demands on patients, their families and the health services. During the 1960s it became clear that such programmes, which aimed at achieving 100 per cent cure, were becoming too expensive and too difficult to implement in most developing countries, and so the search began for shorter courses of chemotherapy that would be designed to achieve less than 100 per cent cure rate with the savings on shorter duration of treatment being traded off against lower total (but still high and acceptable) cure rates. With the introduction of rifampicin in the late 1960s, and advances in understanding the mechanisms and actions of the anti-tuberculosis drugs in experimental murine tuberculosis, the British Medical Research Council and others embarked on large controlled clinical trials in several countries; the results of which form the basis of modern anti-tuberculosis chemotherapy. Some historical milestones in the development of chemotherapy since 1944 are briefly outlined in Table 16.1.

ACTIONS AND EFFECTS OF FIRST-LINE ANTI-TUBERCULOSIS DRUGS

Mycobacterium tuberculosis is an obligate aerobe which grows at a rate proportional to the oxygen tension of its environment. As a result the bacillus multiplies most rapidly in the high oxygen tension

Table 16.1
Some historical milestones in the development of chemotherapy[13, 36]

1944	Discovery of streptomycin.[34]
1948	British MRC report on a controlled trial of streptomycin in tuberculosis.[4]
1950	British MRC report on treatment of tuberculosis with streptomycin and PAS[5] (combined therapy became established).
1952	Isoniazid introduced, British MRC trial showed emergence of resistant bacilli in almost 75 per cent of patients treated with INH alone.[6]
1952	Pyrazinamide introduced as a 'secondary' drug but its bactericidal action was not exploited.[28]
1956–59	Trials showed decisively that chemotherapy eliminated the need for rest and that patients could be treated at home.[30, 38]
1960	High cure rate, low relapse rate of prolonged, combined chemotherapy well established.[12]
1962	Medical Research Council trial established optimum duration of therapy (two years) for cavitary tuberculosis (thus eliminating the need to resect cavities which remained after adequate chemotherapy).[7]
1966	Rifampicin introduced.[39]
1967	Basis for short course chemotherapy (with regimens containing RIF and INH) established in experimental murine tuberculosis.[3, 26, 39]
1968	Ethambutol introduced.[25]
1969	Effectiveness of supervised intermittent chemotherapy (without RIF) established.[32]
1970–7	Effectiveness of 12 and 9 month regimens (without RIF) established.[27, 29]
1973	British MRC trial demonstrated superiority of RIF containing regimens.[8]
1974–81	East African/British MRC trials established effectiveness of short (six months) and ultra-short (four months) courses.[14–20, 35, 37]
1980	American Thoracic Society approval of nine month courses which included RIF and INH.[1]
1990	British Thoracic Society recommendations for chemotherapy and management of tuberculosis in the United Kingdom.[10]

environment of pulmonary cavities and more slowly in solid caseous foci. This feature, together with its overall slow growth rate (mean replication time 20 hours as compared with 20 minutes for *Escherichia coli* and *Staphylococcus aureus*) and its high rate of mutation to drug resistant forms, are characteristics which have important implications for therapy.[24]

Although tuberculosis is the classic model of infectious disease with intracellular bacterial multiplication, the process of caseation releases bacilli into the extracellular compartment where rapid multiplication takes place when liquefaction and cavity formation result in favourable oxygen tensions. At least three populations of bacilli can be identified: one large and made up of actively multiplying bacilli at neutral pH in liquefied caseous material lining cavity walls, and two others, both similar populations with slower growth rates — (i) organisms within macrophages and at an acid pH, and (ii) organisms within solid caseous areas where, despite neutral pH, low oxygen tension permits only intermittent multiplication. A fourth very small, completely dormant, population of bacilli may also exist.

The bacteriological basis of short course chemotherapy for tuberculosis is founded on this concept of there being several populations of mycobacteria on which anti-tuberculosis drugs have differing actions. These data, which have been fully reviewed by Grosset,[24] are briefly summarized in Table 16.2 together with considerations of tissue penetration.

Isoniazid, rifampicin and streptomycin (in that order of potency) act on the large population of actively multiplying extracellular bacilli in aerobic cavitary lesions. Although this large bacillary population contains a significant number of mutants resistant to any single drug, adequate treatment with this combination is strongly bactericidal and contributes to lasting cure by eliminating all extracellular bacilli. Inadequate treatment

Table 16.2
Effects of first-line drugs on various populations of tubercle bacilli and tissue penetration

DRUG	ACTIVITY	TISSUE PENETRATION
	BACTERICIDAL	
Isoniazid	Against populations* (1),(2) and to some extent(3)	Good (including CSF)
Rifampicin	Against populations (1), (2) and especially(3)	Good (but not as well into CSF)
Streptomycin	Against population (1) (at neutral or alkaline pH)	Good into ECF, pleura and peritoneum Decreased into pericardium and CSF when active inflammation has subsided
Pyrazinamide	Against population (3) predominantly (acid milieu)	Good (including CSF)
	BACTERIOSTATIC	
Ethambutol	Against populations (2) and (3)	Good but decreases into CSF when active inflammation has subsided

* Populations of tubercle bacilli:
(1) Large ($1 \times 10^{7-9}$) actively dividing, extracellular population in aerobic cavitary lesions. Contain significant number of mutants resistant to any single drug.
(2) Small ($1 \times 10^{2-5}$) intermittently dividing, extracellular and intracellular population in closed (anaerobic) caseous areas.
(3) Small ($1 \times 10^{2-5}$) occasionally dividing, intracellular population ('persisters').

Table 16.3
Various chemotherapy regimens and some recommendations[11]

		TOTAL DURATION	COMMENTS
	DAILY THROUGHOUT		
1.	• SHR_2 HR_7	9 months	
	• EHR_2 HR_7	9 months	Avoids unpleasantness and toxicity of streptomycin
2.	• $SHRZ_2$ HR_4	6 months	Pyrazinamide provides advantage in situations where initial INH resistance is high
	• $EHRZ_2$ HR_4	6 months	Avoids unpleasantness and toxicity of streptomycin
3.	• $SHRZ_2$ HT_6	8 months	Advantage of much reduced cost
4.	• SHT_{1-2} HT_{12-18}	12–18 months	High non-compliance rate in developing countries
	• SHE_{1-2} HE_{12-18}	12–18 months	(22–72% failure to complete course)
	• SHP_{1-2} HP_{12-18}	12–18 months	
	PARTIALLY INTERMITTENT		
5.	• SHRZ daily for two months SHZ 2 x week	8 months	Suitable for use where in hospital treatment can be given for at least two
6.	• SHRZ daily for two months HR 2 x week	6 months	months and there are only sufficient facilities for intermittent supervision at clinics.
7.	• SHT daily for two months SH 2 x week	12–18 months	
	• SHP daily for two months SH daily 2 x week	12–18 months	
	INTERMITTENT THROUGHOUT		
8.	• SHRZ 3 x week for four months HRZ 3 x week for two months	6 months	Suitable for environments which lack hospital facilities and can only provide supervised therapy less frequently
9.	• EHRZ 3 x week for six months	6 months	than on a daily basis.

S = Streptomycin	H = Isoniazid	R = Rifampicin Z = Pyrazinamide
T = Thiacetazone	E = Ethambutol	P = Para-amino-salicylic acid

leads to treatment failure either as a result of outgrowth of the original sensitive organism or of resistant organisms.

Rifampicin, INH and pyrazinamide (in that order of potency) act on slowly multiplying intra- and extracellular organisms within macrophages and in closed caseous lesions. Adequate treatment contributes to lasting cure by sterilizing the lesion through the elimination of 'persisters', which are slow or intermittently growing organisms.

It is important to note that adequate treatment is dependent both on the *dose* of drugs used and on the *duration* of therapy. Using higher doses of drugs does not permit a significantly shorter duration of treatment (see below), and with adequate doses good results can be achieved, even with intermittent treatment, if given for an adequate period of time. Inadequate treatment leads to the late growth of 'persisters' and consequent clinical relapse.

Isoniazid and rifampicin are the two most useful drugs for the prevention of the emergence of resistant organisms, while rifampicin and pyrazinamide are the two most important sterilizing drugs as they kill semi-dormant organisms which are not affected by INH. The excellent (or at least adequate) tissue penetration of all the first-line drugs (Table 16.2) ensures the potential to cure tuberculosis in any organ with the delivery of adequate doses of drugs in appropriate combinations for an adequate period of time.

TREATMENT REGIMENS

Advances in the understanding of the pathobiology of tuberculosis and of the effects of anti-tuberculosis drugs *in vitro*, together with the results of many carefully designed and well-conducted clinical studies form the basis on which recommendations regarding modern treatment

Table 16.4
Recommendations of the Joint Tuberculosis Committee of the British Thoracic Society for the treatment of tuberculosis in the United Kingdom[10] (reproduced with permission.)

	INITIAL PHASE		CONTINUATION PHASE		TOTAL
	DRUGS	MONTHS	DRUGS	MONTHS	MONTHS
ADULTS					
Pulmonary	RHZE	2	RH	4	6
Non-pulmonary					
Meningitis	RHZ	2	RH	10	12
Pericarditis	RHZ	2	RH	4	6
Lymph node	RHZ	2	RH	4	6
Bone, joint					
Other sites	RHZE	2	RH	4	6
	or RHE	2	RH	7	9
CHILDREN					
Pulmonary	RHZ	2	RH	4	6
	or RH	2	RH	7	9
Non-pulmonary					
as for adults					
Chemoprophylaxis*	H	6		6	
	RH	3		3	

* The author is not aware of any studies adequately documenting the effectiveness of 6 or 3 month regimens of chemoprophylaxis.

S = Streptomycin	H = Isoniazid	R = Rifampicin	Z = Pyrazinamide
T = Thiacetazone	E = Ethambutol	P = Para-amino-salicylic acid	

regimens are made. The sources of information for all these regimens include the various East African/British Medical Research Council Trials, the Hong Kong/British Medical Research Council Trials, the Singapore/British Medical Research Council Trials and the Madras Study. These studies explored the effects of varying drug combinations and of schedules of treatment on the rate at which sputum was rendered smear and culture negative, the proportion of patients who relapsed after stopping treatment and the effect of treatment on natural and acquired resistance. The extent to which the duration of treatment could be shortened and the implications of intermittent drug therapy were also examined. Although his work was not based on scientific study, Pearson drew attention in 1978 to his gratifying four year experience with fully supervised short course chemotherapy in field conditions in the Cape Divisional Council jurisdiction. In successfully applying this regimen he was clearly at the forefront in translating modern advances in knowledge into practical benefit for patients.[31]

The daily, partially intermittent and completely intermittent regimens recommended by Citron and Girling[11] are shown in Table 16.3, and the more recent recommendations of the Joint Tuberculosis Committee of the British Thoracic Society[10] in Table 16.4. It is recommended that all drugs should be taken in a single daily dose half an hour before breakfast.

The standard regimens currently recommended and used in the United Kingdom and other developed countries are often too expensive for many developing countries. An effective and cheaper regimen recommended for use under these circumstances is a combination of streptomycin, pyrazinamide, INH and rifampicin for two months, continuing with INH and thiacetazone for a further six months (total duration of treatment, eight months). Longer courses without rifampicin and with longer duration of INH and thiacetazone are less effective because of poor compliance with longer courses. This is illustrated by surveys of results obtained by routine chest services when treating pulmonary tuberculosis with standard regimens of chemotherapy for twelve months or longer in India and Kenya. These showed that 50 and 72 per cent of patients respectively had stopped attending at one year.[11]

In his review of short course chemotherapy, Fox has emphasized that the role of streptomycin as a fourth drug is relatively minor, and that neither thiacetazone nor ethambutol (both of which are bacteriostatic) contribute much to either bactericidal or sterilizing activity within short course chemotherapy regimens. He also points out that for regimens not containing PZA nine month courses are better than six month courses.[22] The elimination of streptomycin saves considerable resources (drugs, personnel, syringes, and needles) and avoids the unpleasantness of repeated intramuscular injections.

Currently recommended regimens of treatment in South Africa are shown in Table 16.5. The rationale for using rifater is to reduce the number of tablets which need to be taken and to ensure that all three drugs are taken. Given the fact that all treatment should be given under supervision, it is not evident that the greater expenditure on this combination preparation is warranted.

As many developing countries have very much smaller health budgets than developed countries, the use of shorter courses of chemotherapy must be considered despite the fact that the overall cure rate will be lower. Fox points out that while courses of four-and-a-half to five months' duration may be associated with a three per cent relapse rate (compared with one or two per cent for the best regimens), shortening the duration of treatment to four months increases the relapse rate to approximately 12 per cent and shortening the course further to three months (even using streptomycin, INH, rifampicin and pyrazinamide) results in at least a 13 per cent relapse rate. The savings in expenditure may, however, warrant accepting this lower cure rate in some environments.

Where it is anticipated that patients may default and that adequate treatment may only be taken for the initial phase, the combination of rifampicin, INH and

Table 16.5(a)
Recommended regimens for treating adults in South Africa
(Dept. National Health and Population Development 1990)

DRUG	DOSE	DURATION	TOTAL COST OF COURSES
REGIMEN 1			
Rifater	1 tablet/10 kg Average adult dose <50 kg 4 tabs >50 kg 5 tabs	Once daily Monday to Friday 6 months	R304 R383
REGIMEN 2*			
Rifampicin	<50 kg 450 mg >50 kg 600 mg	As above	R139 R171
Isoniazid	300 mg		
Pyrazinamide	1,5 g		
REGIMEN 3*			
Rifampicin	600 mg		
Isoniazid	20 mg/kg body mass	3 (or 2) x/week for 6 months	R120 (R80)
Pyrazinamide	3 g		

* In areas with known high incidence of INH resistance, Ethambutol may be added.

Table 16.5(b)
Recommended regimens for treating children 6 years of age and younger
(Department of National health and Population Development 1990)

	DOSE	DURATION
Rifampicin	10 mg/kg body mass	Once daily, Monday to Friday, 6 months
Isoniazid	8–10 mg/kg body mass	Once daily, Monday to Friday, 6 months
Pyrazinamide	20–25mg'kg body mass	Once daily, Monday to Friday, 6 months

For children 7 years of age and older the following doses apply:

Regimen 1   Rifater 1 tablet/10 kg body mass
Regimen 2   Isoniazid 8–10 mg/kg Rifampicin 10 mg/kg
            Pyrazinamide 20–25 mg/kg Ethambutol 20 mg/kg
Regimen 3   Rifampicin 10–15 mg/kg Pyrazinamide 30 mg/kg
            Isoniazid 20 mg/kg Ethambutol 30 mg/kg

pyrazinamide should be given. Both the large, rapidly dividing and the smaller, slower and intermittently dividing bacillary populations are susceptible to this combination and it is the only regimen capable of producing at least an 80 per cent cure rate if given for three months. This combination of drugs also has the potential to prevent bacteriological failure resulting from the emergence of resistant bacilli during treatment. It has the further advantage of being as effective against strains of bacilli initially resistant to INH, streptomycin (or both) as against organisms that are fully sensitive. If relapse occurs after such a regimen has been given for an inadequate duration, the same drugs can usually be safely used for re-treatment, as this combination does not result in the outgrowth of strains with additional resistance.

Table 16.6
Doses and side-effects of anti-tuberculosis drugs

DRUGS AND SIDE-EFFECTS	DAILY DOSE		INTERMITTENT DOSE (3 x PER WEEK)	
	ADULTS*	CHILDREN	ADULTS*	CHILDREN
Isoniazid (Hepatitis, Peripheral neuritis, Skin reactions)	300 mg	10 mg/kg	15 mg/kg	15 mg/kg
Rifampicin Hepatitis, Febrile reactions, Enhanced metabolism of other drugs, Stains urine and soft contact lenses pink/orange	450 mg 600 mg	10 mg/kg	600 mg 900 mg**	15 mg/kg**
Pyrazinamide Hepatitis Hyperuricaemia Arthralgia Anorexia	1,5 g 2,0 g	35 mg/kg	2,0 g 2,5 g 2,5 g+ 3,0 g+	50 mg/kg 75 mg/kg
Streptomycin Eighth nerve damage Nephrotoxicity, Skin reactions	750 mg 1 g	15–20 mg/kg	750 mg 1 g	15–20 mg/kg
Ethambutol Optic neuritis (rare 15 mg/kg)	25 mg/kg for two months followed by 15 mg/kg or 15 mg/kg throughout		30 mg/kg 35 mg/kg+	30 mg/kg 35 mg/kg+
Ethionamide GIT disturbances in adults Well tolerated by children	750 mg/kg 1 000 mg	15-20 mg/kg given in 3 doses daily		

* Lower doses for adults <50 kg, high doses >50 kg.
+ When given 2 x weekly.
** There remains some controversy regarding the need to use higher doses of rifampicin in intermittent regimens.
NB. Doses must be adjusted in children as they gain weight.

TUBERCULOSIS CONTROL PROGRAMMES IN DEVELOPING COUNTRIES

Aquinas and Todd have outlined some of the particular problems which face tuberculosis control programmes in developing countries.[2] They recommend that tuberculosis programmes should be nationwide, and they express the view (with which the author concurs) that this can only be achieved through the infrastructure provided by an overall general health service which is adequately organized to effectively deal with other common diseases such as malnutrition, malaria, and parasitic infection. The need for government commitment to the programme is emphasized, but the importance of community participation to ensure success is also highlighted. Support from the World Health Organization, the International Union Against Tuberculosis and other organizations makes a major contribution in some countries.[2]

The Department of National Health and Population Development in South Africa recommends that supervised ambulatory care and compliance may be improved by providing a service characterized by:

- *courtesy:* creating a good first impression and maintaining this through friendliness and encouragement;
- *communicativeness:* letting the patient know what is expected and allowing two way communication;
- *continuity:* reinforcement of clear messages through repetition;
- *consistency:* follow-up by the same staff member if at all possible;
- *client orientation:* listening to clients' (patients') feelings about the diagnosis and the problems it may cause; discussing barriers to compliance and helping the patient overcome these;
- *clear contractual arrangements:* preferably in writing with explicitly stated expectations on both sides;
- *community orientation:* eliciting social support for those patients with impaired access to tuberculosis services;
- *convenience:* short clinic waiting times and an appointment system if possible;
- *contact maintenance:* follow-up of non-attendance as soon as possible;
- *caring relationship;*
- *cleanliness* in the clinic as a mark of respect for patients and for the service being offered.

DRUG DOSES AND SIDE-EFFECTS

Doses of drugs recently recommended in the United Kingdom and their side-effects are shown in Table 16.6.[10] The current costs (1990) of anti-tuberculosis drugs in South Africa are listed in Table 16.7.

Adverse drug reactions are relatively uncommon (in less than five per cent of patients), most are mild, but some are potentially life-threatening. Management of such adverse reactions, of relapse, of acquired

Table 16.7
Cost of anti-tuberculosis drugs in South Africa (October 1990)

DRUG	DOSE PER UNIT	PRICE PER DOSE LISTED	PRICE PER DAILY DOSE
Isoniazid	100 mg	1c	3c
Rifampicin	150 mg	24c	72–96c
Pyrazinamide	500 mg	10c	30–40c
Streptomycin	1 g	139c	139c
Ethambutol	100 mg	3c	20c
	400 mg	6,7c	
Rifater	R 120 mg	58c	230–290c
	H 80 mg		
	Z 250 mg		

resistance and the use of second line drugs, have been adequately covered elsewhere,[11, 23] and are not discussed in this chapter.

RECOMMENDED TREATMENT FOR SPECIAL GROUPS OF PATIENTS[9, 10]

Recommendations for chemotherapy in patients with diabetes, liver and other diseases are summarized in Table 16.8. In general terms, few modifications need to be made to the standard recommended chemotherapy, but patients with tuberculosis and other diseases do require closer medical and psychological attention. It should be noted that the British Thoracic Association Trial showed that the addition of PZA to rifampicin and INH does not increase morbidity in patients with underlying liver disease. It is, however, recommended that liver function be regularly monitored in these patients. The induction of microsomal hepatic enzymes by rifampicin reduces the serum half-life of several drugs including warfarin, phenytoin, sulphonylureas, oestrogen oral contraceptives and corticosteroids. Corticosteroid doses should be doubled and other drugs monitored either by serum levels or measurement of their therapeutic effect. Treatment of patients with silicosis and tuberculosis is covered in Chapter 12.

CHANGES IN CHEMOTHERAPY AND THE MANAGEMENT OF TUBERCULOSIS OVER THE LAST FIFTY YEARS

The progressive introduction of the drugs currently used in the treatment of tuberculosis, coupled with a deeper understanding of the pathobiology of tuberculosis and

Table 16.8
Recommendations for treatment of special groups of patients[10, 11]

Diabetes	Standard treatment recommended. RIF interacts with some oral hypoglycaemic drugs; additional care in control of diabetes.
Liver disease	Standard treatment recommended. Addition of PZA to RIF and INH does not increase morbidity. Monitoring of liver function recommended.
Pregnancy	Avoid streptomycin and other aminoglycosides. Ethionamide and prothionamide may be teratogenic. Normal breast feeding recommended while on Rx. Some oral contraceptives have diminished effect when given with RIF.
Renal disease	Reduce dose of aminoglycosides and ethambutol and monitor serum levels. Rifampicin use necessitates doubling dose of steroids if these are being used to treat renal/systemic disease. Drug dose modification required for patients on dialysis.
AIDS	Standard Rx, but duration may have to be prolonged.
Unconscious patient	INH and RIF syrup available. PZA tablets can be crushed and given via nasogastric tube. RIF, INH available for IV infusion. INH, streptomycin can be given IM.
Alcoholics	Standard chemotherapy. Additional attention via Alcoholics Anonymous or other facilities to stop the patient from drinking.

Table 16.9
Comparison between chemotherapy and management of tuberculosis in the 1950s and the 1980s

	1950s	1980s
• Basis for treatment	Early clinical trials	Bacteriological and pharmacological insight and sophisticated clinical trials
• Place of treatment	In hospital and sanatoria	At home or at work
• Duration	Two years or longer	Six months or less
• Drugs	Streptomycin, PAS, INH, Unsupervised	INH, rifampicin. pyrazinamide Supervised
• Surveillance during treatment	Monthly sputum smear, and culture and CxR sensitivity routinely evaluated	Sputum smear/culture CxR at diagnosis and after completion of treatment
• Compliance	A major problem in view of need for prolonged treatment	Remains problematic but with intermittent, supervised short course regimens, this problem can be minimized
• Surgery	Becoming less frequent	Rare
• Follow up	Prolonged	Minimal after adequate treatment
• Social attitude	Stigmatized Little role for education and community involvement	Accepted Education and community involvement valued and widely practised

of the action of individual drugs, have led to a series of changes in the management of tuberculosis between the introduction of anti-tuberculosis drugs in the late 1940s and the establishment of efficacious short-course chemotherapy in the early 1980s. The evolution in management strategies to which these advances have led is striking (Table 16.9). Hospitalization is now only required for a small proportion of patients (those too ill for outpatient treatment, where cooperation or supervision is inadequate, for miliary, meningeal or other complicated cases, drug toxicity or resistance, or when surgery is being considered); high cure rates can be achieved with *supervised* short courses of therapy at relatively low total cost and given to patients while they continue to work; the stigma associated with the disease is considerably reduced; health education plays an important role in the management programme; and long term follow-up is much less necessary. These advances have been more effectively achieved in developed countries, and the challenge to do the same in developing countries remains high.

The search for new drugs, however, continues and is mandated by both increasing resistance to conventional drugs and the potential need for additional drugs in the treatment of tuberculosis complicating AIDS. It has been estimated that in a population of tubercle bacilli, 1 in 10^5 bacilli are resistant to INH, 1 in 10^6 to streptomycin, and 1 in 10^8 to both drugs.[24] The frequency with which drug resistance emerges is determined by the origin of the infecting organism, the size of the bacillary population, the combination of drugs used in treatment and the drug concentration achieved in tuberculous lesions.

Table 16.10
Newer antituberculous drugs[33]

GROUP	DRUGS
4-Quinolones	• Ciprofloxacin
	• Ofloxacin
Rifamycin	• Rifapentine
	• Rifabutin
Macrolides	• Roxithromycin
Phenazines	• Clofazimine
β Lactams	• β Lactamase stable cephalosporins
Miscellaneous	• Fusidic acid
	• Gangamicin
	• Dihydromycoplanecin A

This emphasizes the need for appropriate combinations of drugs in adequate doses especially when treating patients with large bacillary loads. The drugs listed in Table 16.10 are still in early stages of development and use. *In vitro* data is available on their activity but clinical experience with their use is limited.

Further advances in treating tuberculosis in developing countries are more likely to come from effective implementation of current knowledge than from new drugs or different therapeutic regimens. It is important to conclude by stressing that for effective implementation of efficacious regimens *direct supervision* of drug ingestion is *vital*. Such supervision can be arranged at the workplace, school or a community centre using trained (often volunteer) key persons.

REFERENCES

1 American Thoracic Society, 1980. Guidelines for short course tuberculosis chemotherapy. *American Review of Respiratory Diseases*. 121, 611–4.

2 Aquinas M & Todd D, 1987. Particular problems of tuberculosis in developing countries. In: Weatherall D J, Ledingham J G G & Warrell D A (eds). *Oxford Textbook of Medicine*. 2nd edn. Oxford: Oxford University Press.

3 Batten J, 1969. Rifampicin in treatment of experimental tuberculosis in mice. *Tubercle*. 50, 294.

4 British Medical Research Council, 1948. Streptomycin treatment of pulmonary tuberculosis. A Medical Research Council investigation. *British Medical Journal*. 2, 769–82.

5 British Medical Research Council, 1950. Treatment of pulmonary tuberculosis with streptomycin and para-amino-salicylic acid. A Medical Research Council investigation. *British Medical Journal*. 2, 1073–85.

6 British Medical Research Council, 1952. The treatment of pulmonary tuberculosis with isoniazid. An interim report to the Medical Research Council by their Tuberculosis Chemotherapy Trials Committee. *British Medical Journal*. 2, 735–46.

7 British Medical Research Council, 1962. Long-term chemotherapy in the treatment of chronic pulmonary tuberculosis with cavitation. A report to the Medical Research Council by their Tuberculosis Chemotherapy Trials Committee. *Tubercle*. 43, 201–67.

8 British Medical Research Council, 1973. Co-operative controlled trial of a standard regimen of streptomycin, PAS, and isoniazid and three alternative regimens of chemotherapy in Britain. *Tubercle*. 54, 99–129.

9 British Thoracic Association, 1981. A controlled trial of 6-months chemotherapy in tuberculosis. First report, results during therapy. *British Journal of Diseases of the Chest*. 75, 141–53.

10 British Thoracic Society, 1990. Chemotherapy and management of tuberculosis in United Kingdom, Recommendations of the Joint Tuberculosis Committee of the British Thoracic Society. *Thorax*. 45, 403–8.

11 Citron K M & Girling D J, 1987. Tuberculosis. In: Weatherall D J, Ledingham J G G & Warrell D A (eds). *Oxford Textbook of Medicine*. 2nd edn. Oxford: Oxford University Press.

12 Crofton J, 1960. Drug treatment of tuberculosis. 1. Standard chemotherapy. *British Medical Journal*. 2, 370–3.

13 D'Esopo N D, 1982. Clinical trials in tuberculosis. *American Review of Respiratory Diseases*. Koch Centennial Supplement 125(3), part 2, 85–93.

14 East African/British Medical Research Councils, 1972. Controlled clinical trial of short course (6-month) regimens of chemotherapy for treatment of pulmonary tuberculosis. *Lancet*. 1, 1079–85.

15 East African/British Medical Research Councils, 1973. Controlled clinical trial of four short course (6-month) regimens of chemotherapy for treatment of pulmonary tuberculosis. *Lancet.* 1, 1331–8.

16 East African/British Medical Research Councils, 1974. Controlled clinical trials of short term (6–month) regimens of chemotherapy for treatment of pulmonary tuberculosis. *Lancet.* 2, 237–40.

17 East African/British Medical Research Councils, 1974. Controlled clinical trial of four short-course (6-month) regimens of chemotherapy for treatment of pulmonary tuberculosis. Second East African/British Medical Research Council Study. *Lancet.* 2, 1100–6.

18 East African/British Medical Research Councils, 1976. Controlled clinical trial of four, 6-month regimens of chemotherapy for pulmonary tuberculosis. Second report. Second East African/British Medical Research Council Study. *American Review of Respiratory Diseases.* 114, 471–5.

19 East African/British Medical Research Councils, 1978. Controlled clinical trial of five short course (4-month) chemotherapy regimens in pulmonary tuberculosis. First report of the 4th study. *Lancet.* 2, 334–8.

20 East African/British Medical Research Councils, 1981. Controlled clinical trial of four short course (4-month) chemotherapy regimens in pulmonary tuberculosis Second report of the 4th Study. *American Review of Respiratory Diseases.* 123, 165–70.

21 Fox W, 1977. The modern management and therapy of pulmonary tuberculosis. *Proceedings of the Royal Society of Medicine.* 70, 4–15.

22 Fox W, 1981. Whither short course chemotherapy? *British Journal of Disorders of the Chest.* 75, 331–57.

23 Girling D J, 1982. Adverse effects of anti-tuberculosis drugs. *Drugs.* 23, 56–74.

24 Grosset J, 1980. Bacteriologic basis of short course chemotherapy for tuberculosis. *Clinics in Chest Medicine.* 1, 231–41.

25 Grumbach F, 1969. Experimental *in-vivo* studies of new anti-tuberculosis drugs, capreomycin, ethambutol, rifampicin. *Tubercle.* Suppl. 50, 12.

26 Grumbach F & Rist N, 1967. Activite anti-tuberculeuse experimentale de la rifampicine, derive de la rifamycine SV. *Review of Tuberculose Pneumonology.* 31, 749–62.

27 Hong Kong Chest Service/British Medical Research Council, 1977. Controlled trial of 6-month and 9-month regimens of daily and intermittent streptomycin plus isoniazid plus pyrazinamide for pulmonary tuberculosis in Hong Kong. The results up to 30 months. *American Review of Respiratory Diseases.* 115, 727–35.

28 McDermott W, Ormond L, Muschenheim C *et al.*, 1954. Pyrazinamide — isoniazid in tuberculosis. *American Review of Tuberculosis.* 69, 319–33.

29 Mehotra M C, Pande D C, Goover K L & Gautam K D, 1970. Comparison of various drug regimens in domiciliary chemotherapy. *American Review of Respiratory Diseases.* 102, 602–13.

30 Moodie A S, 1956. Ambulatory treatment of tuberculosis in Hong Kong. *Tubercle.* 37, 451–4.

31 Pearson J D, 1978. A short course regimen for the treatment of tuberculosis. *American Review of Respiratory Diseases.* 117, 1143–4.

32 Ramakrishnan C V, Devadatta S, Evans C *et al.*, 1969. A four year follow-up of patients with quiescent pulmonary tuberculosis at the end of a year of chemotherapy with twice-weekly isoniazid plus streptomycin or daily isoniazid plus PAS. *Tubercle.* 50, 115–24.

33 Reynolds J E F, 1989. *Martindale: The Extra Pharmacopoeia.* London: The Pharmaceutical Press.

34 Schatz A, Bugie E & Waxman S A, 1944. Streptomycin, a substance exhibiting antibiotic activity against gram positive and gram negative bacteria. *Proceedings of the Society for Experimental Biological Medicine.* 55, 66–9.

35 Singapore Tuberculosis Service/British Medical Research Council, 1979. Clinical trial of six-month and four-month regimens of chemotherapy in the treatment of pulmonary tuberculosis. *American Review of Respiratory Diseases.* 119, 579–85.

36 Stead W W & Dutt A K, 1982. Chemotherapy for tuberculosis today. *American Review of Respiratory Diseases.* Koch Centennial Supplement 125(3), part 2, 94–101.

37 Tripathy S P, 1979. Madras study of short course chemotherapy in pulmonary tuberculosis. *Bulletin of the International Union of Tuberculosis.* 54, 28–30.

38 Tuberculosis Chemotherapy Center, Madras, 1959. A concurrent comparison of home and sanatorium treatment of pulmonary tuberculosis in South India. *Bulletin of the World Health Organization.* 21, 51–144.

39 Verbist L & Gyselen A, 1968. Anti-tuberculosis activity of rifampicin in vitro and in vivo and the concentrations attained in human blood. *American Review of Respiratory Diseases.* 98, 923–32.

CHAPTER 17

Voluntary organizations in tuberculosis control

K Ginwala and T Collins

In 1982, when the centenary of the discovery of the tubercle bacillus by Robert Koch was celebrated throughout the world, the Director-General of the World Health Organization lamented the lack of progress in the fight against this ancient enemy of mankind, and emphasized that: 'the role of voluntary organizations continues to be extremely important in the prevention and control of tuberculosis'.[14]

To develop an understanding of the contribution made by voluntary organizations in South Africa it is appropriate to deal with this subject in the context of South African welfare policy and ideology; the nature of voluntarism; organized voluntary services; and voluntary organizations themselves.

SOUTH AFRICAN WELFARE POLICY AND IDEOLOGY

The World Health Organization's adoption in the late 1970s of the term 'Health for All by the Year 2000' as a policy for the implementation of health care was based on two assumptions:[3]

- in developing communities health improvements could be brought about through social policy, without general increases in incomes, by improving nutrition, water supply and sanitation;
- these improvements could be effected through a redistribution of resources, increased external assistance, and greater efficiency in the use of resources.

Social welfare may be viewed either as a 'residual' function or as an 'institutional developmental' function. The former implies that intervention will assure a minimal level of personal well-being, assuming that welfare programmes assist in meeting emergency needs through charity, philanthropy, relief and assistance to the sick, disabled and disadvantaged.

This is the traditional role of the South African welfare system for blacks, entrenched more firmly through the adoption of a new social welfare policy (1989) which holds that social welfare institutions should come into play only when the normal defence structures of society, family, community and the market economy break down, or are unable to meet needs.

In the event of an individual or a community being unable to overcome their plight, reliance is placed on voluntary welfare organizations, religious organizations, or private enterprise.

The state's role is minimal; the proportion of national income spent on statutory services is low, the levels of benefit (pensions/grants) are based on race, and the service is coercive and fragmented.

In South Africa social welfare benefits are not regarded as a right and official South African welfare policy entrenches racial differentiation in social services, encourages privatization and is state controlled, but with considerably reduced state financial responsibility. The 'residual' model perpetuates the 'victim blaming' mentality that identifies the individual as being ultimately responsible for his or her own plight.

Social forces influence and have an impact on individuals and communities who will respond in a manner consistent with the prevailing social order. In South Africa the plight of those who are socially dependent has been compounded by the deliberate disintegration of established socio-economic structures by means such as the Bantu Education Act of 1953, Group Areas Act of 1949, relocations, migration and migrant labour (with their effects on urban and rural populations), homelands policy, and the total disregard and neglect of the consequences of the urbanization process on black communities.

By contrast the 'institutional' model finds affinity with a broader concept of social development, its role extending far beyond the provision of services for the needy. The 'institutional' approach recognizes that all citizens require a variety of services, in order to achieve and maintain an optimum standard of well-being and to perform productive roles in society.

It acknowledges that social problems are the result of unhealthy social structures, that a resolution to these problems rests in interventions at various levels, and that social functioning can be improved by a collaborative role with other major social services.[5] Thus, social welfare cannot be seen in isolation from other services such as health or education.

The 'institutional' approach is not primarily a crisis service. There is no victim blaming or stigma attached, and the status of the client population is not necessarily low.

Welfare for whites in South Africa is 'institutional', with state spending being six times higher for whites than it is for blacks. Through the provision of services to meet physical needs, such as nutrition, water, housing and security, and to meet the emotional needs of identification and status, self-actualization and fulfilment are achieved. Through the re-distribution of wealth, social problems affecting individuals, families and communities may be eradicated, and life chances increased through higher standards in health, education and housing. The political support base of whites is thus secured.[6] This does not apply to the black population.

THE NATURE OF VOLUNTARISM

Volunteer effort or voluntarism relates to a belief in the intrinsic value of a human being and a willingness to participate fully and so respond to the economic, social, political and cultural forces within society. In accepting responsibility to participate and respond, the volunteer, or voluntary organization, focuses on preventing human problems and promoting an enhanced quality of life for the common good.

Traditionally this manifests itself in the following ways:

* *good neighbourliness*, which arises spontaneously and expresses itself in some form of loose organization to provide a service (often to meet the call of a disaster);
* *organized philanthropic effort* which aims at assisting disadvantaged groups;
* *mutual aid* which mutually supports and maintains organizations founded for persons suffering from some common affliction, such as tuberculosis or alcoholism.

A wide range of activities sustain the interest of volunteers, including the care of the elderly, the disabled, children without families, families in distress, problems of education, health and housing, the promotion of good working conditions in the workplace, employment opportunities and adequate wages, care of offenders against the law, the provision of legal aid and advice to those without the means to obtain defence in Court or justice.[10]

ORGANIZED VOLUNTARY SERVICES

Organized welfare services are the expression of a community's need and interest in fostering those social and economic resources which are essential for the well-being of a community in accordance with its value and lifestyle.

These services are therefore provided on the initiative of groups or community agencies which carry a delegated responsibility to protect their members from conditions detrimental to the welfare of themselves and the total community. By such means society gives effect to its concern for its own well-being by creating welfare organizations in which resources are brought together to deal with selected problems and to meet perceived needs which threaten the well-being of the community.[15]

Welfare services may be initiated in several ways.

Pioneering

Voluntary organizations can initiate previously unprovided services to meet grassroots needs, of which the state or relevant statutory bodies are either unaware or consider mundane or politically inexpedient. Thus, voluntary organizations can go ahead of public opinion, or even against it, and, in a democracy, convince the state of the appropriateness of its pioneering effort. After a protracted struggle, the state may assume partial responsibility by subsidizing professional posts or by providing grants or taking over the relevant service.

Examples are the present Child Health Services of the Durban City Health Department which was pioneered at the Brook Street Clinic by the Durban Indian Child and Family Welfare Society in 1930 and the efforts in the control of tuberculosis by the Friends of the Sick Association (FOSA) and the South African National Tuberculosis Association (SANTA).

Gap filling service

Voluntary organizations fill gaps in care which the state may not have considered, such as meals on wheels services for the elderly and infirm, or sheltered employment for tuberculosis patients.

In fulfilling this function, voluntary organizations frequently employ social workers who are able to provide professional assistance. Social workers are able to draw on at least three established methods to carry out their tasks.

The case work method has as its central focus the need of the individual client or family who is socially dislocated in a given setting or impoverished environment. An attempt is made through a process of adjustment to convert the dependent state of the client to one of independence and self-direction. The case worker does not attempt to change the environment or to eliminate elements within it which are inimical to the client's interest.

The group work method, which promotes social welfare by improving social relations through groups and through neighbourhood and service functions, such as education and health.

Community planning and organization may evolve from the group work method. This may facilitate the improvement of inadequate social conditions, thereby reducing community needs.

Social action service

Voluntary organizations act as pressure groups to initiate change, the ambit of their activity extending beyond a remedial approach to human problems, to the achievement and maintenance of fundamental human rights. Typically the circumscribed and limited resources of most voluntary organizations prove inadequate to achieve this goal and large scale socio-economic state input is required.

In South Africa, however, the encroachment of a distinctive overtly repressive and discriminatory state ideology into the domain of welfare services, the altruistic nature of the volunteer and the empirically pacifist approach of voluntary organizations have all combined to assign this approach a low priority.

Before 1920 the response to social problems in South Africa came virtually entirely from the churches, religious groups, educational trusts and labour organizations, rather than from health and welfare organizations. In 1920, and again in 1930, a specific state department to deal with welfare matters was created, while a National Council system to deal with specific specialist social problems was not instituted until later.

Voluntary organizations can have a direct or indirect bearing on the control of tuberculosis. Those organizations which have been established specifically for the control of tuberculosis are the Friends of the Sick Association and the South African National Tuberculosis Association, the latter being the national umbrella organization.

Other voluntary organizations, which deal with the impact of social problems, housing and the environment on individual communities, indirectly assist the efforts at tuberculosis control by their demands for improvements to society and for the allocation of greater resources to deprived communities.

'VOLUNTARY' ORGANIZATIONS

History of voluntary organizations

History of the South African National Tuberculosis Association

Voluntary organizations have been active in South Africa from the earliest days of the epidemic. As far as can be ascertained, the first public meeting convened for the purpose of organizing local community effort against tuberculosis took place in Cape Town on 3 June 1904.[7] These voluntary organizations functioned locally and independently until 1947, when they united under the umbrella of the South African National Tuberculosis Association (SANTA).

Matters discussed at the 1904 meeting included notification and the practical application of disinfection. The meeting registered its regret at the Government's decision to confine the regulation which prevented spitting in public places to male adults only and not to the general population. Subsequently substantial pressure was placed on the railways to place spittoons in carriages.

Later there were long-drawn-out negotiations in attempts to find a suitable site for a sanatorium for early cases of consumption, but these came to naught because of 'lack of funds and a parsimonious and unconvinced government'.

'The Association for the Prevention of Consumption' provided financial assistance for the establishment of the first Sunshine Home for child contacts of tuberculosis families in 1929, and actively assisted in this respect for 10 years until the 'South African Christmas Stamp Fund' took over full control.

Other voluntary bodies with similar interests had come into existence in the meantime. In June 1936, at a joint meeting, a co-ordinating body called the 'Cape Province Tuberculosis Council' was constituted on the basis of the former association, and its aims included closer liaison with the 'Care Committee for Tuberculosis Patients'. Dr Karl Bremer was elected first Chairman of the Council.

Mrs Elizabeth Pitt, a founder member of the Care Committee and later of the Council, became the first voluntary tuberculosis visitor in Cape Town in 1917 — and probably the first in the country. Affectionately known as 'Ma Pitt', she retired from active work in the field of tuberculosis in 1975 at the age of 86 years, and a fitting tribute was paid to her by Dr F K Mitchell when she died in April 1982. She persuaded the Cape Town Medical Officer of Health to start the first tuberculosis clinic, situated in Newmarket Street, because most of her patients could not afford a doctor's visit, which cost two shillings and sixpence. Patients did not want to go to the City Hospital which at that time was a collection of tin shanties.

On 4 May 1933 the 'Natal Anti-Tuberculosis Association' (NATBA) was formed in Durban with somewhat grandiose objectives incorporated into its Memorandum of Association. These included the employment of medical, surgical and other officers, nurses and staff and the necessary equipment for proposed Sanatoria. It was largely due to the influence of NATBA that the government built the King George V Silver Jubilee Hospital for tuberculosis in Durban, and later acquired the Springfield Military Hospital for the same purpose. Pressure exerted by NATBA was responsible wholly or in part for the appointment of Dr B A Dormer as Tuberculosis Officer for Natal and later as adviser for the Union, the construction of tuberculosis clinics in Durban and Pietermaritzburg, the initiation of the King George V Silver Jubilee Fund for assistance to patients and their families, and for the acceptance by the government of tuberculosis as a disability qualifying the sufferer and family for disability benefits.

In 1934 the foundation stone of the Christmas Stamp Fund Preventorium was laid on a six hectare site in Pietermaritzburg. Years later, with the advent of modern drugs and other progress in the management and prevention of tuberculosis, this Preventorium and the other Sunshine Homes built and managed by the Fund became redundant and were sold. Committee members were understandably disappointed when the time came for these visible monuments to their dedication to be closed, but they continue to sell Christmas Stamps and channel the funds raised in this way into other aspects of tuberculosis control.

Soon after its formation in 1947 SANTA was approached by the Department of Health to establish settlements for convalescent patients on the basis of a pound-for-pound government contribution towards capital costs and payment of a daily patient tariff. It was not long before these settlements were obliged to admit acute patients, and they then became known as SANTA centres. In the first decade of its existence SANTA built, equipped and staffed 35 of these centres throughout South Africa, with a total of 7 200 beds. They were built to serve for 10 years only, but 22 are still in operation, having been upgraded from time to time.

SANTA's objectives, as set out in its constitution may be briefly summarized as being to support anti-tuberculosis work and the spread of information aimed at the eradication of the disease; to promote the prevention and treatment of the disease; and generally to be concerned with all matters relating to the care of patients, their dependants and contacts. These aims are carried out through the management committees of centres and the many branches and care groups, supported by paid staff at the national office in Johannesburg and other staff who operate in the field.

The organization remains true to its objectives as described in its very first publication, a striking pamphlet that reads as follows:

In dealing with tuberculosis, an infectious disease, the mere provision of curative medical services, necessary though they are, without preventing people from becoming diseased is a waste of money. Logically and economically, prevention is the goal at which to aim, and to which the efforts of the various agencies, official and voluntary should be geared.[7]

Tuberculosis treatment centres

Towards the middle of this century close on 400 notifications of newly-diagnosed tuberculosis per 100 000 population were being recorded, and the prevalence of the disease was probably three times as high. Mortality at that time was estimated to exceed 40 deaths daily. It was during this crisis period that SANTA, with its convalescent settlements built to a standard design at a cost of approximately 150 pounds per bed, came to the rescue of the Department of Health whose new state hospitals cost nearly 2 500 pounds per bed.

Inevitably, because of the great demand, these settlements were forced to accept acute cases, and a process of upgrading in terms of nursing and general facilities was undertaken, sometimes with the support of Rotary and other service clubs. Following the advent of modern chemotherapy and the acceptance of the safety and effectiveness of supervised regular ambulatory treatment, the number of centres gradually decreased.

Today the largest of these is the East Rand SANTA Centre, with 550 registered beds. Originally a disused mine compound with accommodation totally unsuitable for nursing acutely ill patients, it has in recent years been transformed into an institution of acceptable hospital standards, thanks to a generous grant from Rotary International. It now has its own x-ray department, extensive occupational facilities, physiotherapy, a social worker, recreational facilities and other amenities — better in some respects than those of many state hospitals.

The recent upsurge in tuberculosis, particularly in the western Cape, has given rise to the criticism that the closure of some centres was premature, and a former centre in that area is now being renovated to provide additional accommodation.

Apart from the increase in the number of tuberculosis sufferers in recent years, ambulatory management of the disease has not proved entirely successful as patients in general fail to take their treatment regularly unless they are strictly supervised. This has given rise to a steadily growing number of treatment failures and states of chronicity with drug-resistant organisms, for which institutional treatment is generally necessary.

An on-going public awareness campaign has done much to counter the stigma still attached to tuberculosis and to reduce the ignorance of the disease that has hindered efforts at control. SANTA has also become an increasingly powerful pressure group, able to bring deficiencies in infrastructure and services, and the many other problems encountered by patients to the attention of responsible authorities. This role has become vitally important with the fragmentation of health services into some 16 separate ministries and the further delegation of responsibility within South Africa to four provincial administrations which in turn are burdened with questions of 'own' and 'general' affairs.

Training of health advisers

Following the closure of the Sunshine Homes and the end of their activities in the interest of prevention of tuberculosis in children, the Christmas Stamp Fund, in consultation with the Department of Health, agreed to provide financial support for the training of health advisers who could be specifically involved in tuberculosis education. It also paid for the erection and equipping of a large training centre with accommodation and catering facilities for groups of students.

A tripartite agreement between the Department of Health, the Stamp Fund and SANTA was entered into, under which SANTA undertook to train and supervise health advisers, with the Department contributing seven-eighths of their salaries, transport and other costs. Unfortunately, however, with the multiplication of governments and health departments in South Africa and the resultant restraints on health spending, state subsidization for this venture has been progressively reduced. SANTA has thus been obliged to undertake the total support of many of the trainees in recent years, with some further financial input coming from the Stamp Fund. It has also trained persons employed by local authorities, industrial concerns, and by some of the national and independent states.

The training centre has in addition been made available to other organizations for short courses designed to meet their own specific needs; yet the number of health advisers available for community work remains totally inadequate if a significant impact on the tuberculosis situation is to be made.

Supervision of ambulatory treatment

The safety and effectiveness of ambulatory treatment for all patients who are not seriously ill or suffering from complications is now generally accepted. Self-administered treatment is, however, frequently irregular, and is causing a problem of increasing secondary drug resistance which is often multiple and involves all of the major agents. Even worse is the spectre of primary drug resistance that is being increasingly seen in susceptible young contacts who develop tuberculosis disease after being infected.

Health advisers are involved in a two-pronged campaign designed to prevent this primary drug resistance. The first aspect of the campaign is to enlist the support of employers in keeping tuberculosis patients at work and in designating a motivated and reliable person whose task it is to ensure that the prescribed medication is actually seen to be swallowed on a regular basis on working days. Secondly, they are enrolling carefully selected members of the community to undertake this task on a voluntary basis for unemployed patients, and they are providing them with sufficient basic information about the disease to ensure that they perform this vital task satisfactorily. The number of these health advisers is, however, totally inadequate.

Prevention of tuberculosis in children

From a conventional perspective little can be done by a voluntary organization to alleviate the socio-economic circumstances that play such a prominent role in the epidemiology of tuberculosis. SANTA is therefore firmly committed to applying specific medical interventions that are calculated to reduce the toll of suffering and death exacted by this disease, and that cannot be provided for in the restricted budgets of responsible authorities. BCG vaccine continues to be supplied by such authorities and is promoted by health advisers for the limited protection it does confer, particularly in young children.

So-called secondary chemoprophylaxis (or treatment of infection before disease results) is a controversial matter in South Africa. In any case it cannot at this stage be accommodated in the official control programme because the funds available are wholly consumed by case finding and treatment of those already diseased. SANTA, however, utilizing money specially donated for this purpose by individuals and corporate bodies, embarked on a tuberculin testing campaign in schools in 1984, followed by treatment of infected (but as yet healthy) individuals with short-course multi-drug preventive chemotherapy under the supervision of previously motivated teachers.

There is documented evidence that this form of preventive treatment (60 doses of a triple-drug combination administered Monday to Friday) will be effective in healthy infected subjects harbouring small numbers of tubercle bacilli, and the concept has been endorsed by the Tuberculosis Division of the Centers for Disease Control in the United States. Nevertheless, a scientific study including an untreated control group, who will be closely monitored, is being undertaken in coloured primary school children in the western Cape, since all previous studies involved the prolonged use of isoniazid alone.

Primary schools for coloured children in that area have been chosen because of the documented increasing incidence and prevalence of the disease in this group, and the evidence provided by age-specific notifications that 80 per cent are 15 years of age and above.

Meanwhile, the programme is continuing on a routine basis elsewhere when certain requirements can be met. These include careful motivation and acceptance by the responsible health and educational authorities, school teaching staff, pupils and the community — the latter being involved in attempts to improve the quality of life (and in particular nutrition), through self-help efforts. Home contacts of infected children are investigated for undiagnosed source cases and any children (whether infected or not) showing signs of illness at any time are referred to the local clinic for examination.

The risk of developing disease after infection in South African coloured and black people has not been determined, but is likely to be nearer to the risk of 40 per cent detected in Eskimos some 40 years ago or the 50 per cent in Indians in India to-day,

than to the misleading figure of 5 to 15 per cent in well-fed and well-housed Americans and Europeans so frequently quoted by detractors of this prevention programme.

In any case, bearing in mind that very many patients are diagnosed after considerable permanent lung or other damage has already occurred and the problems associated with ensuring regular treatment which in turn gives rise to chronicity and the secretion of drug-resistant organisms, as well as the suffering and high mortality that continue to occur, SANTA believes it is well worth while to treat a certain number of children unnecessarily in order to prevent even a few tragedies. The organization is dedicated to the people who continue to suffer and die and does not consider the issues as just an abstract 'problem'. For this humanitarian approach it is receiving increasing support from individuals, commerce and industry and other bodies.

History of the Friends of the Sick Association (FOSA)

Natal was the birthplace of another splendid organization that harnessed community activity in the fight against this disease. Early in 1941 five men of different racial backgrounds (two Indians, two whites and one black) met to discuss the terrible threat that tuberculosis posed for the Indian community. They were members of the Society of Servants in South Africa, formed in 1939 as an offshoot of the original society in India.

The main aims of the Society were to widen and deepen the spirit of service among all races and especially among the Indians of Natal; and to bring into being organizations to deal with any aspect of social or humanitarian work *for which no machinery appeared to exist.*[20]

In this second category the Society identified tuberculosis, adult literacy and temperance. They decided that while the tuberculosis problem was rightly one for the state, the community itself could do much to help through Care Committees. Known as the 'Friends of the Sick Association' (FOSA), their aim was 'one friend for each sick person', at a time when the mortality rate from tuberculosis amongst Indians in

South Africa was not much less than 400 per 100 000 population.

The founder of the new organization, Paul Sykes, had in 1939 temporarily acted as research assistant to Professor Raymond Burrows of the Department of Economics at the University of Natal. Sykes was thus exposed to the living conditions in the Durban Corporation's Magazine Barracks which housed municipal workers. The Barracks consisted of old mule stables which had been partitioned off with no lighting or proper sanitation and no privacy.[2]

In the 1940s the Indian community had little knowledge and a superstitious fear of tuberculosis, and this led to poor reporting of cases within families. The difficulties were compounded by threats from health inspectors who condemned shacks in the face of an acute housing and accommodation shortage.

Following the depression of the 1930s and the Second World War, there was an influx of hundreds of thousands of people of all race groups into the towns, and large families, unemployment and poor wages served as breeding ground for tuberculosis. Even until the present day local authorities have refused to face and remedy the problems as being due to urbanization. White attitudes and official government ideology have continued to exacerbate these issues through racial interventions.

From its inception FOSA was open to all races, and worked through Care Committees established as far afield as Stanger and Dannhauser. The philosophy behind FOSA was 'one friend, one case' and the Standard of the Association was the Lorraine Cross.[18] The task of the 'Friend' was to give confidence to a tuberculosis sufferer, to explain the nature of the disease and to advise on nutrition, ventilation, 'isolation', and cleanliness.

The cultural background, beliefs, fears, and prejudices were considered and obstacles to compliance and acceptance of the disease removed, and treatment instituted.

Through its Care Committees, 'friends' took the service to the people without any apparent social distance between the server and the served. Contacts were screened, the sick referred for treatment, children sent to clinics, and grants, relief and aid obtained. In order to improve the socio-economic situation of contact families and convalescents and to retain the integrity of the family, the concept of a Settlement was established in 1945. The existing sanatoria were for white patients only and most required payment. At FOSA the patient was treated within the family group and was not removed from the nuclear family.

FOSA Settlement consisted of cottages for families of tuberculosis patients, a children's hospital, a children's school and sheltered employment for chronic tuberculosis and ex-tuberculosis patients who were incapable of competing for employment on the open labour market. There were vegetable gardens, a poultry section and a weaving school. The Settlement was originally intended to provide accommodation for tuberculosis contact families in which the wage earner had died or was in hospital for a lengthy period, but two years after its establishment FOSA admitted the first child patients at a state-subsidized daily tariff of four shillings and sixpence.

Today the whole of Natal is honeycombed by Area Care Committees born spontaneously out of a desire to find tuberculosis and to fight it where it occurs.[19] The committees are served by dedicated men and women who give freely, voluntarily and without stint of time, their services and their ability to search for tuberculosis and to attempt to destroy it.

Comprehensive care of tuberculosis by voluntary organizations

The key to Health for All by the year 2000 is Primary Health Care (PHC). The definition of PHC as enunciated at Alma Ata has been articulated and interpreted in various forms by different bodies, including the Department of National Health and Population Development.

The most fundamental and crucial part of the definition for all those responsible for the provision of health care is that 'PHC forms an integral part both of the country's health system of which it is the central function and main focus and of the overall social and economic development of the community'.[22] Health workers and social workers cannot divorce themselves from their commitment towards social and eco-nomic development of their patients or clients.

The top-down approach to community development and the insidious intrusion of

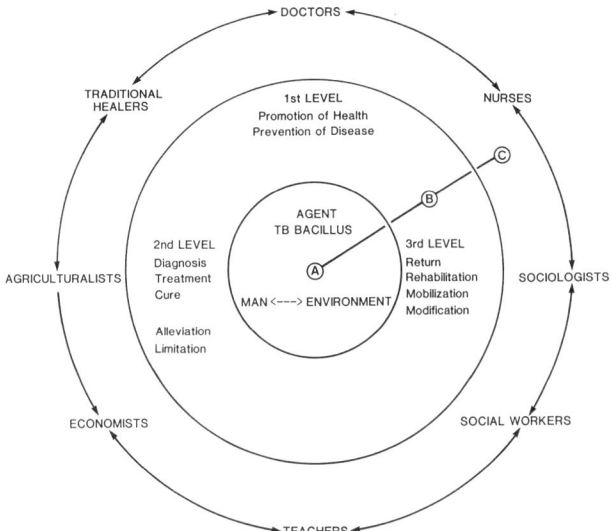

Figure 17.1. The essentials of comprehensive health care. A. Consideration of the interaction of the agent causing the illness, the environment and the health status of the individual. B. Promotion of health, diagnosis, treatment, cure and rehabilitation. C. The need for medical practitioners, social, and health care workers to work in multi-disciplinary teams.

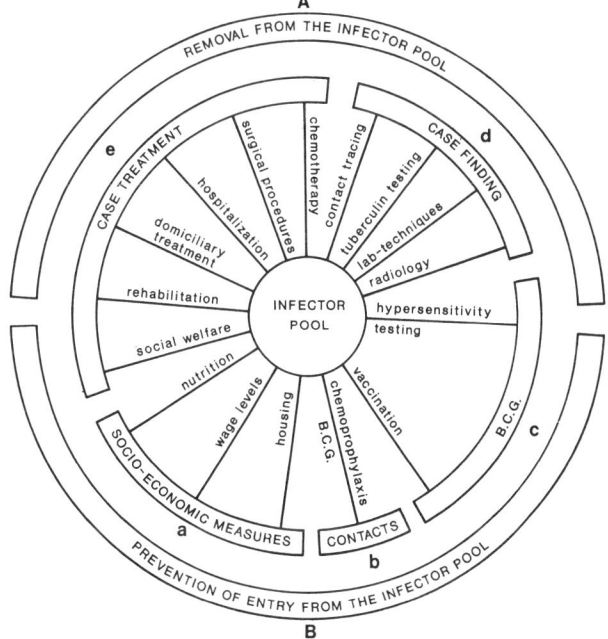

Figure 17.2. The levels of intervention in the control of tuberculosis.[21]

the population development programme into existing local community structures has had a negative effect and aroused resentment among communities. Overall social and economic development requires major financial input and redistribution of resources by the state, but South Africa's response has increasingly been the privatization of health and welfare, and with it the denial of financial responsibility for the nation's health care in situations of utter deprivation.

The comprehensive practice of medicine takes into consideration the interaction of the agent causing illness (*Mycobacterium tuberculosis*), the environment and the health status of the individual[21] (Figure 17.1(A)). Health cannot be viewed in isolation from social 'well-being' — the provision of welfare, nutrition, clothing, shelter, education and employment are all inter-related and are essential components of total or holistic health and social welfare delivery.

Comprehensive health care incorporates the three levels of medical responsibility:

• promotion of health, prevention of illness;
• diagnosis, treatment, cure or alleviation; and
• rehabilitation (Figure 17.1(B)).

At the first level of care, through their education programmes, training of health advisers and contact tracing efforts, SANTA and FOSA respond to the promotive and preventive aspects of health in areas where they operate. The provision of preventive services in terms of the Health Act (63 of 1977) is, however, designated as a local authority function.

At the second level of diagnosis and treatment, SANTA and FOSA have rendered sterling service through their treatment centres, settlements and Sunshine Homes in treating acute and chronic patients as well as those with re-activation. By providing beds for acutely ill patients, voluntary organizations fulfilled a responsibility which in terms of the Health Act was essentially that of the state.

At the third level of care, SANTA and FOSA supervise, monitor and rehabilitate patients discharged from hospital. In a limited way the philosophy of FOSA as

expressed through health education and health promotion at the Settlement has assisted in improving sanitation and hygiene.

The need for medical practitioners, social workers and health care workers to work in multi-disciplinary teams is essential (Figure 17.1(C)).

Intervention by voluntary organizations in the control of tuberculosis

Tuberculosis is a socio-economic disease which spreads easily in overcrowded and deprived communities. Consequently, the role of voluntary organizations in the actual control of tuberculosis is limited at an interventive level.

In Figure 17.2 the levels of intervention in the control of tuberculosis are identified.[21] At the core, spreading the disease, is the pool of infected patients excreting active bacilli. Limitation of spread clearly entails preventing the entry into the infector pool of new patients (B) and the removal or egress of those cured or treated (A). The responsibility of SANTA and FOSA at the first and second level (case finding and case treatment) has been noted, but their role in undertaking the socio-economic measures required or in institutional social welfare is very seriously restricted.

The incidence of tuberculosis will not be reduced substantially unless socio-economic measures in the form of adequate wage levels, housing and nutrition are improved.

The Report of the National Health Commission, 1942–4[17] (the Gluckman Commission) was critical of the financing, legislation and administration of South Africa's Health Services. Its findings included a lengthy account of the deficiencies in housing, nutrition and wage levels, and recommendations were made for a National Health Service.

Similarly in evidence before the Natal Judicial Commission in 1944[16] the Friends of the Sick Association (FOSA) submitted the following *inter alia*:
• tuberculosis is the major health problem in the Indian community;
• there is no other known disease that is so disruptive of normal social and economic

life; recovery is seldom complete and the danger of recurrence is high;

• it is evident that because treatment and recovery are a long drawn out process, only those with considerable means can meet the financial implications of a long period of income loss;

• the majority of sufferers, being wage earners, cannot ride the storm of tuberculosis unless they are borne financially by a service with very considerable money resources;

• if the incidence of tuberculosis is high in a given community, it imposes so substantial a burden on health services as to necessitate its acknowledgement as a national and not simply a local or regional obligation. To the extent that tuberculosis, under the Public Health Act (1919), was recognized as being 'the responsibility of the Union Government', acknowledgement of the national character of the response to tuberculosis had indeed been recorded, noted FOSA.

FOSA recommended the following:[16]

(a) *nutrition*: subsidization of essential and protective foodstuffs by the government;

(b) *housing*: the community should be adequately housed with consideration being given to locality, security of tenure, construction materials, adequacy of light, size and number of rooms, and sanitary and cooking arrangements.

These recommendations continue to be echoed 45 years later throughout the length and breadth of South Africa by, *inter alia*, voluntary organizations involved in child and family welfare, housing action groups, housewives' leagues and the Urban Foundation. As shown below those social conditions which render communities vulnerable to tuberculosis persist to the present day.

The present position

Tuberculosis

According to SANTA an estimated 12 million people in South Africa had dormant tuberculosis in 1988, and an estimated 15 per cent of these would contract a full-blown form of the disease, resulting in a daily death rate of between 10 and 20.[1] Figures for the disease in the western Cape according to the Medical Officer of Health of the Regional Services Council (RSC) were amongst the highest in the world.[1]

The large pool of dormant tuberculosis is a consequence of the increasing numbers of relapse cases resulting from poor compliance to treatment, distances from clinics, poor and inadequate facilities for radiology, and poor laboratory facilities outside the urban centres, and the socio-economic conditions and deprivation of the majority of South Africans.

Malnutrition

Malnutrition, especially the more severe forms such as kwashiorkor and marasmus, is an emotionally charged issue in South Africa. Government representatives go to great lengths to minimize the prevalence of protein-energy malnutrition (PEM), but there is absolutely no question that large numbers of black children in the country have the condition. Two quasi-national[8, 12] and a number of regional and local studies suggest the following:

• protein-energy malnutrition is a major health problem in South Africa, especially among black, coloured, and, to a lesser extent, Indian pre-school children;

• chronic PEM (as shown by reductions in height or stunting) is widespread among rural black pre-school children with a prevalence of between 25 and 41 per cent; about 12 per cent of urban blacks have stunting;

• about 31 per cent of rural black pre-school children are underweight; the figure for peri-urban blacks is between 10 and 15 per cent;

• roughly 20 per cent of coloured pre-school children are stunted and 48 per cent are underweight;

• about six per cent of Indian pre-school children are stunted and 35 per cent are underweight.

Housing

The position in respect of housing is no better. The South African government no longer builds family housing units for blacks in the non-independent homelands, whilst the housing shortage in 1988 in South Africa (including the 10 homelands) was estimated at between 1,1 and 1,8 million units[1] (Table 17.1).

The shortage exacerbates the extensive overcrowding in black homes. According to a Council for Scientific and Industrial Research (CSIR) report in 1985,[9] 6,3 million blacks were crammed into an estimated 486 000 relatively small dwellings in the white-designated areas, representing an average of 13 people per house.

The CSIR reported a projected housing shortage of 3 413 000 houses in the year 2000 (Table 17.2).

RESTRAINTS

Voluntary organizations cannot, of course, be accountable for the lack of a state urbanization policy, nor for the malnutrition and prevalence of tuberculosis. They operate on the one hand within the requirements and demands of their particular constituency to provide the best holistic care of their clients that they can with the resources available (Figure 17.3); on the other hand, several external restraints exist beyond these internal constraints.

Political commitment and legislative constraints

Political commitment can be measured by the extent to which socially relevant development strategies of health and welfare are actually being implemented and accompanied by explicit and adequate resource allocation by the state.

Political commitment should be articulated by a declaration of the right of the citizen in respect of health and welfare, endorsed by health policy action in a Bill of Rights and complemented by the allocation of adequate resources. The primary health

Table 17.1
Housing shortages in South Africa, 1988

RACE	GOVERNMENT ESTIMATES	URBAN FOUNDATION ESTIMATES
Coloured	100 000	—
Indian	48 747	800 000
Black:	—	—
White designated areas	702 750	—
Non-independent homelands	185 578	892 000
'Independent' homelands	125 150	125 000
Total	1 162 225	1 817 000

Source: South African Institute for Race Relations survey 1989

Table 17.2
Projected housing shortage in South Africa: 1990 and 2000

RACE	1990	2000
Coloured	77 000	176 000
Indian	53 000	87 000
Black	2 107 000	2 969 000
White	+ 4 000	181 000
Total	2 133 000	3 413 000

The surplus of white housing in 1990 will change to a shortage by the year 2000.[8]
Source: South African Institute for Race Relations survey 1989

COMPONENTS OF CARE

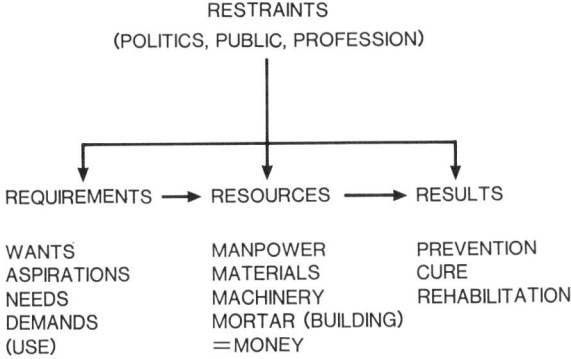

Figure 17.3. Restraints on the provision of health care.

care approach is a multi-sector approach and includes activities in many different sectors which are health related, such as education, community development, water supply, sanitation, housing and nutrition. This is the commitment the state must endorse. On the part of individuals, health workers, and social workers, there must be a dedication to change and the provision of alternative, democratically initiated and promoted structures.

Some of the legislative restraints to socio-economic development in respect of the vast majority of the people in South Africa are listed in Table 17.3 — these have bedevilled voluntary organizations over the years.

The public is denied the right of true and unbiased information on which to form judgements because of restrictions on a number of basic human freedoms, such as the press, association, expression and movement.

Public restraints

Beyond the stigma which continues to be attached to tuberculosis by an unaware public, there exist cultural and social barriers between health workers and social workers and patients. In addition there is a need for increased public awareness that the cure of tuberculosis requires a holistic approach, and that the medical practitioners' role is minimal.

Professional restraints

Professional autonomy and jealousy can have serious effects on the overall health, welfare and development of individuals and communities.

The current method and content of medical and social work training in South Africa is, for the greater part, based on inappropriate models developed in the richer countries. Little attention is given by academic institutions to problem-solving community-based and self-directed learning skills.

There is a lack of involvement of the medical fraternity in the non-medical determinants of public health, and a tendency towards detachment from the community's major socio-economic and inter-related political processes, policies and programmes. There is a need to emphasize the practice of teamwork and multi-disciplinary effort.

There must be an honest commitment to primary health care (Alma Ata), allocation of adequate financial resources and redistribution of wealth for social and economic development. The 40 000 odd family planning clinics and service points throughout the country must be geared to providing comprehensive health care and to monitoring patients with tuberculosis.

Analysis and evaluation

Given their vigorous and sustained efforts, and the widely-acknowledged gains made by SANTA and FOSA, it is important to critically analyse their role as voluntary organizations.

- They have been effective in pioneering services that meet grassroots needs which the state and statutory bodies have failed to address. For example, after a prolonged struggle, the state assumed partial financial responsibility for meeting individual appeals and for capital development of the Sunshine Homes.

- Both organizations have filled essential gaps in the system of health care. They have assisted individual patients and their families to make reasonably satisfactory adjustments to their illness and environments, and they have accepted responsibility (which they did not invite) for the provision of beds for acutely ill patients.

- Voluntary organizations have however been weak in pressurizing for change. Traditionally, voluntary organizations and professional social workers have a responsibility to society and public welfare as well as to individual clients.[4] In their social action role as pressure groups, voluntary organizations can call into question the adequacy and good faith of the institutions of society and government for societal conditions, as they, not individuals or families, are at the root of many human problems. When limitations and impediments exist to measures undertaken to redress the conditions of those that are afflicted, voluntary organizations have an obligation and a role to promote political and social action; this is even more the case if, as in South Africa, the conditions are a result of politics and racism.

The 1936 National Conference of Social Work was told:

To assist and resettle an afflicted family is laudable but in the long run it is both poor case work and poor health work merely to improve particular families and do nothing toward changing the conditions out of which you have taken them and into which others will move.[11]

A number of factors have an influence on the utilization of health services,[13] and so the processes by which people actively seek and further comply with treatment are numerous. These are dependent on the geographical accessibility to health care, the financial burden imposed by seeking it, the cultural and social barriers between health workers and patients, and the characteristics of consumers.

The greater portion of resources are concentrated and distributed in urban areas and are monopolized by those who may have fewer needs than their less demanding and less vocal rural counterparts. Thus, the redistribution of resources and an equitable development of services can redress the barriers of distance, travel, time and means of transport.

Voluntary organizations have an obligation to take into account and address the factors which influence utilization of their services.

CONCLUSION

To be relevant and effective a voluntary organization requires:

- a grassroots knowledge of the community it serves, its demography, power structures, environment and resources; it also needs to have a mandate from the community to operate;

- an awareness of community needs and an assessment of the extent to which these can be met, given the possible restraints which may impede progress;

- an acceptance of the need for multi-disciplinary initiatives, involvement and teamwork;

- the ability to adapt, while yet being persuasive about making desired changes for a holistic approach to care;

- accountability to the community through a process of monitoring and evaluating the relevance of its service;

- legitimacy and credibility with the community it serves; and

- a commitment to progressive political change.

Throughout South Africa in recent times community initiatives have come about as a

Table 17.3
Restrictions to black development

1. The Bantu Education Act of 1953 placed black education under state control. The quality of education militated against normal education development and skills.

2. Prevention of socio-economic development and the settlement of blacks in urban areas through the bantustan policy. The National States Constitution Act of 1971.

3. The Republic of South Africa Constitutional Act of 1982 heralded the tri-cameral system and its multiplicity of authorities.

4. The Group Areas Act of 1966, the Black Land Act of 1913 and the Development Trust and Land Act of 1936, which prevented blacks from occupying or owning land outside the black townships, bantustan and South African Development Trust (SADT) areas.

5. The Prevention of Illegal Squatting Act of 1951, which provided for the summary eviction of persons unlawfully occupying land, and for the demolition of informal structures.

6. The Trespass Act of 1959, which provided for the arrest of persons entering or remaining on property without the permission of the lawful occupier, and for sentence on conviction of a fine of up to R2 000 or imprisonment for up to two years, or both.

7. The Health Act (63 of 1977), which empowered local authorities to prohibit and prevent possible health risks, to ensure 'satisfactory living conditions' and to combat overcrowding. The standards for satisfactory living conditions were often unrealistically high.

8. The Slums Act of 1979, which empowered authorities to order the demolition of buildings without compensation to the owner or occupant, if the premises were deemed unsafe, injurious to health, over-crowded, or if there was an inadequate water supply or inadequate lavatories. Demolition often contributed to further informal structures.

9. The Black Local Authorities Act of 1982, which enabled black local authorities to make bylaws relating to, *inter alia*, the control of slums in black townships. Bylaws were often not uniform and of inappropriately high standards.

10. The Black Communities Development Act of 1982, which empowered the Minister of Constitutional Development and Planning to disestablish any town or portion of a town (including a black township) if he thought that the residents were living under conditions which endangered the health or safety of any group of persons. The Department of Development Planning was empowered to demolish any structure for such purposes without paying compensation.

11. Public Health and Slum Control regulations were promulgated by local authorities which empowered them to demolish structures considered to be unsightly or dilapidated, or which failed to comply with minimum standards of hygiene.

response to the perceived needs and experiences of people regarding their poor health, welfare and education status. Community exposure to injustices and inequalities have led to an understanding of the root causes of social ills; through grassroots structures and mass mobilization people are being empowered to determine and chart alternative structures in health, education and welfare for the future.

Voluntary welfare organizations may well borrow a lesson from organized religion which encourages believers to distinguish the compassionate role (or altruism) from the protective role:

A minister may be priest or prophet; at best he is both, but rarely are these talents combined in one holy person. As priest he counsels, he comforts, he reconciles, he listens, he accepts, … he plays out a ritualistic role. As prophet … he has a harder role to play. He holds up absolute standards against which the sins of man and the shortcomings of the world may be measured and judged; his cry is less for charity and compassion than for justice.

REFERENCES

1 Anon., 1989. *Race Relations Survey.* Johannesburg: South African Institute of Race Relations (SSIV).

2 Brian J B, 1988. Paul Carton Sykes 1903–1983. *The Fosalink.* 27, 1.

3 Camper G, 1985. Economic development, health services and health. In: Lee K & Mills A (eds). *The Economics of Health in Developing Countries.* Oxford: Oxford University Press.

4 Chambers C A, 1962. *An Historical Perspective on Political Action versus Individualized Treatment. Current Issues in Social Work seen in Historical Perspective.* New York: Council on Social Work Education.

5 Chetty T D, 1989. *Approaches to Welfare.* Discussion paper presented at a Workshop on an Alternate Welfare Policy for South Africa, 23 January 1989.

6 Chetty T D, 1989. *Towards a Non-racial Welfare Movement.* Paper presented at the Biennial General Meeting of Regional Forums, 30 September 1989.

7 Collins T F B, 1987. The birth of SANTA. A short history of the voluntary organizations in the fight against tuberculosis in South Africa. *SANTA News.* pp 3, 4, 7–8.

8 Department of National Health and Population Development, 1987. First RHOSA Nutrition Study. Anthropometric assessment of nutritional status in black under-fives in rural RSA. *Epidemiological Comments.* 14, 1–37.

9 *Financial Mail.* 3 June 1987.

10 Ginwala K N, 1972. *Organized Voluntary Care in Relation to Community Needs.* Address to Annual General Meeting of Durban Indian Child and Family Welfare Society, May 1972.

11 Hall H, 1936. The consequence of social action for the group-work agency. *Proceedings of the 1936 National Conference of Social Work.* 235–7.

12 Kotze G P, Williams W N, McIntyre N, De Hoop M E *et al.,* 1986. Anthropometric and dental data on different population groups in South African primary schools. *South African Journal of Science.* 82, 329–34.

13 Lee K, 1985. Resources and costs in primary health care. In: Lee K & Mills A (eds). *The Economics of Health in Developing Countries.* Oxford: Oxford University Press.

14 Mahler H, 1982. *Koch 100. Defeat TB Now and Forever.* (Information kit). International Union against Tuberculosis and World Health Organization.

15 Naidoo B A, 1972. *Some Aspects of Voluntary Effort in the Field of Child Welfare.* Paper presented at a training course for volunteers by the Stanger Child Welfare Society, 19 November 1972.

16 Natal Indian Judicial Commission, 1944. *Memorandum by Friends of the Sick Association, 15 July 1944.* Durban: Fosa.

17 National Health Commission, 1944. *The Report of the National Health Commission (1942–1944).* The Gluckman Commission Report. Pretoria: Government Printer.

18 SANTA News, November 1982. 21, 11.

19 SANTA News, December 1982. 21, 12.

20 Satchell W H, 1947. *Ashrain Review.* Poona: Aryabhushan Press.

21 Spencer I W F, 1980. *Principles and Relationships of Epidemiology, Comprehensive Medicine and Community Medicine in Community Health: Community Health.* Pietermaritzburg: Shuter and Shooter Pty Ltd.

22 World Health Organization, 1978. *Declaration of Alma Ata.* World Health Organization/Unicef International Conference on Primary Health Care.

CHAPTER 18

Tuberculosis control in South Africa

T Lee and E Buch

INTRODUCTION

The natural cycle of tuberculosis and its risk factors,[118] as well as measures for its control are shown in Figure 18.1. The control measures are aimed at reducing infection and reactivation, essentially by socio-economic improvement and by utilizing an effective health service with a good Tuberculosis Control Programme (TBCP).

Socio-economic advancement will help prevent infection (or reinfection) through improved, less crowded, living conditions, and will help prevent reactivation by reducing the stresses of poverty. The health service can contribute to the prevention of infection by effective case-finding and case-holding, through good coverage with BCG vaccination, and to the prevention of active disease through the selective use of secondary chemoprophylaxis and through BCG vaccination.

In spite of knowing the measures needed to control tuberculosis and the availability of the necessary technology, tuberculosis control in South Africa remains unsatisfactory.[5, 7, 33, 46]

Mortality figures reflect a failure of case-finding and/or case-holding. In 1988 there were 5 563 registered tuberculosis deaths in blacks, 1 270 in coloureds, 88 in whites and 35 in Indians[19, 20] compared to 2 309 notified tuberculosis deaths.[37] However, as there is under-reporting of deaths and misclassification of the causes,[117] particularly in blacks,[10] and because the registered data exclude the 'independent' homelands*, both figures are conservative.

In 1987, the RSA TBCP incidence rates per 100 000 were: coloured 519, black 335, Indian 59 and white 18.[34] There is a rising incidence in coloureds and blacks in the western Cape.[106]

In 1988 there were 58 898 new RSA cases reported to the TBCP[36] (giving an incidence of 290 per 100 000), compared to the 49 500 that were notified.[37] Due to underdiagnosis, under-notification (an estimated one-third to one-half of tuberculosis cases are not notified),[12, 33, 60] and under-reporting, multiplying either of these figures by two or three gives a more accurate idea of the number of cases.

Only 11 964 cases were notified from the 10 homelands in 1988,[37] suggesting considerable under-notification. In fact, there appear to be considerably more tuberculosis inpatients in homeland hospitals than are reflected in notification data.[108] The Transkei, known for its high rates of tuberculosis, reported an incidence of only 2,13 per 100 000 in 1988.[37]

The risk of infection is the best single indicator for an evaluation of the tuberculosis situation and its trend.[94] It is independent of changes in the proportion of cases found or of the quality of routine surveillance data. While the risk of infection in South African children is generally decreasing, there is no change in coloureds in the western Cape, which means that the actual number of infections is increasing each year.[106] Also, the gap in the risk of infection between blacks and coloureds on the one hand, and whites and Indians on the other,

---

* Apartheid policy has led to the creation of 4 'independent' and 6 'self-governing' national states. The authors oppose this policy but as it has impacted on TB control and since state data are presented in this way, we have used this classification. In this chapter, where possible figures are presented for the whole country (SA) but where figures represent the seven health regions and exclude the homelands, this is denoted as RSA.

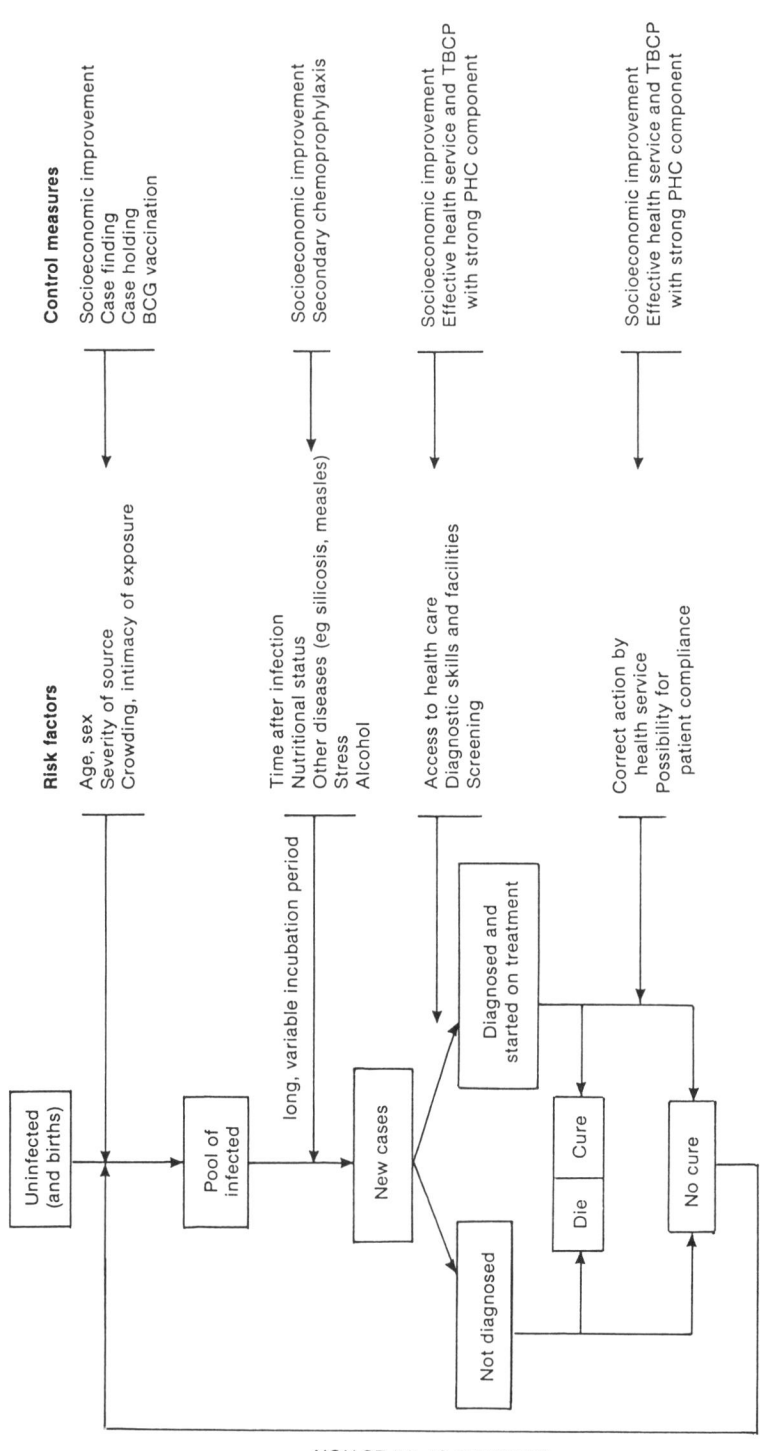

Key: TBCP — Tuberculosis Control Programme; PHC — Primary Health Care

Figure 18.1. Simplified model of tuberculosis – its natural cycle, risk factors and control measures.

is increasing. Developed countries have shown an annual 11–13 per cent decrease in the risk of infection,[94] a figure for which the TBCP should aim (personal communication, Professor Glatthaar). South African figures do not approach this. The annual change in risk was –6,2 per cent for coastal blacks, –7,9 per cent for inland blacks, –2,2 per cent for coloureds and approximately –11 per cent for Indians and whites.[106]

The data confirm that tuberculosis control in South Africa is not satisfactory. There is a pool of up to 10 million infected persons[42] with a 5–10 per cent (or possibly higher)[52] risk of developing active disease later in life. More than 100 000 people have active tuberculosis.

The dramatic increase in tuberculosis in South Africa coincided with the discovery of gold on the Witwatersrand in 1886,[30, 77, 102] but since then the decline of tuberculosis in whites has paralleled that of developed countries in the nineteenth century where the decline occurred before the advent of anti-tuberculosis drugs.[25, 71] Yet tuberculosis remains inadequately controlled in black South Africans in spite of chemotherapy and BCG vaccination, a paradox which can be explained by the link between TB and socio-economic conditions.[7, 57, 65, 66]

Black poverty in South Africa arose as a result of particular political and socio-economic conditions, culminating in the apartheid policy of 1948. South Africa now has the highest inequality in income distribution of the 57 countries for which data are available.[87]

Blacks in the rural interior (on white-owned farms and in small villages), the homelands,[108] and the urban squatter areas bear the brunt of this poverty — poverty which is linked to the risk factors for tuberculosis (Figure 18.1). These include overcrowding, alcoholism, silicosis, undernutrition, viral infections (such as measles), and other stresses. While not exclusive to the poor, these risk factors obviously impact more on the lives of the poor.

Household contacts of a tuberculosis case are at the highest risk of being infected.[53] As infectiousness is associated with closeness of contact, duration of exposure and the bacillary sputum load,[26] the over-

crowding in the townships and squatter areas due to the severe housing shortage[101] is thought to be associated with a higher rate of tuberculosis. However, the South African studies on this are not conclusive.[17, 22, 92] An attempt has been made to optimize tuberculosis case-finding by identifying high risk socio-economic groups. Migrant workers,[85] farm workers,[55] families who have been relocated[80] (and who need to commute daily for up to six hours[48]), or who live in the homelands (with low annual income[68] and mass unemployment) provide examples of the physical and emotional stresses faced by many blacks. It has particularly been suggested that the stress of long term separation contributes to reactivation of latent infection.[27]

A significant number of urban blacks consume a large amount of alcohol daily,[86] probably as a result of both the stresses placed on them and alcohol marketing strategies. An association between alcohol problems and tuberculosis has been found locally.[22]

Tuberculosis, although less serious than before, remains a major occupational hazard in the mines,[58] and in particular in silica-using industries,[39] where dust levels remain high.[84] Lack of state or employer commitment to occupational health[29] compounds this.

The effect of the above socio-economic factors, combined with the effects of malnutrition[54] and measles[41] in poor communities, means that children in South Africa carry a high tuberculosis burden.[35, 56]

All of these points illustrate why tuberculosis is so aptly called a disease of poverty. Yet South Africa has sufficient resources to significantly alleviate poverty, if only it were to embark on socially just policies. Beyond this, the impact of an inefficient health service on tuberculosis and the management of the Tuberculosis Control Programme (TBCP) itself present added problems. It is these that are explored further in this chapter, in which tuberculosis services are considered in the light of the thinking of the International Union Against Tuberculosis (IUAT) and the World Health Organization (WHO) study group,[111, 113, 114] the Primary Health Care (PHC) approach as outlined in the Alma Ata declaration,[109] the South African national tuberculosis policy of 1979,[33] local literature, and personal experience.[13, 14, 64]

HEALTH SERVICE FACTORS AFFECTING TUBERCULOSIS CONTROL IN SOUTH AFRICA

The 1979 tuberculosis policy, which is the basis of the TBCP, is in line with internationally recommended tuberculosis policies. Its stated objectives are:

> *To reduce the risk of contracting a tuberculosis infection to 0,3 per cent and below for all population groups in the Republic of South Africa; and to ensure effective treatment of all tuberculosis disease that occurs and is diagnosed.*[33]

The TBCP, explained in a later document,[47] is seen to have two phases. The first phase aimed to reduce the infectious pool through active and passive case-finding and supervised short course therapy, and to offer protection against infection through BCG vaccination. The second phase aims to reduce the infected pool and endogenous reactivation and to protect against infection. This would be achieved by secondary chemoprophylaxis of positive tuberculin reactors, improvement of socio-economic and other stress conditions (the 1979 policy did not make reference to this), BCG vaccination and continuation of the methods used in phase one. The tuberculosis policy accorded tuberculosis health education first priority, followed by supervised therapy, active and passive case-finding and BCG administration. Community involvement was required to assist with case-finding and supervised ambulatory care (SAC).

The selective distribution of socio-economic resources in South Africa has also been applied to the health service,[6, 11, 69] and this, together with a number of structural and centrally controlled factors, has undermined the TBCP. These factors include:

- the fragmented health service, a weak PHC system, and inadequate central coordination of tuberculosis control;
- an insufficient welfare system; and
- a lack of community involvement.

Over and above their own effects, these factors combine to impact on the implementation of services at the local level. The results are:

- inadequate support and referral systems;
- inappropriate health education;
- inadequate integration of peripheral health workers; and
- insufficient evaluation.

All of these factors are interlinked and it is their combined effect on tuberculosis control that is of concern. However, for the purpose of explanation it is useful to consider them separately.

Structural and centrally controlled factors affecting the TBCP

The fragmented health service

Preventive and curative health services have always been separated in South Africa. Apartheid led to racially segregated facilities and to the establishment of fourteen Departments of Health, one for each homeland and one each for coloured, Indian and white South Africans as well as one general affairs department. This fragmentation created an unequal, inefficient, wasteful and irrational health service.[31, 82]

Communication and coordination between the different health authorities is inadequate,[64, 120] jeopardizing the referral of patients from one authority to another and wasting resources. One report has indicated that a tuberculosis service was not allowed to follow up 43 per cent of their patients or their families or to organize SAC for them, simply because they came from a different homeland to the one in which the hospital was situated:

> *If the patient defaults on our doorstep, it must be reported to our head office who report it to the other head office, who then inform their nearest hospital superintendent, who must ask his public health nurse to travel about 40 km to take the patient to a hospital far from home.*[15]

Problems of this nature affect black workers on white-owned farms as well,[15] as one 'country's' staff and vehicles may not enter another.

The expanding private sector, encouraged by the state policy of privatization, has led to further fragmentation.[81] The use by the state of private contractors to run tuberculosis hospitals outside the homelands is an example. This has led to maldistribution of tuberculosis beds, and, in the case of for-profit contractors, appears to have led to an increased emphasis on hospitalization, there being a financial incentive to retain the inpatients for as long as possible. This undermines the role of SAC, and therefore, although there is a reported reduction in inpatient day costs compared to state-run hospitals, privatization does not appear to be cost-effective for the TBCP as a whole.

The solution to fragmentation, and its impact on tuberculosis control, is a unitary health service, which has been called for on previous occasions.[8, 75]

The recent devolution of day-to-day tuberculosis care from the Department of National Health to provinces and local authorities is a positive move. Also, the respective Departments of Health have agreed to treat patients freely, regardless of where they come from, but some peripheral personnel have resisted this. Although the important step of desegregating services became policy in 1990, conditions have not changed much in practice. Nevertheless, the political direction of the country bodes well for the removal of fragmentation.

The primary health care system

South Africa has had no national commitment to the Alma-Ata approach.[109] There is presently some interest in PHC in the Department of National Health, but as yet there is little evidence of concrete changes. The PHC system has not been the main focus of the health service, which is inadequately funded and staffed, and does not provide adequate essential health care.[62] The service lacks support (for instance, there is an inadequate drug supply)[16, 63] and it has severe material constraints (such as a lack of equipment).[93]

The weak PHC system affects both tuberculosis staff and patients. Rural clinic sisters feel unable to cope with their present load[63] and are reluctant to take on an added tuberculosis responsibility, or else they give it low priority.[120] For many tuberculosis patients the service is not accessible,[120] affordable, appropriate, available, or acceptable. The advanced stage of tuberculosis disease at diagnosis further reflects poor access. One study found that more than 50 per cent of tuberculosis patients had problems in getting their treatment, distance from the clinic being an important factor.[99]

It is now accepted that the complexity of integrating the tuberculosis service into the PHC system has been underestimated,[111] and integration will be difficult to achieve.[115] Nevertheless, sustained efforts to do so must continue as it is at the primary level that case-finding, treatment and immunization should occur.[111] Every primary health service point should become a tuberculosis service point. However, the vertical nature of the tuberculosis service means that fixed and mobile clinics in some areas do not dispense tuberculosis drugs or perform tuberculin tests. Instead patients have to travel, often long distances, to the district hospital.

Central coordination of the TBCP

Decentralization is a crucial step in the development of health services, but this must be accompanied by strong central coordination and programme development.[59] This has not occurred in South Africa, with the result that there are many gaps in the implementation of the TBCP.

The recent devolution of executive functions by the Department of Health to second and third tier health authorities is logical, but still does not appear to have been accompanied by the necessary central infrastructure for coordination and development. For example, the Department has limited information on expenditure on tuberculosis control.[36] The TBCP has also been compromised by insufficient and irregular funding.[46]

Clear guidelines for the practical implementation of the tuberculosis policy have been lacking, but this is presently being worked on. While the use of *ad hoc* circulars has been confusing to tuberculosis workers, the lack of guidance for treatment of HIV-positive patients and of prisoners has been particularly noted. There has also been a call for clear policy objectives.[97]

Inadequate central coordination has had many effects at the periphery. Management of tuberculosis by health workers and authorities has been haphazard and fragmented.[46, 98, 120] Incorrect implementation of policies on bacteriological diagnosis, standardized treatment, SAC and contact tracing have been shown.[98] There has been a lack of development of SAC services[46, 98] — at least 50 per cent of all newly diagnosed patients are hospitalized,[46] while much ambulatory care is not adequately supervised. Natal treats mostly on an inpatient basis,[23] and Ciskei policy has been to admit as many tuberculosis patients as possible.[97] The varying management practices of 29 local authorities in the western Cape identified the need for clear notification criteria and for clear definitions of patient compliance and defaulting.[119]

The lack of effective middle level management is recognized internationally as being an important inhibitor of health programmes.[112] Tuberculosis middle management, dependent on a wide range of staff, is underdeveloped. There are only one or two tuberculosis regional medical officers in each of the seven health regions of RSA, making each responsible for too vast an area. Also, as their role is not clearly delineated, they lack the authority needed for coordination of the TBCP. Middle managers have complained that Health Departments do not consult them enough, are insufficiently responsive to their needs, and do not play a strong coordinating role.

There has been a call for a tuberculosis task force,[7] needed to facilitate central coordination and to develop a cadre of skilled and motivated regional and local tuberculosis managers, who can develop the TBCP at district PHC and hospital levels. In this way vertical coordination of decentralized services would occur.

The welfare system

Much criticism has been levelled at the social welfare services in South Africa.[67, 70, 79] In tuberculosis care health workers have to be particularly concerned about income while the patient is unable to work. The lack of job security[50] and unemployment benefits, the inadequate funds for and inordinate delays in receiving welfare grants, and the prolonged hospital care are thought to contribute to absconding. A breadwinner may have no income for up to six months. Fifty-one out of 100 randomly selected hospitalized tuberculosis patients were their families' major breadwinners. Six were paid by their employers while in hospital (personal communication, Dr M Westaway).

The finding that compliance levels are lowest amongst blacks[4] and the unemployed[4, 119] underlines the importance of social support. Poverty-related problems such as unemployment, lack of disability grants and lack of food are reported by health authorities in the Cape and Ciskei as having compromised tuberculosis care.[97]

Clearly, the above and other welfare needs of tuberculosis patients must be addressed, particularly to improve caseholding.

Community involvement

Lack of community involvement has been cited as being the most important reason for failure in the TBCP.[46] While community involvement in health has been difficult to achieve worldwide,[112] the political situation of South Africa has made it even more difficult, interventions from the state being commonly viewed with suspicion and treated as if they were further elements of repression.

At the local level there is little evidence of effective mass-based community involvement. Community involvement, unless it empowers the community itself, is not necessarily community supportive.[103] Too often it means the State shifting its responsibility onto a community which can ill afford it.[110] The tuberculosis policy has seen community involvement in South Africa limited to assisting in case-finding and SAC. There are, however, a few examples of more successful community involvement, through the South African National Tuberculosis Association (SANTA) branches (who have trained local workers and initiated 'Help Yourself To Better Health Programmes'), by state services,[105] and by non-government health projects.[1, 28] These may offer models for the future, but the complexity of developing and sustaining such efforts should not be underestimated.

The high degree of recent political violence may also have led to a decrease in patient attendance and in contact tracing.[116]

The important changes taking place in the country open up possibilities for better community involvement. A clear strategy is needed to ensure the involvement of broader representative structures and community development projects.

Factors affecting implementation of TB control

Support and referral systems

Any health service, including the TBCP, requires an effective support system.[2] On the positive side, rifampicin is widely available, but, given the nature of the health system it is not surprising that there are problems with referral procedures, vehicles and their kilometre allowances, radiology and laboratory facilities, reference texts and teaching aids. These problems are greater in rural areas.

Referral of suspected tuberculosis cases for further investigation is made difficult by distance and cost. Referral for continuation of care (which occurs frequently as a result of migrant labour) is also problematic. It is often unclear where to refer a patient to, and posting a referral letter or giving it to the patient often amounts to sending him or her into a 'black hole', as follow-up is difficult due to the lack of coordination between services,[64] and the complexities of migrancy and the uncertainty of end addresses.

Vehicles are essential for tuberculosis care. Contact and defaulter tracing and SAC are dependent on transport. In rural areas there are too few vehicles, and many of those available are poorly serviced and not sturdy enough for the roads.[64] Restrictions on the distances that staff may travel, for example in farm (section 30) areas, also limits tuberculosis work.[13] Radiological and laboratory facilities are lacking in many peripheral areas.[46, 97] Despite an emphasis in the tuberculosis policy on diagnosis by sputum cultures, these are not widely enough available. Quality control and rapport between laboratory personnel and others in the tuberculosis team[61] needs improving.

Health education

The tuberculosis policy states:

Health education shall form an integral, essential component of the total endeavour. It will be directed at the community with the aim of inculcating an awareness of the disease so that the community becomes involved in a practical sense, assisting especially in case-finding and treatment control.[33]

These goals have to a large extent not been met.

In practice there has been a lack of support and funding for health education, resulting in insufficient time, skill, teaching aids and health educators.[64] A lack of any prior tuberculosis education is found in tuberculosis patients when they present to the health service.[64, 99]

The gap between improving knowledge and actually influencing behaviour is well recognized. Measures that address the latter in mass media, small group or individual tuberculosis education are not well practised. Too often an approach of condescending lecturing, rather than a dialogue using adult education methods, is applied. Teaching is not innovative enough, participants are expected to be passive, technical language is used without adequate explanation, and the key messages are unclear.[13]

The result of this is that tuberculosis patients' knowledge of and attitudes towards the disease have been poor. Denial of risk and misconceptions on hospitalization and treatment time[104] and on the causes of tuberculosis[72, 73, 90] have been reported. The stigma related to tuberculosis remains.[104]

In spite of many efforts, including those of SANTA, studies have concluded that tuberculosis health education in South Africa has not been sufficiently effective.[73, 90, 99]

Health workers

Many staff are unable to adequately carry out all the activities of the first phase of the TBCP. There is insufficient staff dedicated to tuberculosis work and too few PHC personnel to include adequate tuberculosis work in their day. Medical[5, 50] and nursing staff need more training[120] and supportive supervision in order to improve their skills and morale. Peripheral staff, in particular, feel isolated and require more motivation.[64, 120] There is a lack of incentives for tuberculosis work.

Patients have at times complained of the inaccessible attitudes of health workers, finding them harsh and in too much of a hurry.[73] Training must include the development of empathy and the avoidance of victim-blaming.[13] It must also be noted that many peripheral workers have been observed to show greater care than might have been expected in difficult circumstances.[13, 14, 64]

Studies have indicated the importance of general practitioners[60] and traditional healers[38] at the primary level, but at present, as there are insufficient links between the TBCP and these practitioners, their potential contribution has not been adequately tapped. Concern has been expressed about private practitioners prescribing incorrect regimens and durations of treatment, not notifying tuberculosis patients, and failing to trace contacts. While there have been calls for closer cooperation between the health system and traditional healers,[109] numerous obstacles still need to be overcome.[45, 49]

Evaluation

Prevalence surveys in South Africa provide useful information, although their interpretation has been criticized.[77]

Routine data are well analysed once they reach the Department of National Health. However there is considerable under-reporting,[60, 98, 117] misclassification,[10] and insufficient local use and regional feedback. There is no national register of patients.

Studies have shown poor record-keeping,[64, 98, 120] as local staff have inadequate recording skills and there is little standardization of data-capturing forms.[98, 120] A positive step has been the development of uniform data-capturing forms for the country, but the problems of fragmentation have resulted in these forms not being fully implemented in the homelands.[23]

The need for evaluation of the TBCP at all levels has been stressed.[111] Health systems[96] and operations[9] research could provide invaluable information on how to improve the TBCP. This field is extremely underdeveloped. Research on topics such as the duration of illness before patients are diagnosed, the factors inhibiting them from seeking care, the reasons for absconding from tuberculosis hospitals, the effectiveness of SAC, and the impact of intensive local education and case-finding efforts are urgently needed, as is process evaluation of interventions.

Implementation of specific TBCP measures

The TBCP, in addition to health education, has correctly emphasized the prevention of infection through effective case-finding, curative treatment and good coverage with BCG vaccination, while preventing active disease through the selective use of secondary chemoprophylaxis and through BCG vaccination. However, the problems of the health service factors as already described undermines these specific measures.

Case-finding

A significant proportion of new cases in South Africa (more than 50 per cent in one estimate[7]) are not diagnosed annually. Weaknesses in both passive (the patient presents to the health service) and active (the health service looks in the community) case-finding and in contact tracing[98] contribute to this.

The real obstacles to passive case-finding are knowledge and beliefs about tuberculosis[100] and health service accessibility. Many patients believe that western care is not appropriate for tuberculosis and choose to consult traditional healers. Assuming a person does want to attend the formal health service, distances to a clinic, the cost of care, the opening times of the service and the attitudes of health workers towards them are all recognized as being barriers to accessibility, particularly for farm labourers and homeland dwellers.[14] Delays at hospital outpatients and x-ray departments may be a factor in urban areas. Although health workers are aware of tuberculosis, the proportion of cases that are missed in primary care settings is likely to be over 30 per cent.[12]

The tuberculosis policy states:

The pool of infectious cases shall be reduced drastically by intensive case-finding.[33]

However, in practice, active case-finding, including seeking chronic coughers and following up families with children who have strongly positive tuberculin tests, is not much used.

Tracing individuals in semi-urban townships[50] and rural areas is difficult because of inadequate transport, kilometre restrictions, poor communication and inadequate address systems. Contact tracing is probably more adequate in urban and more affluent areas, now assisted by the scrapping of influx control legislation, making the index case more willing to come forward.

Indiscriminate mass radiography is no longer practised in South Africa, and this seems appropriate given its low case yield compared to other case-finding techniques[91] However, no alternative has replaced it. Given the high prevalence of tuberculosis, selective active case-finding (either through radiology and bacteriology or bacteriology alone) among symptomatic people in defined high-risk groups should be used.[74] This should be preceded by an intensive health education campaign in the target area to encourage those symptomatic and at risk to present themselves.[13] Similar recommendations were made in the 1979 tuberculosis policy, but were insufficiently implemented. Of note, the Johannesburg SANTA branch does radiological screenings of all employees at factories. Contrary to the tuberculosis policy, these appear to be at the request of the employer and not co-ordinated by the Regional Tuberculosis Medical Officer.

Curative treatment

The tuberculosis policy states:

All patients diagnosed to be suffering from active tuberculosis shall be given effective treatment, including the use of rifampicin where indicated.[33]

The recommended drug regimens (all short term therapy with rifampicin) are appropriate and are generally applied in the RSA. However, some of the homelands, because of budgetary constraints, are still using suboptimal regimens. Some Transkei health wards use a rifampicin-containing regimen for two months and then isoniazid and thiacetazone alone (personal communication, Dr T F B Collins).

The main problem facing curative care is case-holding. Of the patients with known outcome, the percentage cured and discharged declined from 78 per cent in 1985 to 74 per cent in 1988, while the percentage of absconders rose from 16 to 21 per cent.[36] This is a minimum estimate of the problem, as it excludes the 36 per cent of patients with unknown outcome, in whom the cure rate is almost certainly lower. Even in 1978, in urban Soweto, only 28 per cent of patients received 80 per cent or more of their required treatment.[88] Two local studies have shown that 36[50] and 26[40] per cent respectively of patients had been previously treated for tuberculosis. It is estimated that 38 per cent of all patients in hospitals are relapsed cases.[46]

Further evidence of the problem of case-holding comes from the increasing frequency of drug resistance. Primary INH resistance is 15 per cent and acquired INH resistance has increased to 50 per cent in many rural areas.[44]

The reasons for this inadequate case-holding are rooted in the health service factors affecting tuberculosis control that have been outlined earlier in this chapter. Beyond this, improved case-holding requires improving the patient-health worker relationship, hospital procedures and SAC services. Attention to these has been shown to improve outcome.[15]

Hospital procedure is still too much like that of an isolation institution treating patients who are perceived as unable to look after themselves, even though the patients are non-infectious and most could be on SAC if arrangements were made. A more open ward policy, patient participation in managing their own ward, and greater attention to patients' social and economic problems could all contribute to case-holding. Patients should be encouraged to elect representatives to meet with hospital management. Admission interviews should be more standardized and should include exploring the possibility of an SAC arrangement and the risk factors for absconding. Patients should become adult partners in their own care.[13, 15]

The tuberculosis policy states that:

Every effort shall be made towards establishing ambulatory/domiciliary treatment for the majority of patients in the Republic ... All treatment must be given under full supervision.[33]

There are a few sites where innovative health workers have succeeded in developing SAC services[15, 105, 107] (personal communication, Dr E Brandes), but the programme has failed at a national level.[46] One reason is that the SAC policy was implemented without the prior setting up of the necessary support structures. As a result, at least 50 per cent of patients are still hospitalized and there are doubts that 25 per cent of patients on ambulatory therapy receive supervised treatment.[46] The latter has raised major doubts about drug compliance, and has encouraged calls for institutionalized care for all tuberculosis patients.

Yet SAC has the advantages that the patient is able to continue with schooling or work, and family life is less disrupted. For the health service SAC is potentially more cost-effective at R400 for clinic care versus R2 800 for hospital care (1986 costs).[23] Approximately two-thirds of the TBCP budget is allocated for hospitalization.[32]

The need to ensure curative treatment could well rank as the greatest priority in tuberculosis control in South Africa today. The solution is multifaceted and will take some effort, but we cannot sit back in the 1990s and rely on socio-economic advancement to control tuberculosis, nor can we justify major case-finding initiatives if we have not established a treatment system that is effective.

Bacille Calmette-Guérin vaccine (BCG)

Although the efficacy of BCG immunization is controversial,[3] it does help protect against tuberculosis in children.[21, 78] The policy and administration of BCG vaccination at birth is well established, but published information

on vaccination coverage in South Africa is lacking[43] and concerns have been expressed over unreliability of the data.[56] However there are enough immunization coverage and BCG scar surveys to support the Tuberculosis Research Institute estimate that more than 80 per cent of infants in South Africa receive a BCG vaccination.[43] This figure is satisfactory at a national level, but the extensive pockets of poorer coverage, the number receiving their immunization later than at birth (in some areas 10–40 per cent of births occur at home), and the inability to reach many of the missed children, reflects on the availability and affordability of maternal and child health services. Poorer coverage tends to occur in the areas where the children most need the protection afforded by BCG immunization. This, together with concerns about the maintenance of the cold chain, means that there is no room for complacency.

Therefore, although the reported BCG coverage is satisfactory, the poor case-holding and case-finding results indicate that the TBCP is not achieving its first phase aim of reducing the infectious pool and thereby reducing the risk of infection to a minimum.

Secondary chemoprophylaxis

The role of secondary chemoprophylaxis for tuberculosis control in South Africa is controversial. The TBCP places it at a second phase level, giving case-finding and treatment the first priority in the light of limited resources. Added arguments against the widespread use of secondary chemoprophylaxis include drug toxicity, INH resistance, low cost effectiveness, the high risk of reinfection and the loss of immunity against tuberculosis. These arguments have all been challenged.[24] While the debate continues, there are two points worth noting: SANTA is proceeding with chemoprophylaxis in black and coloured children, and lifelong chemoprophylaxis for HIV-positive patients is needed.[18]

The implication of AIDS for tuberculosis control

Predictions have put the potential number of HIV-infected adults at about 2,5–7,5 million by 2005 (personal communication Dr N. Padayachee) and of diseased adults at

850 000.[89] Given that approximately 10 million South Africans have tuberculosis infection today, that AIDS will rapidly increase the number of tuberculosis cases[95] (conservatively estimated to treble the present incidence),[76] and that the tuberculosis services are not adequate at present, there is an urgent need to improve the TBCP to cope with the impending large case-load.

CONCLUSION

This chapter has provided some evidence that the TBCP in South Africa is inadequate. It has contended that the problem is rooted in the socio-economic system and in the nature of the health service.

It follows that political change leading to a redistribution of the country's resources and a growth economy is the most important intervention in tuberculosis control.[7, 111] This should also lead to a unitary health system with a more rational, effective and even distribution of health services, and a genuine commitment to the PHC approach.[109] The important changes happening in the country, following years of popular struggle, augur well for this.

However, these changes will not in themselves ensure adequate tuberculosis control. Specific efforts are needed to develop the TBCP, with strong central coordination and effective decentralization of the tuberculosis service into district programmes and into the PHC system.

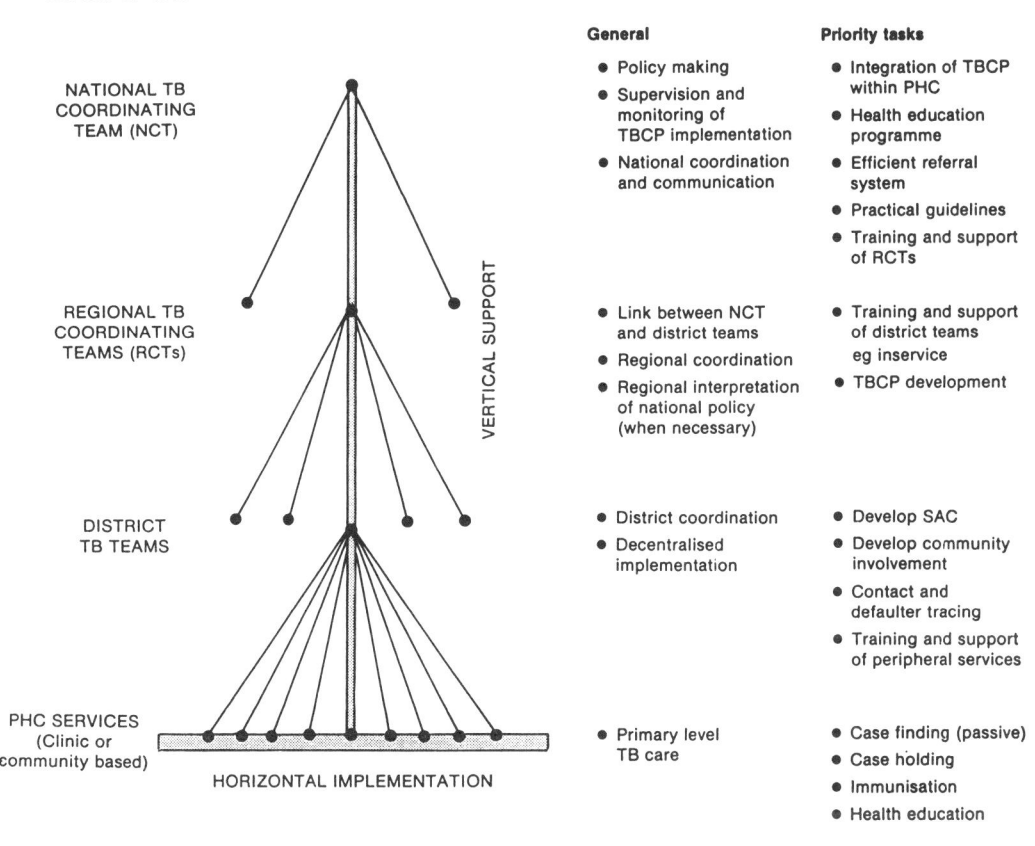

Figure 18.2. Proposed model for a Tuberculosis Control Programme.

A proposed structure for the TBCP is shown in Figure 18.2. There is the need for a national tuberculosis coordinating team[7] which, enabled by the changing political situation, would liaise with other countries in southern Africa. However, a priority task is to find practical, effective ways of integrating the TBCP into the PHC system.[113] The regional coordinating teams would serve rational, as opposed to racial or tribal, areas and would provide a dynamic link between the national tuberculosis coordinating team and the local district teams. They would be responsive to regional needs, interpreting national tuberculosis policy when necessary (e.g. SAC arrangements to suit local conditions), but will ensure that anarchic implementation of the TBCP[46, 98, 119] no longer occurs. The regional coordinating team would help with problems encountered by local authorities[119] in implementing policy. District tuberculosis teams will require managerial and evaluative skills for the coordination of the TBCP at local level.

In this way a degree of verticality will be maintained (there will be a chain of specialized tuberculosis workers from national to local level), ensuring proper coordination and expertise, combined with the development of the WHO/IUAT proposed integration of case-finding, treatment and other measures into the role of peripheral health workers.[111] Successful integration of the TBCP into PHC will certainly enhance tuberculosis control,[113] but a concerted effort is needed. The World Health Organization cautions that success in decentralization also depends on peripheral services being readily accessible.[111]

There are many pressing reasons for improving our TBCP, not the least of which is the suffering that patients and their families endure. Also, a poor TBCP can actually slow down the natural decline of the disease,[51] and will fail to meet the threat that AIDS poses for a dramatic increase in active tuberculosis cases. Finally, in many ways the tuberculosis situation serves as a social barometer of the country — the potential for change is better now than at any time this century. It is to be hoped that this potential is realized by the country, its health service and its TBCP.

Acknowledgements

We would like to thank the following who gave either technical advice or valuable commentary on early drafts of this chapter: Dr T F B Collins, Prof E Glatthaar, Dr D Kritzinger, Dr S Naidoo, Dr N Padayachee, Dr J Seager and Dr M Westaway. These individuals do not necessarily endorse the views expressed in this chapter, for which the authors take responsibility.

REFERENCES

1 Abdool Karim S S (ed), 1987. *Primary Health Care. Reports Presented at a Consultative Meeting.* Cape Town: National Medical and Dental Association.

2 Amonoo-Lartson R, Ebrahim G J, Lovel H J & Ranken J P, 1984. *District Health Care: Challenges for Planning, Organisation, and Evaluation in Developing Countries.* London: Macmillan.

3 Baily G V J, 1980. Tuberculosis prevention trial, Madras. *Indian Journal of Medical Research.* 72, 52–74.

4 Bell J & Yach D, 1988. Tuberculosis patient compliance in the western Cape, 1984. *South African Medical Journal.* 73, 31–2.

5 Benatar S R, 1982. Tuberculosis in the 1980s with particular reference to South Africa. *South African Medical Journal.* 62, 359–64.

6 Benatar S R, 1986. Medicine and health care in South Africa. *New England Journal of Medicine.* 315, 527–32.

7 Benatar S R, 1989. The Tuberculosis Control Programme — a time to re-evaluate? *South African Medical Journal.* 76, 639–40.

8 Benatar S R, 1990. A unitary health service for South Africa. *South African Medical Journal.* 77, 441–7.

9 Blumenfeld S, 1985. *Operations Research Methods: A General Approach in Primary Health Care.* Chevy Chase, Maryland: Primary Health Care Operations Research, Centre for Human Services.

10 Botha J L & Bradshaw D, 1985. African vital statistics – a black hole? *South African Medical Journal.* 67, 977–81

11 Botha J L, Bradshaw D, Gonin R & Yach D, 1988. The distribution of health needs and services in South Africa. *Social Science and Medicine.* 26(8), 845–51

12 Bradshaw D, *et al,* 1987. *Review of South African Mortality (1984) (Technical Report No. 1).* Cape Town: South African Medical Research Council.

13 Buch E, 1985. *Tuberculosis Services in the Southern Transvaal.* A Report to the Regional Director, Department of National Health and Population Development.

14 Buch E, 1986. *Aspects of Rural Health Services Development Experience from Work in Mhala in the Eastern Transvaal 1982–4.* Johannesburg: Health Services Development Unit, Department of Community Health, University of the Witwatersrand.

15 Buch E, Johnson K & Mashabane R, 1984. *Can Good Tuberculosis Care be Provided in the Face of Poverty?* Paper presented to the Second Carnegie Inquiry into Poverty and Development in Southern Africa. Cape Town: SALDRU, University of Cape Town.

16 Buch E, Stephenson D & Evian C, 1984. *How Well do our Rural Clinics Function?* Paper presented to the Second Carnegie Inquiry into Poverty and Development in Southern Africa. Cape Town: SALDRU, University of Cape Town.

17 Burney P G & Sittampalam Y, 1984. The social parameters of tuberculosis infection among children in the Transkei. *Tropical Geographical Medicine.* 36(1), 37–43.

18 Centers for Disease Control, 1989. Tuberculosis and human immunodeficiency virus infection: recommendations of the Advisory Committee for the elimination of Tuberculosis (ACET). *MMWR.* 38, 236–50.

19 Central Statistical Service, 1988. *Report No. 03.09.01 (1988) — Deaths of Whites, Coloureds, Asians 1988.* Pretoria: Government Printers.

20 Central Statistical Service, 1988. *Report No 03.10.01 (1988) — Deaths of Blacks 1988.* Pretoria: Government Printers.

21 Coetzee L & Fourie P B, 1986. Efficacy of BCG vaccination. *South African Journal of Science.* 82, 388–89.

22 Coetzee N, Yach D & Joubert G, 1988. Crowding and alcohol abuse as risk factors for tuberculosis in the Mamre population: Results of a case-controlled study. *South African Medical Journal.* 74, 352–4.

23 Collie A & Kustner H G V, 1989. The Tuberculosis Control Programme, 1985–6. *South African Medical Journal.* 76, 676–80

24 Collins T F B, 1981. Applied epidemiology and logic in tuberculosis control. *South African Medical Journal.* 61, 566–9.

25 Collins T F B, 1982. The history of southern Africa's first tuberculosis epidemic. *South African Medical Journal.* 62, 780–8.

26 Comstock G W, 1982. Epidemiology of Tuberculosis. *American Review of Respiratory Diseases.* 125(3), 8–15.

27 Comstock G W, Edwards L B & Livesay V, 1974. Tuberculosis morbidity in the U.S. Navy: its distribution and decline. *American Review of Respiratory Diseases.* 110, 572–80.

28 Critical Health Editorial Collective, 1986. Community health projects. *Critical Health.* Numbers 16 and 17.

29 Davies J C A, 1988. *A Time to Speak.* Inaugural lecture. Johannesburg; Witwatersrand University Press.

30 De Beer C, 1984. *The South African Disease — Apartheid, Health and Health Services.* Johannesburg: South African Research Services.

31 De Beer C, Buch E & Mavrandonis J, 1988. Fragmentation and political disorganisation of health care in South Africa. *In: A National Health Service for South Africa. Part 1.* Johannesburg: The Centre for the Study of Health Policy, University of the Witwatersrand.

32 Department of Finance, 1987. *Estimates of Expenditure to be Defrayed from the State Revenue Account for the Year ending 31 March 1988.* Pretoria: Government Printer.

33 Department of Health, 1979. *Policy Statement: Tuberculosis Control in the Republic of South Africa.* Pretoria: Department of Health.

34 Department of National Health and Population Development, 1988. Tuberculosis Control Programme — 1987. *Epidemiological Comments.* 15(11), 20–36

35 Department of National Health and Population Development, 1989. *Epidemiological Comments.*

36 Department of National Health and Population Development, 1990. Tuberculosis Control Programme — 1988. *Epidemiological Comments.* 17(1), 3–13.

37 Department of National Health and Population Development, 1990. *Epidemiological Comments* 17(1), 22.

38 Edwards S D, 1986. Traditional and modern medicine in S. Africa: a research study. *Social Science and Medicine.* 22, 1273–6.

39 Ehrlich R I, Rees D & Zwi A B, 1988. Silicosis in non-mining industry on the Witwatersrand. *South African Medical Journal.* 73, 704–8.

40 Felten M K & Kahler R, 1987. *Estimated Rates of 'Relapse' and 'Failure' in Tuberculosis Hospitals.* TBRI Symposium on Tuberculosis in Southern Africa, May 1987.

41 Ferrinho P, 1991. (Dissertation in preparation) *Measles in South Africa, A Community Health Interpretation of the data.* Johannesburg: University of the Witwatersrand.

42 Fourie P B, 1985. Current concepts in tuberculosis epidemiology. Paper presented at the First Tuberculosis Research Institute Symposium, *Current Views on Tuberculosis,* Pretoria, August 1985.

43 Fourie P B, 1987. BCG vaccination and the EPI. *South African Medical Journal.* 72, 323–6.

44 Fourie P B & Knoetze K, 1986. Tuberculosis prevalence and risk of infection in Southern Africa. *South African Journal of Science.* 82, 387.

45 Freeman M & Motsei M, 1988. *Is There a Role for Traditional Healers in Health Care in South Africa?* Johannesburg: The Centre for the Study of Health Policy, University of the Witwatersrand.

46 Glatthaar E, 1982. Tuberculosis control in South Africa 'Where have we gone wrong' and 'A look at the future'. *South African Medical Journal.* Special Issue, 17 November, 36–41.

47 Glatthaar E, 1982. *Tuberculosis: Basic Perspectives.* Pretoria: Medunsa.

48 Goldblatt D, 1986. The night riders of KwaNdebele. *In:* Badsha O. *South Africa — The Cordoned Heart.* Cape Town: Gallery Press, S A Photographic Gallery Series 3.

49 Green E C, 1988. Can collaborative programs between biomedical and African indigenous health practitioners succeed? *Social Sciences and Medicine.* 27(11), 1125–30.

50 Griffiths M L, Makgothi M M & Nordesjo G, 1981. Tuberculosis management in a rural community — factors in failure. *South African Medical Journal.* 61, 14–16.

51 Grzybowski S, 1982. The value of different diagnostic treatment and preventive programmes. *South African Medical Journal.* Special Issue, 17 November, 6–8.

52 Grzybowski S, 1983. *Tuberculosis and its Prevention.* Missouri: Warren Green.

53 Grzybowski S, Barnett G & Styblo K, 1975. Contacts of active pulmonary tuberculosis. *Bulletin of the International Union on Tuberculosis.* 50, 90–106

54 Hansen J, 1984. *Food and Nutrition Policy with Relation to Poverty: The Child Malnutrition Problem in South Africa.* Paper presented to the Second Carnegie Inquiry into Poverty and Development in Southern Africa. Cape Town, SALDRU, University of Cape Town.

55 Hendrie D, Adams A & Arafdien Y, 1986. *Saldru Handbook of Labour and Social Statistics.* Cape Town: SALDRU, University of Cape Town.

56 Ijsselmuiden C B, Kustner H G V, Barron P M & Steinberg W J, 1987. Notification of five of the EPI target diseases in South Africa. An assessment of disease and vaccination reporting. *South African Medical Journal.* 72, 311–7.

57 Kark S L, 1974. *Epidemiology and Community Medicine.* New York: Appleton-Century-Crofts.

58 Kielkowski D & Murray G, 1991. *Pathology Division Report, Demographic Data, Silicosis and Tuberculosis Rates 1989/1990.* Johannesburg: National Centre for Occupational Health, Report No.1.

59 Kleczkowski B M, Roemer M I & Van Der Werff A, 1984. *National Health Systems and their Reorientation towards Health for All. Guidance for Policy-making.* Geneva; World Health Organization.

60 Kleeberg H H, 1982. The dynamics of tuberculosis in South Africa and the impact of the control programme. *South African Medical Journal.* Special Issue, 17 November, 22–3.

61 Kleeberg H H, 1986. TB bacteriology and the laboratory situation. *South African Journal of Science.* 82, 394–5.

62 Knight S & Buch E, 1988. *A Study to Investigate the Primary Health Care Service in the Northern Region of Kwazulu.* Presented to the Seventh Epidemiological Conference, Warmbaths.

63 Lee T, Buch E & Peden C (in press). Support systems, facilities and staffing of clinics in Mhala: Are they adequate? *South African Medical Journal.*

64 Lee T, Price M & Wynne J, 1991. *An Evaluation of the Kangwane Tuberculosis Programme,* in *A Review of Health Services in Kangwane and the South-eastern Transvaal,* Vol. 11. Johannesburg: Centre for Health Policy, University of Witwatersrand.

65 Lister S, 1932. *Tuberculosis Research Committee Report 1932. 5 (30)*. Johannesburg: South African Institute of Medical Research.

66 Lowell A M, Edwards L B & Palmer C E, 1969. *Tuberculosis*. Cambridge: Harvard University Press.

67 Lund F, 1990. Welfare under pressure: financing South African social welfare. *Transformation*. 13, 67–80.

68 McGrath M, 1984. *The Determinants of Poverty: A Theoretical Analysis*. Paper presented to the Second Carnegie Inquiry into Poverty and Development in Southern Africa. Cape Town: SAL-DRU, University of Cape Town.

69 McIntyre D E & Dorrington R E, 1990. Trends in the distribution of South African health care expenditure. *South African Medical Journal*. 78, 125–9.

70 Mckendrick B W, 1990. Future of social work in South Africa. *Social Work — Maatskaplike Werk*. 26(1), 10–18.

71 Mckeown T & Lowe C R, 1974. *An Introduction to Social Medicine*. Oxford: Blackwell.

72 Metcalf C A, Bradshaw D & Stindt W W, 1990. Knowledge and beliefs about tuberculosis among non-working women in Ravensmead, Cape Town. *South African Medical Journal*. 77, 408–11.

73 Moloantoa K E M, 1982. Traditional attitudes towards tuberculosis. *South African Medical Journal*. Special Issue, 17 November, 29–31.

74 Myers J, 1986. Tuberculosis screening in industry. *South African Medical Journal*. 70, 251–2.

75 National Health Services Commission, 1944. *Report on the Provision of an Organised National Health Service for all the Sections of the People of South Africa (U.G. 30)*. Pretoria: Government Printer.

76 Nunn P & Odhiambo J, 1990. Tuberculosis and HIV infection. *Lancet*. 1044.

77 Packard R, 1989. *White Plague, Black Labour, Tuberculosis and the Political Economy of Health and Disease in South Africa*. Los Angeles: University of California Press.

78 Pan American Health Organization, 1986. *Tuberculosis Control: A Manual on Methods and Procedures for Integrated Programs (No. 498)*. Washington: Pan American Health Organization.

79 Patel L, 1987. Towards a critical theory and practice in social work with specific reference to South Africa. *International Social Work*. 30(3), 222–35.

80 Platzky L & Walker C, 1985. *The Surplus People — Forced Removals in South Africa*. Johannesburg: Ravan Press.

81 Price M & de Beer C, 1988. Can privatization solve the problems in the health sector? *In: A National Health Service for South Africa, Part 1*. Johannesburg: The Centre for the Study of Health Policy, University of the Witwatersrand.

82 Price M, Steinberg M & de Beer C, 1985. The new constitution and health. *In:* Zwi A B & Saunders L D (eds). *Towards Health Care for All. Namda Conference 1985*. Johannesburg: NAMDA.

83 Reichman L B & O'Day R, 1978. Tuberculous infection in a large urban population. *American Review of Respiratory Diseases*. 117, 705–12.

84 Rendall R E G & Paidas D, 1987. Environmental conditions in factories. *South African Journal of Science*. 83, 6–8.

85 Reynolds P F, 1984. *Men without Children*. Paper presented to the Second Carnegie Inquiry into Poverty and Development in Southern Africa. Cape Town: SALDRU, University of Cape Town.

86 Rocha-Silva L, 1989. *Drinking Practices, Drinking-related Attitudes and Public Impressions of Services for Alcohol and Other Drug Problems in Urban South Africa*. Pretoria: Human Sciences Research Council.

87 Roukens de Lange R & van Seventer D E, 1986. *Implications and Implementation of Income Redistribution: An Investigation Based on Social Accounting Matrix*. Second Carnegie Inquiry into Poverty and Development in Southern Africa, Post-Conference Series. Cape Town: SALDRU, University of Cape Town.

88 Saunders L D, Irwig L M, Wilson T D, Kahn A & Groeneveld H, 1984. Tuberculosis management in Soweto. *South African Medical Journal*. 66, 330–42.

89 Schall R, 1990. On the maximum size of the AIDS epidemic among the heterosexual black population in South Africa. *South African Medical Journal*. 78, 507–10.

90 Seager J R, 1986. Health Education in TB hospitals. *South African Journal of Science*. 82, 389–90.

91 Seager J R, 1986. Tuberculosis case-finding. *Tuberculosis Research Institute Bulletin*. 7(1), 10–1.

92 Seager J R, Schoeman J H, Wilkinson I S & Westaway M S, 1987. *An Attempt to Optimize Tuberculosis Case-Finding by Identifying High Risk Socio-economic Groups*. Second TBRI Symposium on tuberculosis in South Africa, 1987.

93 Solleder G, 1987. Material constraints at rural clinics in Transkei. *South African Medical Journal*. 72.

94 Styblo K, 1980. Recent advances in epidemiological research in tuberculosis. *Advances in Tuberculosis Research.* 20, 1–63.

95 Styblo K, 1989. The potential impact of AIDS on the tuberculosis situation in developed and developing countries. *Bulletin of the International Union Against Tuberculosis.* 63(2), 25–8.

96 Taylor C E, 1984. *The Uses of Health Systems Research.* Geneva: World Health Organization.

97 Thomson E M & Myrdal S, 1986. Regional variations in tuberculosis policy in the Cape and Ciskei. *South African Medical Journal.* 70, 253–7.

98 Thomson E M & Myrdal S, 1986. The implementation of tuberculosis policy in three areas in South Africa. *South African Medical Journal.* 70, 258–62.

99 Thomson E M & Myrdal S, 1986. Tuberculosis — the patients' perspective. *South African Medical Journal.* 70, 263–4.

100 Tintswalo Hospital Primary Health Care Nursing Class of 1982, 1982. *Beliefs and Knowledge about TB in the Mhala District.* Paper presented to the conference 'Health Realities in Africa', Garankuwa, 1982.

101 Urban Foundation. 1990. *Housing For All, Proposals for a National Urban Housing Policy.* Johannesburg: Urban Foundation.

102 Webster D, 1982. *Capital, Class and Consumption: A Social History of Tuberculosis in South Africa.* Paper presented to U.C.T. Medical Student Conference, 'Consumption in the Land of Plenty — TB in South Africa'. Cape Town: Medical Students Council, University of Cape Town.

103 Werner D, 1980. Health care and human dignity — a subjective look at community based rural health programmes in Latin America. *Contact.* No. 57.

104 Westaway M S, 1989. Knowledge, beliefs and feelings about tuberculosis. *Health Education Research.* 4(2), 205–11.

105 Westaway M, Conradie P W & Remmers L (in press). Supervised out-patient treatment for tuberculosis: Evaluation of a South African rural programme. *Tubercle.*

106 Weyer K & Fourie P B, 1989. Die epidemiologie van tuberkulose in Suider-Afrika. *CME.* 7(3), 239–47.

107 Whitehouse A B. The modern management of tuberculosis in a rural area. *South African Medical Journal.* 60, 695–6.

108 Wilson F & Ramphele M, 1989. *Uprooting Poverty: The South African Challenge.* Cape Town: David Phillip.

109 World Health Organization, 1978. *Alma-Ata 1978: Primary Health Care.* Geneva: World Health Organization.

110 World Health Organization, 1981. *National Decision-making for Primary Health Care.* Geneva: World Health Organization.

111 World Health Organization, 1982. *Tuberculosis Control. Report of a Joint IUAT/World Health Organization study group.* Geneva: World Health Organization.

112 World Health Organization, 1988. *From Alma-Ata to the year 2000: Reflections at the Midpoint.* Geneva: World Health Organization.

113 World Health Organization, 1988. *Tuberculosis Control as an Integral Part of Primary Care.* Geneva: World Health Organization.

114 World Health Organization, 1991. *Tuberculosis Control and Research Strategy for the 1990s.* Geneva: World Health Organization.

115 Yach D, 1986. Problems associated with integrating tuberculosis control and primary health care. *South African Journal of Science.* 82.

116 Yach D, 1987. *The Impact of Political Violence on Health and Health Services in Cape Town 1986.* Parow, Cape Town: Institute for Biostatistics, Medical Research Council.

117 Yach D, 1987. Tuberculosis deaths in South Africa. *South African Medical Journal.* 72, 149–51.

118 Yach D, 1988. Tuberculosis in the Western Cape Health Region of South Africa. *Social Sciences and Medicine.* 27(7), 683–9.

119 Yach D, Hoffman M & Van Herzeele A, 1988. Western Cape local authority compliance with tuberculosis policy, 1984. *South African Medical Journal.* 73, 33–35.

120 Yeats J R, 1986. Attendance compliance for short-course tuberculosis chemotherapy at clinics in Estcourt and surroundings. *South African Medical Journal.* 70, 265–6.

Index

abdominal distension, frequency of 103
abdominal lymph node enlargement 100
abdominal masses, frequency of 103
abdominal pain, frequency of 103
abdominal TB
    conditions confused with 10
    diagnosis 117
    epidemiology 68
    historical synonyms 7
    in adults 116-17
    in children 91, 99, 101-3
    mortality 103, 117
    post-mortem findings 104
    symptoms 103
    treatment 117
    see also gastrointestinal TB
abducens nerve 153
abortion, TB and 94
abscesses, subcutaneous 142
abscesses, tuberculous 138, *160,* 157, 163-4, 175, *175*
acid-fast bacilli 121, 153-4, 196, 246
acquired resistance *93*
    see also acquired *under* immunity
ACTH gel 158
activity, assessment of 220-1
acute progressive tuberculosis 7
ADA 117, 251
Addison's disease 92, 107, 119
adenitis, lymph- *see* lymphadenitis
adenoids, tuberculosis of the 104, 106
adenopathy, extra-abdominal (symptom) 103
adenopathy, lymph- *see* lymphadenopathy
adenosine deaminase activity 117, 251
adhesions *149,* 152
adjuncts to treatment 225
adjuvant therapy 159
adrenals 92, 107
adults, TB in 63, 64, 68, 111-21
    differences between childhood TB and 92-3, 172-3
    recommended regimens for treating 264
    see also specific types of TB
aetiology 69-76; *see also* risk factors; risk ratios
AFB investigation 153-4, 246
Africa, TB in 15-16
age factors 18, 59-63, 67, 70, 78-9, 93, 113, 118, 215-16, 247-8, 277
    immunity influenced by 224, 236

    see also adults; children
aged *see* elderly
agglutination technique 250
agricultural reforms and TB 19
AIDS and TB 65, 71-2, 82-3, 84-5, 109, 113, 119-21, 191, 225, 238, 296
    chemotherapy 267, 296
    diagnostic factors 245-6
    radiographic manifestations 120-1, 216-17
alcohol and TB 72, 181, 185, 214-15, 289
alcoholics, treatment of 267
allergic reaction 96
Alexander of Thalles 8
Allan, Peter 27 *bis,* 46
altitude therapy 15, 25
ambulant therapy 50, 190-1, 275, 290, 296
    see also supervised ambulatory care
amenorrhoea 107, 246
Americas, TB in 3-5, *5, 6,* 9, 10, 16
anergy 103, 108, 225, 231, 233-4, 237, 238
angiograms 162
Anglo-Boer War and TB 26
animal husbandry risk 183
ankle, tuberculosis in the 173, *174*
ankylosis 169, 172
annual risk of TB infection 61, 62, 112
anorectal lesion 116
anorexia 99, 113, 125, 153
anosmia 162
anthropometric status 72
antigens 224-9 *passim,* 233, 250-1
    detection 155-6, 225, 250
    presentation 229
    processing 228-9
apartheid 43, 47-55, 289
apathy 108
apicolysis 38
appetite, loss of 108, 118
APT (Artificial pneumo-thorax) 36-8, *37,* 40
Arabian accounts of TB 8
arachnoiditis 151 *bis,* 152, 165
areflexia 165
Aretaeus 8
ARI 61, 62, 112
Aristotle 8
art, evidence of TB in 4-5, *4-6, 32*
arteritis 145
artery territory infarcts scan 156
arthritis 98, 169
    acute and chronic 169